Health Communication in the New Media Landscape

Jerry C. Parker, PhD, received his training in the field of psychology, earning a master's degree from Xavier University and a PhD from the University of Missouri. He is currently associate dean for research and clinical professor of physical medicine and rehabilitation, School of Medicine, at the University of Missouri. Dr. Parker is also director of the Missouri Arthritis Rehabilitation Research and Training Center. At the national level, Dr. Parker has served on the NIH National Advisory Board for Arthritis and Musculoskeletal and Skin Diseases and was a member of the NIH Consensus Panel on Traumatic Brain Injury. He also has served on national peer review panels for the NIH, the National Institute for Disability and Rehabilitation Research, and the Arthritis Foundation. Dr. Parker's research has focused on clinical problems and the translation of clinical research into improved health outcomes. This research, which has been funded by the NIH, the National Institute on Disability and Rehabilitation Research, and the Arthritis Foundation, has resulted in a series of randomized clinical trials examining various self-management interventions for persons with rheumatoid arthritis. As director of the Missouri Arthritis Rehabilitation Research and Training Center, Dr. Parker has overseen a comprehensive research program in the area of arthritis rehabilitation, which involves projects in aerobic fitness, online self-management programs, workplace adaptation, support systems for juvenile arthritis, musculoskeletal problems of seasonal and migrant farmworkers, and strategies for use of the mass media for improving health communication. In 1990, Dr. Parker received the Merit Award from the Arthritis Health Professions Association in recognition of "outstanding clinical scholarship in rheumatology."

Esther Thorson, PhD, is professor, associate dean of the School of Journalism, and director of research for the Reynolds Journalism Institute at the University of Missouri. Dr. Thorson has published more than 100 scholarly articles and books on news effects, advertising, media economics, and health communication and has edited six books. She has headed grant and research contracts totaling nearly $3 million. She is the only female fellow of the American Academy of Advertising. She applies research, both hers and that of her colleagues, in newsrooms and advertising agencies across the United States and abroad. She serves on eight journal editorial boards. She has advised more than 35 doctoral dissertations, and her former students hold prestigious professorships throughout the United States and Asia. She is the recipient of the American Advertising Federation's Distinguished Advertising Education Award, the American Academy of Advertising Outstanding Contribution to Research Award, a Missouri Alumni Association Faculty Award, and the Missouri Curator's Award for Scholarly Excellence. Dr. Thorson has two central management goals: first to integrate theory and practice in graduate journalism and persuasion education, and second to bring scholarly research to bear on the news and advertising industries. Her research (with Professor Duffy) for the Newspaper Association of America has been presented in national forums throughout the United States.

Health Communication in the New Media Landscape

JERRY C. PARKER, PhD
ESTHER THORSON, PhD
Editors

SPRINGER PUBLISHING COMPANY

NEW YORK

Springer Publishing Company, LLC
11 West 42nd Street
New York, NY 10036
www.springerpub.com

Acquisitions Editor: Jennifer Perillo
Production Editor: Julia Rosen
Project Manager: Julia Rosen
Cover design: Joanne E. Honigman
Composition: Apex Publishing, LLC

12 13 14 15 / 5 4 3

Library of Congress Cataloging-in-Publication Data

Health communication in the new media landscape / [edited by] Jerry Parker, Esther Thorson.
    p. ; cm.
  Includes bibliographical references and index.
  ISBN 978-0-8261-0122-8 (alk. paper)
  1. Communication in medicine.   2. Mass media in health education.   I. Parker, Jerry C. (Jerry Calvin), 1947–   II. Thorson, Esther.
  [DNLM: 1. Delivery of Health Care—trends. 2. Communication. 3. Consumer Participation. 4. Medical Informatics—methods. W 84.1 H437413 2008]
  R118.H434 2008
  610—dc22   2008024572

Printed in the United States of America by Gasch Printing

This book is dedicated to my wife, Jane, and our sons, Aaron and Adam,
who are the inspiration for all I do.
—Jerry C. Parker

This book is dedicated to my daughter, Kylie, who is on the brink of
discovering just how special she is. And to Margaret Duffy, who never
fails to share a great idea and a laugh—or two.
—Esther Thorson

Contents

Contributors

Suzanne A. Boren, PhD, MHA, is an assistant professor of consumer health informatics in the Department of Health Management and Informatics in the School of Medicine at the University of Missouri and a research health scientist with the Health Services Research & Development Program of the Harry S. Truman Memorial Veterans' Hospital in Columbia, Missouri. Her major research interest is the appropriate use of information technology to facilitate evidence-based self-care behavior change in chronic illness.

Gordon Brown, PhD, is professor in the Department of Health Management and Informatics in the School of Medicine at the University of Missouri. He teaches and carries out research in work design and organization and process change in health organizations and systems. From 1997 to 2007, he was chairman of the Department of Health Management and Informatics, which included on-campus and executive master's programs in health services management and health informatics, a nationally recognized postdoctoral training program in medical informatics funded by the National Library of Medicine, and a doctoral program in health informatics. During this time, the department built a strong research program in health outcomes and community-based health services. Dr. Brown holds an MA and PhD in health administration from the University of Iowa, and a BS in industrial administration from Iowa State University. He is recognized internationally for his leadership in health administration education and has served as chairman of the Accrediting Commission on Education for Health Services Administration and chairman of the Board of the Association of University Programs in Health Administration. From 1999 to 2007, Dr. Brown served as a senior fellow at the Center for Health Care Quality, a center for health quality research at the University of Missouri. He served as a scientist with the World Health Organization on the development of integrated regional health systems and on the faculties at the University of Iowa, Pennsylvania State University, and the Universidad del Valle in Cali, Colombia, prior to coming to the University of Missouri. Dr. Brown has conducted research and authored numerous articles and book chapters in addition to consulting nationally and internationally in the areas of managing information technology, quality improvement, organization strategy, integrated health delivery systems, and health administration education.

Glen T. Cameron, PhD, is the Maxine Wilson Gregory Chair in Journalism Research and co-founder of the Health Communication Research Center at the Missouri School of Journalism. The author of nearly 300 books, chapters, articles, and convention papers, he has received numerous national awards for individual research projects as well as the Baskett-Mosse and Pathfinder awards for his entire body of work. Dr. Cameron has extensive experience and proficiency in survey research, experimental design, content analysis, and qualitative techniques such as focus groups and in-depth interviewing. At Missouri, Dr. Cameron has contributed to over $20 million in external funding from sources such as the NIH, the National Cancer Institute, the Missouri Foundation for Health, the USDA, the CDC, the NIDRR, the U.S. Department of Defense, and Monsanto.

Alwyn T. Cohall, MD, is an associate professor at Columbia University's Mailman School of Public Health and New York Presbyterian Hospital, where he is the director of the Harlem Health Promotion. He is also the director of Project STAY (Services to Assist Youth)—a clinical program that provides comprehensive medical and psychosocial services to high-risk and HIV-infected youths. Through the Morgan Stanley Children's Hospital of New York Presbyterian, he has developed a private practice devoted to the health and wellness of adolescents and young adults. Dr. Cohall has authored several scientific papers in peer-reviewed journals, coauthored a reference book for adolescents and parents on common teen health problems, and coedited a recent edition of *Adolescent Medicine: State of the Art Reviews* on the use of technology to enhance adolescent health promotion.

Katherine Downey, MD, joined the University of Missouri Department of Physical Medicine and Rehabilitation in July 2007. She received her medical degree from the University of Missouri–Kansas City in 2004 and in 2007 completed a residency in physical medicine and rehabilitation at the University of Missouri, where she served as co-chief resident from 2006 to 2007. Dr. Downey works with traumatic brain injury and general rehabilitation inpatients at the Rusk Rehabilitation Center. She has presented regionally and is currently a member of the American Academy of Physical Medicine and Rehabilitation.

Margaret E. Duffy, PhD, is chair of strategic communication and a faculty and associate professor at the Missouri School of Journalism. She is also principal investigator for the Missouri Arthritis Rehabilitation Research and Training Center. Dr. Duffy was associate professor at Austin Peay State University in Clarksville, Tennessee, before joining the Missouri School of Journalism faculty in August 2001. At Austin Peay State University, Duffy taught graduate and undergraduate courses in organizational communication, marketing communication, consumer behavior, public relations, advertising, integrated marketing communication, and media business management and was the creator and director of the university's Institute for Corporate Communication. Her research focuses on how individuals choose media; with Esther Thorson, she developed a model that helps health communicators, media companies, and advertisers create products and services tailored to customer needs and interests. She has presented her research to academics, advertisers, and news groups in the United States, China, Thailand, Germany, South Africa, Canada, and Italy. Professionally, she was previously a marketing, advertising, and public relations executive for GTE Corporation, now Verizon Corporation. In 1995, Duffy earned her PhD in mass communication from the University of Iowa.

Mohan J. Dutta, PhD, is associate professor of health communication, public relations and mass media in the Department of Communication, and affiliate faculty member of Asian Studies, the Center for Education and Research in Information Assurance and Security, the Discovery Learning Center, the Burton D. Morgan Center for Entrepreneurship, and the Regenstrief Center for Healthcare Engineering at Purdue University. Professor Dutta is the 2006 Lewis Donohew Outstanding Scholar in Health Communication and has received multiple research and teaching awards for his scholarly contributions. At Purdue University, he is a service learning fellow and a fellow of the leadership academy. He teaches and conducts research in the areas of health communication theory, the culture-centered approach to health communication, health care disparities, and health campaigns.

Petya Eckler, MA, is a doctoral student of Internet health communication at the Missouri School of Journalism. Her research interests include health communication, strategic communication, new media, and international health communication. She has worked in the areas of tobacco control, breast cancer, cancer, and arthritis. Prior to joining the doctoral program, she had professional experience in both journalism and public relations. She received a bachelor's in journalism and political science from the American University in Bulgaria and a master's in journalism from the University of Missouri.

Marianne Farkas, ScD, a research associate professor, is currently the director of training, dissemination, and technical assistance at the Center for Psychiatric Rehabilitation, Boston University. In this role she is currently the co-principal investigator of the Rehabilitation Research and Training Center on Recovery for People with Mental Illnesses and the co-principal investigator of the Innovative Knowledge Dissemination and Utilization for Disability and Professional Organizations and Stakeholders, working on developing a process for knowledge translation in the disability research field. For more than 25 years, Dr. Farkas has worked in various capacities in the field of psychiatric rehabilitation and has been recognized for her contributions to the field with various awards. Among her many roles, Farkas was in charge of the World Health Organization Collaborating Center in Psychiatric Rehabilitation, providing training, consultation, and research expertise to the WHO network around the globe. She has served on a committee for the WHO to develop methods of categorizing evidence-based and promising practices in the context of international literature. She has developed training, consultation, and organizational change methodologies to support programs and systems in their efforts to adopt psychiatric rehabilitation and recovery innovations. Dr. Farkas is the current president of the National Association of Rehabilitation Research and Training Centers and the vice president of the World Association of Psychosocial Rehabilitation.

Robert L. Glueckauf, PhD, is professor in the Department of Medical Humanities and Social Sciences at the Florida State University College of Medicine. Before moving to Florida State University in August 2003, he directed the Center for Research on Telehealth and Healthcare Communications at the University of Florida. Dr. Glueckauf obtained his MS and PhD in clinical psychology at Florida State University. He is former president of the American Psychological Association's Division of Rehabilitation Psychology and served as associate editor of the division's journal, *Rehabilitation Psychology*. Dr. Glueckauf has authored over 80 empirical and theoretical articles, books, and chapters in the field of health care and rehabilitation and has been the recipient of numerous federal and state grants. His research and clinical interests lie in the development and evaluation of telehealth delivery systems for underserved individuals with chronic illnesses and their family caregivers, the measurement of rehabilitation and health outcomes, and family systems interventions for persons with severe disabilities.

Paul R. Gully, MB, ChB, FRCPC, FFPH, is senior adviser to the Assistant Director of General Health Security and Environment at the World Health Organization in Geneva, Switzerland. He has an interest in risk communication and policy issues related to avian influenza and pandemic preparedness and emerging diseases. Up to April 2006, he was deputy chief public health officer for Canada responsible for infectious diseases and emergency preparedness and has held various posts in Health Canada since 1990. Prior to that he worked in public health at the local and regional level in Canada, the United Kingdom, and Zambia. Dr. Gully is a physician with specialty training in public health in the United Kingdom and Canada and has held honorary and adjunct academic positions in the United Kingdom and Canada.

Kristofer J. Hagglund, PhD, ABPP, is the associate dean of the School of Health Professions at the University of Missouri. He co-directs the Center for Health Policy, a non-partisan research and policy analysis organization committed to improving health care. He also serves as interim director of the master of public health program at the University of Missouri–Columbia. Dr. Hagglund's current projects include grants from the Missouri Foundation for Health to increase health literacy and reduce health care disparities, and the Health Care Foundation of Greater Kansas City to expand health equity collaboration. His recent articles explore the financing and delivering of personal assistant services. In 2006, he coedited a book entitled *Handbook of Applied Disability and Rehabilitation Research*. Dr. Hagglund obtained a BA in psychology from Illinois State University and a PhD in clinical (medical) psychology from the University of Alabama at Birmingham. He is a diplomate of the American Board of Professional Psychology and a fellow of the American Psychological Association. He was a 2000–2001 Robert Wood Johnson Health Policy fellow in the office of Senator Tom Harkin (D-IA), where he worked on legislation addressing patients' rights, mental health parity, rural health care, the health professions workforce, community health centers, and the National Health Service Corps.

Muhiuddin Haider, PhD, is an associate professor of global health at the School of Public Health at the University of Maryland. He also serves as adjunct faculty at Johns Hopkins University's School for Advanced International Studies and as a visiting professor in health communication at the James P. Grant School of Public Health at BRAC University in Bangladesh. He has served as an associate professor in global health and international affairs in the Department of Global Health at the School of Public Health and Health Services and in the Elliott School of International Affairs at George Washington University. He has worked in Asia, the Middle East, sub-Saharan Africa, and Latin America to strengthen the health systems of developing nations. Among his areas of expertise are health communications, infrastructure development, training, capacity building, and health care reform, with an emphasis on reproductive health, family planning, AIDS prevention, maternal and neonatal health, child survival, and water management.

Eric S. Hart, PsyD, is a clinical assistant professor in the Department of Health Psychology in the University of Missouri School of Health Professions. He received his BS in psychology from Illinois State University, his MA in clinical psychology from Eastern Illinois University and his MA in counseling psychology and his PsyD in clinical psychology from the Adler School of Professional Psychology in Chicago, Illinois.

Brian K. Hensel, PhD, MSPH, is a National Library of Medicine postdoctoral fellow in health informatics at the University of Missouri. Dr. Hensel's research interests include health communication via informatics applications in supporting chronic disease management and health behavior change, and in improving long-term care provision. His doctoral training at the Missouri School of Journalism focused on health communication. He achieved a master of science in public health, with a focus in health administration, in 1987 also from the University of Missouri. Prior to entering his doctoral program, Dr. Hensel was a health care administrator for 15 years, overseeing home health, hospice, and long-term care services. He has served on the board of the Kansas Hospice Association and as a preceptor for the Xavier University graduate program in hospital and health administration. Dr. Hensel is a fellow of the University of Missouri Interdisciplinary Center on Aging.

Bradford W. Hesse, PhD, is chief of the Health Communication and Informatics Research Branch at the National Cancer Institute. Trained as a psychologist, Dr. Hesse has spent most of his career working to improve the ways in which mediated communication environments can be utilized to support behaviors in positive ways. His work has taken him into the areas of human-computer interaction, medical informatics, health psychology, media psychology, interpersonal communication, health communication, and artificial intelligence. Dr. Hesse currently serves as program director for the Health Information National Trends Survey (a biennial survey of adults' use of health information technologies), the Centers of Excellence in Cancer Communication Research, and he has accumulated a rich portfolio of basic science communication projects and grants. Dr. Hesse also serves in an advisory capacity for the National Cancer Institute's User-Centered Informatics Research Laboratory and is a standing member of the American Psychological Association's Electronic Resources Advisory Committee.

María E. Len-Ríos, PhD, is an assistant professor of strategic communication in the Missouri School of Journalism. Len-Ríos's research focuses on health communication and underserved audiences, public relations campaigns and crisis communication, and how social groups are represented in the mass media. Her work has been published in the *Newspaper Research Journal, Journalism & Mass Communication Quarterly*, the *Journal of Promotion Management, Public Relations Review*, and *Public Relations Quarterly*.

Mia Liza A. Lustria, PhD, is assistant professor at the Florida State University College of Information, where she teaches information science, information architecture, and health informatics courses for the undergraduate IT program. Dr. Lustria earned her BS and MS in development communication from the University of the Philippines, and her PhD in health communication at the University of Kentucky. She has expertise in consumer health informatics, particularly in designing, implementing, and evaluating interactive behavior change technology systems for health communication and education. Dr. Lustria is currently the principal investigator on a project involving the design and evaluation of an informatics system to support rural health care providers' capacities to provide timely referrals for breast cancer screening and adjuvant therapies in rural Florida. This 3-year study is funded through a $348,000 grant funded by the Department of Health Bankhead Coley Cancer Research Program. In addition, Dr. Lustria has expertise in diabetes and behavioral cancer control research, online health information seeking, use of Web 2.0 technologies for health communication, computer tailoring, and health literacy issues.

Janet M. Marchibroda, MBA, is the chief executive officer of the Washington, DC.–based eHealth Initiative and its foundation, national nonprofit organizations that aim to improve the quality, safety, and efficiency of health care through information and information technology. She previously served as the executive director of Connecting for Health, a public-private sector initiative funded and led by the Markle Foundation and supported by the Robert Wood Johnson Foundation. She cofounded and served as chief operating officer of two health care information organizations that focused on the provision of compliance information to physicians to support patient safety and the provision of electronic publishing services to the payer community to support member information needs. She also served as the interim chief operating officer for the National Coalition for Cancer Survivorship and as the chief operating officer of the National Committee for Quality Assurance, an organization devoted to evaluating and improving the quality of health care for Americans. She holds an MBA with a concentration in organizational development from George Washington University. In 2005, she was recognized as one of the top 25 women in health care by *Modern Healthcare* and in 2006 received the Federal Computer Week Top 100 Award.

Jordan G. McCall, BS, BA, is an MPH candidate at the University of Missouri–Columbia and a graduate teaching assistant in the School of Health Professions. As a graduate research assistant at the Center for Health Policy at the University Missouri, his primary research interest is health literacy among older adult populations.

Wendy Meltzer, MPH, is the managing editor of the *Journal of Health Communication: International Perspectives,* a scholarly peer-reviewed journal that presents the latest developments in the field of health communication, including research in social marketing, communication (from interpersonal to mass media), psychology, government, and health education in the United States and the world. With a focus on promoting the vital life of the individual as well as the good health of the world's communities, the journal presents research on progress in the areas of technology and public health, ethics, politics/policy, and the application of health communication principles. Ms. Meltzer has managed the journal since 2001. Previously, Ms. Meltzer was an editor and writer for several consumer-oriented health advocacy publications. Ms. Meltzer holds an MPH from the George Washington University School of Public Health and Health Services.

Mary E. Northridge, PhD, MPH, is currently professor of clinical sociomedical sciences at the Mailman School of Public Health at Columbia University. She is also editor-in-chief of the *American Journal of Public Health*. She currently serves as a faculty member and thesis advisor for the urban planning program at the Graduate School of Architecture, Planning and Preservation, the evaluator of the ElderSmile Program at the College of Dental Medicine, and a co-investigator at the Harlem Family Asthma Center. She is involved in community-based participatory research on environmental and social determinants of health, scholarly and practical applications of joint urban planning and public health frameworks, health initiatives designed to mitigate asthma and its triggers, and advocacy and teaching concerning environmental and social justice issues. She has cotaught an interdisciplinary course now titled Interdisciplinary Planning for Health that stresses sustainable community-level interventions. She earned a BA in chemistry at the University of Virginia; an MPH in environmental health at Rutgers, the State University of New Jersey/University of Medicine and Dentistry of New Jersey; and a PhD in epidemiology at Columbia University.

Andrew Pleasant, PhD, is actively involved in health literacy research and practice. He currently has projects ranging from topics such as HIV/AIDS in Kenya to improving practice in clinical care settings in the United States. He is a coauthor of one of the best-selling books on health literacy, *Advancing Health Literacy: A Framework for Understanding and Action* (2006), has authored numerous peer-reviewed journal articles, and constantly gives keynote presentations, grand rounds, and training seminars on health literacy in the United States and internationally.

He has designed, led, and participated in research projects in the United States, Kenya, South Africa, Ghana, China, India, and Mexico.

Scott C. Ratzan, MD, MPA, is vice president of Global Health, Government Affairs & Policy, at Johnson & Johnson, and editor-in-chief of the *Journal of Health Communication: International Perspectives.* He was the founder and director of the Emerson-Tufts Program in Health Communication, a joint master's degree program between Emerson College and the Tufts University School of Medicine. He continues to maintain faculty appointments at the Tufts University School of Medicine and George Washington University Medical Center as well as the Cambridge University–Judge Business School and the College of Europe in Belgium. In addition, he was the senior technical adviser in the Bureau of Global Health at the United States Agency for International Development, where he developed the global health communication strategy for U.S.-funded efforts in 65 countries. His publications include *The Mad Cow Crisis: Health and the Public Good* (1998), "Attaining Global Health: Challenges and Opportunities" (2002), and *AIDS: Effective Health Communication for the 90s* (1993). He has appeared on *Good Morning America* and *Nightline* and has published articles in the *New York Times, Wall Street Journal,* and *Financial Times.* Dr. Ratzan received his MD from the University of Southern California; his MPA from the John F. Kennedy School of Government, Harvard University; and his MA from Emerson College.

E. Sally Rogers, ScD, is director of research at the Center for Psychiatric Rehabilitation at Boston University, where she has conducted mental health and vocational research since 1981. She is also a research associate professor for the university's Sargent College of Health and Rehabilitation Sciences, where she has taught master's- and doctoral-level research courses and seminars She currently serves as coprincipal investigator of a Research and Training Center grant that allows her to carry out research studies on the recovery of individuals with mental illness, another grant to culturally adapt a measure on recovery for Spanish-speaking mental health clients, and a postdoctoral fellowship award from the National Institute on Disability and Rehabilitation Research. She was the principal investigator of a multisite grant to study consumer-operated services funded by the Center for Mental Health Services of the Substance Abuse and Mental Health Services administration. Dr. Rogers has written over 50 peer-reviewed papers on topics related to the vocational rehabilitation, assessment, and recovery of persons with severe psychiatric disabilities and has developed instruments currently used by research studies and service organizations. In 2007, she received the Loeb Research Award from the International Association of Psychosocial Rehabilitation Services. She is a licensed psychologist in the state of Massachusetts.

Juan D. Rogers, PhD, is associate professor of public policy at the School of Public Policy, Georgia Institute of Technology. He received his PhD in science and technology studies from Virginia Polytechnic Institute and State University, and an EE from the University of Buenos Aires, Argentina. Dr. Rogers teaches science and technology policy, information management and policy, knowledge management, logic of policy inquiry, and bureaucracy and policy implementation. His current research interests include modeling the research and development process; assessment of research and development impacts, especially in the formation of scientific and technical human capital, technology transfer; and research and development policy and evaluation. He has been principal investigator and coprincipal investigator in projects funded by the U.S. Department of Energy and National Science Foundation to develop methods of assessment of research and research impacts, including the flow of knowledge across institutional and sector boundaries. He has been a consultant on the evaluation of publicly funded research and development for agencies in the United States and South America.

Cheryl L. Shigaki, PhD, is an assistant professor in the Department of Health Psychology at the University of Missouri. Dr. Shigaki has published in the areas of rehabilitation, including brain injury; access to health care among people with disabilities; and the role of psychologists in shaping Medicaid health care policy. Other areas of interest include aging and chronic illness, health literacy, and adjustment to chronic conditions and disability following cancer. Dr. Shigaki currently provides psychological services to the Geriatric Inpatient Team of the Rusk Rehabilitation Center. Dr. Shigaki obtained her PhD in clinical psychology from the University of Florida in Gainesville. She completed her predoctoral psychology internship at the Internship Consortium at the University of Missouri–Columbia, and a two-year NIH T-32 postdoctoral fellowship through the Department of Health Psychology at the University of Missouri. Dr. Shigaki currently serves as chair of the American Psychological

Association Committee on Disability in Psychology and is a member of the University of Missouri Committee for Persons with Disabilities and the School of Health Professions Research Committee.

Rubiahna L. Vaughn, MPH, graduated from Columbia University's Mailman School of Public Health in 2008. She is currently a medical student at the University of Washington in Seattle. She earned her bachelor's in human biology from Stanford University. She is a Henry Luce scholar and a Jack Kent Cooke scholar.

Rebecca L. Woelfel, BJ, is senior information specialist for the Missouri Arthritis Rehabilitation Research and Training Center in the Missouri School of Journalism. The focus of her current work is a civic journalism strategic communication campaign to improve U.S. media coverage of rheumatic diseases. She also promotes an interactive Web site to coordinate care for children with juvenile arthritis. Woelfel has produced a streaming video series for public school educators and administrators on pediatric rheumatic diseases. Woelfel holds a bachelor of journalism from the Missouri School of Journalism.

Gregory M. Worsowicz, MD, MBA, received his medical degree from the University of Florida School of Medicine in 1986 and completed a residency in physical medicine and rehabilitation at Baylor College of Medicine in Houston, Texas, in 1990. After his residency he practiced in both academic and private practice settings. He was on the faculty of the University of Medicine and Dentistry of New Jersey's Department of Physical Medicine and Rehabilitation, serving as the director of satellite services until 2002, when he was named chairman of the Department of Physical Medicine and Rehabilitation at the University of Missouri–Columbia School of Medicine and medical director of the HealthSouth Howard A. Rusk Rehabilitation Center. In addition, he is presently the chair of University Physicians at the University of Missouri, which includes 400 practicing physicians. His clinical and research interests include the cost-effective systems of care/program development, health care policy, and geriatric rehabilitation. He currently is a coprincipal investigator for the Missouri Arthritis Rehabilitation Research and Training Center, which is federally funded by the National Institute on Disability and Rehabilitation Research. He has presented regionally and nationally on practice management and systems of post-acute care. He has served as a member of the board of directors for both the Association of Academic

Physiatrists and American Congress of Rehabilitation Medicine and is currently the chair of the American Academy of Physical Medicine and Rehabilitation's Health Policy and Legislative Committee.

Kevin B. Wright, PhD, is an associate professor in the Department of Communication at the University of Oklahoma, where he earned his PhD in 1999. He is the author of three books and over 30 journal articles and book chapters. The bulk of his research examines the relationship between the communication of social support and health outcomes in computer-mediated support group contexts among individuals dealing with health issues. His other research interests include communication among individuals with cancer and their caregivers, hospice and palliative care, provider–patient interaction, health promotion campaigns, aging and health, and face-to-face support groups for people facing health issues such as substance abuse, HIV, and eating disorders.

Christina Zarcadoolas, PhD, is associate clinical professor in the Department of Community and Preventive Medicine at Mount Sinai School of Medicine. She is a sociolinguist nationally known for her work in health and environmental literacy. She works at the intersection of linguistics and cultural studies, focusing on analyzing and closing the gaps between expert knowledge and public understanding of health and environmental issues. Prior to coming to the Mount Sinai School of Medicine, she spent 15 years on the faculty of Brown University. Dr. Zarcadoolas is the lead author of *Advancing Health Literacy: A Framework for Understanding and Action* (2006), a critically acclaimed textbook that presents a multidimensional model of health literacy that includes the domains of fundamental literacy, science literacy, cultural literacy, and civic literacy. The *New England Journal of Medicine* recently called the book "required reading" for public health professionals.

Foreword

Advances in communication technology offer new and exciting opportunities to empower individuals and groups in relation to their health, to significantly enhance the quality of practice of health care and public health professionals, and to address inequities in people's access to health information and services. In order to ensure these results, however, the use of these technologies must be managed and directed appropriately, and technological tools must be made equitably available.

Communication is at the heart of health care and health promotion. Given that most people are driven by the need to influence factors that affect their lives (see "Enhancing Consumer Involvement in Health Care" by Hesse in this volume), it can be assumed that they will, where possible, respond to improved access to health information to make better-informed decisions. For their part, health professionals understand that the information that an individual needs is not limited to that provided in a clinic or hospital. More equal access to information, advice, and support through electronic means can be the foundation of partnerships that lead to higher-quality care and improved public health.

Through enhanced availability of health information, rapid advances in digital technology should promote greater equity and increased opportunities to make informed decisions. However, the products of technology have to be available in a form that is appropriate to the needs of those wanting to promote their own health or the health of others. There must be coherence between these needs and the tools available. For example, the Web will work for some, while e-mail, text messaging, video clips, telephone calls, and even reminders sent by mail will work for others. If the appropriate tools do not exist, they should be developed in partnership with the health consumer. Empowerment means linking the needs of people to the right tools and enabling participation in their development. Not only is access to information required, but a level of "health literacy" is needed, and the means to acquire this is also not always equitable.

Health is also influenced by factors that cannot be easily changed by personal decisions, and the means to take action to mitigate risk from lack of clean water, sanitation, safe food, and a clean and secure environment vary widely across societies and the globe. However, even where there is a lack of basic services, wireless technology may be used to notify authorities of outbreaks of disease, which will enable more rapid containment and alert populations as to external threats. In addition, the Internet has great utility in enabling access to information or technology, for example through telemedicine, in situations where there is absence of or limited access to professionals.

The Internet can also enable access to social networks for the purpose of support or as an aid in health promotion. Personal contact with peers, friends, family, and the health professions will remain important but can be complemented by electronic ways of securing advice and support. This can translate into availability of knowledge and access to virtual communities, even where health care and public health services are not optimal.

Along with these benefits, rapidly developing communications technology brings real challenges for both health professionals and the public. The huge number of research findings published, disseminated, and reported on daily have to be interpreted by one and understood appropriately by the other. The creation and widespread availability of new knowledge is way ahead of the means to make use of that knowledge. The science of informatics can assist in the presentation of information, but translation of knowledge is necessary. There is now greater access to health portals, reviews, and authoritative advice, and decision makers at all levels of government will need assistance in translating this knowledge to help them make the most appropriate policy decisions.

There are also other forces at play that can easily negate efforts to improve health. We cannot ignore the negative influences of the new media in promoting unhealthy foods and tobacco, for example. We can look to the social sciences to assist us in understanding why such efforts are effective and perhaps use the same methods for a positive effect on health.

Given the high prevalence of chronic diseases in many populations, small reductions can result in major advances in population heath status. In addition, acceptance of public health strategies such as immunization can prevent acute disease, which puts extra strain on overburdened health systems. Communication of risk during acute events is a fundamental part of public health practice and enables individuals and decision makers to make appropriate decisions at times of crisis as well as helping health or emergency response authorities to better manage an event. Opportunities offered by the new media can be used as an additional means to influence avoidable mortality and morbidity, which should not be ignored.

This book is a glimpse into the world of the new media; the authors present analyses of evidence of the utility of new opportunities in a wide variety of health environments. The chapters predominately focus on health issues in the United States, but evidence of the usefulness of new media and the needs of individuals and communities can and should be considered by those with an interest in health promotion, care, and treatment around the globe. In this volume there are examples of how advances in technology not only empower individuals in their interactions with a health system but also enable health professionals to better tailor their work and time for the benefit of patients and clients.

Computers, which dominate our lives, should augment, not replace, human thought (see "Enhancing Consumer Involvement in Health Care" by Hesse in this volume). Our goal should be to promote the equitable distribution of tools so that we use advancing technology—the new media—to benefit health for all.

Paul R. Gully, MB, ChB, FRCPC, FFPH
Senior Adviser to Assistant Director-General
Health Security and Environment
World Health Organization
Geneva, Switzerland

Preface

In recent decades, the growth in medical knowledge has been dramatic. Over 10,000 randomized, clinical trials are conducted annually, and the budget of the National Institutes of Health has grown to over $30 billion. Innovative research in areas such as genomics, cell restoration, diagnostic imaging, prosthetics, and rehabilitation all hold the potential to greatly improve health and to reduce disability for millions of people across the globe. Yet compelling evidence suggests that the rapid scientific advances in the fields of health care and medicine are not being effectively translated into improved health outcomes.

Unfortunately, these well-documented failures are occurring at a time when health care demands are expanding. Citizens in both developed and developing countries are living longer, and the percentage of the global population older than age 65 is rapidly increasing. As a result, a higher percentage of the population is living with one or more chronic diseases—many of which would be potentially preventable if evidence-based public health information were effectively translated into practice. Currently, the diffusion of information into the awareness of the general public (including health care practitioners) is frequently passive and even serendipitous. Health-related research is typically presented at professional conferences and published in scientific journals, but only a fraction of this information finds its way into the mainstream, public media on the basis of selected stories that journalists and editors deem newsworthy. Equally problematic, the news reports on scientific research are often exceedingly narrow and do not effectively place new research findings into an appropriate scientific context. In short, news reports to the public generally do not provide a framework for behavior change or for immediate application; they also are often contradictory. Furthermore, the uneven adoption of evidence-based, health-related research across racial and socioeconomic groups contributes to disparities in health care outcomes.

Digital technologies appear to present tremendous opportunities for the dissemination of health-related and rehabilitation information. Indeed, the transformation of the spectrum of human communication as a result of advances in electronic media capability is occurring in dramatic fashion. E-mail, digital commerce, online television, cell phones, iPods, and the general integration of all traditional modes of mass communication onto the Internet have resulted in fundamental changes in how the citizens of the world approach their basic communication needs; the rapid adoption of electronic communication is reflected by instant messaging, blogging, photo sharing, social networking, and video downloads, among other digital capabilities.

This dramatic change in human behavior which is occurring as a result of the new media landscape also poses many challenges. Certainly, the new media landscape raises fundamental questions about how people interact with communication systems. For example, what will be the role and meaning of "news" in the new landscape? How will people's perceptions of what is important and what is valued be altered? How will people learn about health-related issues and health care? How will persons with chronic diseases learn about resources, support systems, and rehabilitation? What will be the impact of the new media landscape on health care providers and on health care policies? This text seeks to summarize what is known about these compelling questions.

Jerry C. Parker, PhD
Esther Thorson, PhD

Acknowledgments

Without Becky Woelfel, this book would never have come into being. Ms. Woelfel organized the conference that spawned the book. She pulled together the book proposal and helped us find the delightful Jennifer Perillo at Springer Publishing. Ms. Woelfel supported every author through the process of submissions, edits, and reedits. She reminded us of deadlines and never lost sight of the end goal. Every single detail was on her radar, and her goal was always to "do it perfectly." All this was accomplished with the warmest and most supportive attitude imaginable. No one ever dreaded an e-mail from WoelfelB! We thank this solid-gold individual from the bottom of our hearts. We also would like to express our heartfelt appreciation for the contributions of Kimberli Holtmeyer, Katrina Rowland, Deborah Taylor, and Erin Willis—all of whom played key roles in the development of this project. In all respects, their insightful, strategic, and well-coordinated support has been greatly appreciated, and their kindness, good humor, and creativity have contributed immeasurably to the pleasure of this work. In addition, the authors of the individual chapters, in all respects, were exceptionally responsive and dedicated to this project, and their scholarly efforts were central to an edited work of this type. Lastly, the authors would like to acknowledge that the seminal ideas for this book were spawned in a state-of-the-science conference funded by the National Institute on Disability and Rehabilitation Research (NIDRR) within the U.S. Department of Education (#H133B031120). The purpose of the conference was to explore the role of health communication for improving health care and rehabilitation services for persons with disability, and the support from NIDRR was deeply appreciated.

Health Communication: Current Status and Trends

PART
I

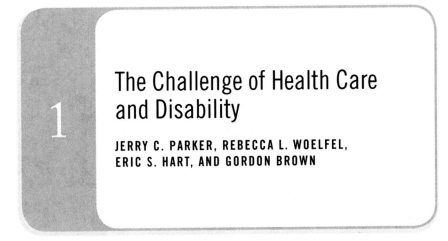

The Challenge of Health Care and Disability

JERRY C. PARKER, REBECCA L. WOELFEL, ERIC S. HART, AND GORDON BROWN

With few exceptions, the delivery of health care and the reduction of disability are challenges for all nations and cultures. In the developing world, access to health care is often severely limited, and programs for reducing disability are, likewise, often unavailable. Even in developed nations, systems for delivering health care and reducing disability are frequently fraught with problems, although the nature of the problems and the strategies used to solve them vary widely.

Indeed, each nation or society defines "health care" in its own way and develops its own diagnostic and treatment theories, practices, and tools to provide services that may range from cures to rehabilitation to stabilization to the provision of comfort and palliative care (Jonas, Goldsteen, & Goldsteen, 2007). The sum of all programs and institutions that promote the work of diagnosis and treatment in a given society can be labeled the health care system for that society (Jonas et al., 2007).

To understand the challenges of health care and disability, an appreciation of the concept of health is necessary. According to the World

Preparation of this chapter was partially supported by the National Institute on Disability and Rehabilitation Research (NIDRR) within the U.S. Department of Education (#H133B031120). The views expressed in this chapter do not necessarily represent the views of NIDRR and are the sole responsibility of the authors.

Health Organization (1946), "Health is a state of complete physical, mental and social well-being and not merely the absence of disease or infirmity." Jonas and associates (2007) discuss a similar definition put forth by the International Epidemiological Association that describes health as "A state characterized by anatomical, physiological and psychological integrity, ability to perform personally valued family, work, and community roles; ability to deal with physical, biological, psychological and social stress; a feeling of well-being; and freedom from the risk of disease and untimely death" (p. 3). These particular definitions of health, and many others, are exceedingly broad. Health care systems are rarely able to promote health and well-being in this idealized manner.

Any definition of health begets the question of what determines health. Jonas and associates (2007) describe the key determinants of health as genetic inheritance, physical environment, social environment, health behavior, and adequacy of health care. A similar framework for the determinants of health has been provided in *Healthy People 2010*, which is a comprehensive plan for promoting healthy living and reducing health disparities in the United States (U.S. Department of Health and Human Services, 2000); a schematic diagram of the determinants of health is shown in Figure 1.1. In the figure, the individual is depicted in the center; the health of a given individual is shown to be directly influenced by biology (e.g., genetic inheritance, unique biological functioning) and by personal behaviors that have relevance for health (e.g., diet, physical activity, substance use, tobacco use, sexual behavior, risk-taking behaviors). The diagram also conveys that an individual resides within unique physical and social environments that can exert an influence on health status. The physical environment may affect health status in numerous ways (e.g., air quality, sanitation, health hazards/violence, presence of toxins), whereas the social environment may influence health status through mechanisms such as the degree of social support, the magnitude of interpersonal stress/conflict, and the level of socioeconomic well-being.

Figure 1.1 also conveys that health status is determined by access to appropriate health care (or lack thereof), including the availability of primary, secondary, and tertiary health care services. Similarly, the policies and conventions within a given health care system can exert an influence on the health status of an individual (e.g., magnitude of health care expenditures, decisions regarding health care priorities). Although the *Healthy People 2010* model for the determinants of health was conceptualized in the context of the U.S. health care system, the general framework

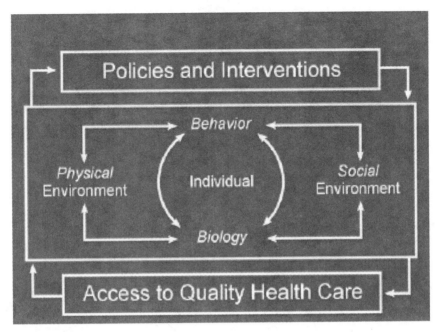

Figure 1.1 Determinants of Health

appears to have relevance for other nations, societies, and cultures. This chapter will examine the challenge of health care and disability in the United States and abroad from the standpoints of chronic disease, access to care, quality of care, and macroeconomics and will introduce the potential contributions of health communication technologies.

ASSESSING THE HEALTH OF NATIONS

A comparative analysis of the performance, outcomes, and quality of international health care systems is exceedingly complex, and an in-depth discussion of this literature is well beyond the scope of this chapter. Yet assessments of the health of nations have been performed, and those nations that spend the most on health care are not necessarily the same ones that achieve the best outcomes for their citizens. For example, Nolte and McKee (2008) conducted analyses that were based on the construct of "amenable mortality," which refers to deaths that occur as a result of causes that would not be expected to result in death if timely and effective health care were available.

Specifically, Nolte and McKee (2008) compared the United States to 14 European nations, Canada, Australia, New Zealand, and Japan between 1997 and 1998 and again between 2002 and 2003, analyzing trends in amenable mortality in persons under age 75. Between the two assessments, there was an average decline of 16% in amenable mortality across all nations. However, the United States was a statistical outlier with a decline of only 4%; the data revealed that the United States did not experience a decline in amenable mortality at the same pace as other industrialized nations. Furthermore, the data suggested that the relative failure of the United States to reduce amenable mortality was associated with a lack of progress in reducing deaths associated with ischemic heart disease and other circulatory diseases, especially stroke. Nolte and McKee observed that the lack of progress in reducing amenable mortality coincided with an increase in the uninsured population of the United States. Although all nations face unique health care challenges, the United States is an example of a health care system for which the magnitude of the financial investment has not yielded the desired outcomes.

OVERVIEW OF HEALTH STATUS IN THE UNITED STATES

Burden of Chronic Diseases

One indisputable fact is that everyone will die of something—so why be concerned about deaths from chronic disease? The reality is that, by definition, deaths from chronic disease are not quick; these deaths are often protracted, painful, and premature. Furthermore, deaths from chronic disease typically take an enormous toll on the affected individuals, their families, and the economic systems in which they live.

According to data from 2001, chronic disease claims the lives of more than 1.7 million Americans each year (Centers for Disease Control and Prevention, 2004). Specifically, five chronic diseases account for more than two-thirds of all deaths in the United States; these five diseases are heart disease, cancers, stroke, chronic obstructive pulmonary diseases, and diabetes. A survey by the Kaiser Family Foundation in 2005 found that 44% of the U.S. population lives with a chronic health condition such as heart disease, cancer, asthma, diabetes, or other handicaps/disabilities that affect daily functioning (Kaiser Family Foundation, 2005). Recent data from the Centers for Disease Control and Prevention (2005a) indicated that more than 90 million persons in the United

States are living with a chronic health condition. As might be expected, persons with chronic diseases encounter difficulty obtaining appropriate health care due to the high costs associated with these conditions, and they are more likely to report financial burdens as a result of overdue medical bills (Kaiser Family Foundation, 2005).

Chronic diseases are the greatest contributors to mortality in the United States. In 2004, cardiovascular diseases accounted for over 872,000 deaths in the United States, which represented 36% of all deaths in the nation (U.S. Department of Health and Human Services & National Institutes of Health, 2007). Cerebral vascular disease alone was the third-leading cause of death in 2004 and accounted for approximately 150,000 lost lives (U.S. Department of Health and Human Services & National Institutes of Health, 2007). In 2001, approximately 550,000 deaths in the United States (23% of all deaths) were due to cancer (Centers for Disease Control and Prevention, 2004); 30% of these deaths could be attributed directly to smoking, and all smoking-related deaths are potentially preventable (Centers for Disease Control and Prevention, 2004). Approximately 18 million Americans have diabetes, and roughly 5 million of these persons are not even aware that they have the condition (Centers for Disease Control and Prevention, 2004). In 2001, diabetes was the sixth-leading cause of death in the United States and accounted for approximately 71,000 lost lives; deaths from diabetes may be underestimated because secondary complications are commonly listed as the cause of death on death certificates.

Risk Factors for Chronic Disease

To a great extent, chronic diseases are a reflection of the behaviors that Americans engage in (or do not engage in) as they go about their daily lives. The behaviors that are the most damaging to the health of Americans and that contribute the most to chronic diseases include tobacco use, failure to engage in sufficient physical activity, and failure to adhere to healthful dietary practices (Centers for Disease Control and Prevention, 2004). Specifically, the tendency for Americans to be overweight has emerged as a major public health issue; a survey conducted during 1976–1980 and followed up in 2002 found that the prevalence of obesity in the United States had doubled (Centers for Disease Control and Prevention, 2005b).

This trend toward obesity starts early in life. Ogden, Flegal, Carroll, and Johnson (2002) found that 15% of 6- to 19-year-olds were overweight;

10% of 2- to 5-year-olds were found to be already overweight. The National Health Nutrition Examination Survey shows that the percentage of overweight children and adolescents tripled from 5% in 1980 to 15% in 1999–2000 (Ogden et al., 2002). These trends appear to be a result of both unhealthy dietary habits and insufficient physical activity; 300,000 deaths per year in the United States are associated with unhealthy eating habits and sedentary lifestyles. In 2002, over 75% of U.S. adults reported not eating the recommended daily quantities of fruits and vegetables (Centers for Disease Control and Prevention, 2004). Based on data from the 2006 National Health Interview Survey, 62% of adults reported not engaging in vigorous leisure-time physical activity of 10 minutes or more per week, although 24% did report engaging in such activity three or more times per week (Pleis & Lethbridge-Cejku, 2007). Using body mass as the criteria, the survey categorized 35% of adults as overweight (but not obese) in 2006, and 26% as obese (Pleis & Lethbridge-Cejku, 2007).

In the United States, approximately 45 million persons smoke tobacco products (Centers for Disease Control and Prevention, 2007). The data also reveal that the rate of decline in smoking among young people has largely stalled, and approximately 3,900 young people initiate smoking activity each day in spite of the extensive evidence linking smoking and adverse health consequences (Centers for Disease Control and Prevention, 2005c). Accordingly, approximately 8.6 million Americans suffer from the consequences of tobacco use, including heart disease, emphysema, and other smoking-related conditions and approximately 440,000 Americans die each year as a result of diseases that are attributable to smoking (Centers for Disease Control and Prevention, 2005c). Nearly 10% of these smoking-related deaths are due to secondhand smoke (Centers for Disease Control and Prevention, 2005c). An inverse relationship exists between smoking and educational level; people with less education are more likely to use tobacco products (Centers for Disease Control and Prevention, 2007).

Health Care Access

Access to health care is a major issue for many U.S. citizens under the age of 65 and for those who are not eligible for public assistance. Specifically, in 2006, nearly 44 million people in the United States (14.8%) were without health insurance (Cohen & Martinez, 2007), which severely restricts their access to care in the context of rising health care costs. Not surprisingly, persons who do not have health insurance are less likely to receive recommended health services; analyses of the 2002 Behavioral Risk Factor Surveillance System revealed decreased use of cancer prevention services, cardiovascular risk reduction services, and diabetic management among persons without health insurance compared to those with health insurance (Ross, Bradley, & Busch, 2006). Even among persons with higher incomes, lack of health insurance coverage was associated with decreased use of preventive health care services (Ross et al., 2006).

Iglehart (2002) found that the relative contribution of employers to health care is decreasing and that the contributions of workers are rising. Thus, out-of-pocket health care expenditures are creating a major financial burden for many Americans.

Indeed, financial concerns are a major barrier to care for persons with major health conditions. A Kaiser Family Foundation survey in 2005 found that 24% of persons with major health conditions, as opposed to only 14% of healthy persons, reported that health care costs were their biggest monthly expense after rent or mortgage. In addition, 29% of persons with chronic health conditions, as opposed to only 16% of healthy persons, reported having an overdue medical bill. Of those with chronic health conditions, 28% reported not being able to afford health care, even though 62% had some form of health insurance. The greatest cause for concern was that 29% of those who could not afford medical care reported skipping medical treatment, cutting pills, or not having a prescription filled as a result of limited funds.

Even for persons who are fully employed, health care in the United States is often not affordable. Specifically, high deductibles, gaps in coverage, and an unfortunate pattern of claims denials can place the working poor on the brink of financial disaster (Shipler, 2004). Access to health care also is not equal for all segments of American society; race, culture, and socioeconomic class play undeniable roles in numerous ways, including the responsiveness of providers, the ability to communicate health care needs, and the potential for mistrust on the part of underrepresented minorities. These health care disparities have been well documented in the IOM report *Unequal Treatment: Confronting Racial and Ethnic Disparities in Health Care* (Smedley, Stith, & Nelson, 2002).

Health Care Quality

According to the Institute of Medicine, health care quality is defined as "the degree to which health services for individuals and populations increase the likelihood of desired health outcomes and are consistent with current professional knowledge" (Institute of Medicine & Committee to Design a Strategy for Quality Review and Assurance in Medicare, 1990, p. 21). However, the assessment of health care quality represents a major challenge that can be approached from the standpoints of populations, individual health outcomes, clinical effectiveness, and patient safety. Strategies for improving health care quality often involve information technology and the communication of critical information to providers and/or consumers. For example, research in the area of clinical effectiveness frequently results in the publication of evidence-based practice guidelines, but such guidelines must be effectively communicated and ultimately adopted by practitioners if improved outcomes are to accrue.

Similarly, there is a growing awareness that medical errors are a major problem that compromises health care quality; the IOM report *To Err Is Human* (Kohn, Corrigan, & Donaldson, 1999) estimated that nearly 100,000 deaths occur annually in the United States as a result of mistakes associated with health care services. Medication errors alone have been estimated to account for over 7,000 deaths annually (Phillips, Christenfeld, & Glynn, 1998). Surprisingly, in 1998, more people died as a result of errors in the U.S. health care system than from motor vehicle accidents (43,458), breast cancer (42,297), or AIDS (16,516) (Martin, Smith, Mathews, & Ventura, 1999). The root causes of medical errors vary, but one key component involves inadequate clinical information systems that inhibit access to timely and complete patient information. In fact, Woolf, Kuzel, Dovey, and Phillips (2004) examined a series of anonymous medical error reports and found that 67% of the cases were set into motion by errors in communication; they describe numerous examples of miscommunication, including information breakdown among colleagues and/or with patients, misinformation in the medical record, mishandling of patient requests/messages, inaccessible medical records, and inadequate reminder systems. Compelling evidence exists that inadequate communication systems play a key role in many of the errors of diagnosis and treatment that occur in health care settings.

Disability in America

The Americans with Disabilities Act defines an individual with a disability as someone who has a physical or mental impairment that substantially limits one or more major life activities, has a record of such an impairment, or is regarded as having such an impairment. A sizable portion of U.S. citizens are living with some form of disability that affects their daily functioning and has the potential to alter their quality of life. The 2006 Disability Status Report for the United States (Rehabilitation Research and Training Center on Disability Demographics and Statistics, 2007) found that the prevalence of disability for persons ages 21 to 64 years was nearly 13%. For persons ages 65 to 74 years, the prevalence of disability was over 30%; for persons over age 75, the prevalence of disability was nearly 53%.

Disability confers major disadvantages in areas related to income, employment, and overall financial well-being. In 2006, the employment rate for adults with disabilities between the ages of 21 and 64 years was only 38%, which is far less than the national average. In 2006, the median annual household income of working-age persons with disabilities in the United States was $36,300, and the poverty rate was over 25% (Rehabilitation Research and Training Center on Disability Demographics and Statistics, 2007). Not surprisingly, these types of socioeconomic disadvantages for persons with disabilities create secondary stressors in many areas, including access to health care.

In fact, access to health care is a profound problem for persons with disabilities. Shigaki, Hagglund, Clark, and Conforti (2002) found that 74% of persons with disabilities who reported needing health care services encountered difficulty accessing at least one service; persons with spinal cord injury reported the greatest difficulty accessing health care services (87%), followed by persons with brain injury (79%) and persons who had experienced stroke (65%). They reported that dental services were the most difficult to access, but that problems also were encountered accessing personal care attendants, medical supplies, eyeglasses, durable medical equipment, physical therapy, and specialty medical care, among numerous others.

A common reason for failure to access health care was found to be limitations in Medicaid coverage (Shigaki et al., 2002). Many persons with a disability face employment challenges and transportation barriers and, accordingly, have limited incomes. Gaps in Medicaid coverage and other components of the U.S. health care "safety net" create profound problems for many Americans who do not have health insurance or substantive financial resources, but this is particularly the case for persons with disabilities.

Health Care Expenditures

Recent data from the Center for Medicare and Medicaid Services indicate that $1.9 trillion was spent on U.S. health care in 2004; this translates to $6,697 per person (U.S. Department of Health and Human Services, Centers for Disease Control and Prevention, & National Center for Health Statistics, 2006). Health care spending accounted for 16% of the U.S. gross domestic product in 2004, which was greater than for any other developed country participating in the data collection of the Organization for Economic Cooperation and Development. Personal health care expenditures, including spending for hospital care, physician services, nursing home care, dental care, and other medical services, accounted for 83% of the $1.9 trillion spent on health care in 2004.

The U.S. Department of Health and Human Services, the Centers for Disease Control and Prevention, and the National Center for Health Statistics (2006) have provided data on the sources of funding and the categories of expenditures for health care in 2004. Thirty-six percent was paid by private health insurance, 34% by the federal government, 11% by state or local governments, 15% in out-of-pocket spending, and the remainder from other private funds. With regard to categories of expenditures, 37% was paid for hospital care, 26% for physician care, 12% for prescription drugs, 7% for nursing home care, and 18% for other personal care, such as visits to nonphysician medical providers, and medical supplies. Hospital care expenditures declined by 9% from 1980 to 2004 (due to efforts to reduce bed days of care), whereas prescription drug expenditures doubled.

Reports from the Centers for Disease Control and Prevention (2005a) have shown that escalating health care expenditures cannot effectively be addressed without recognition of the costs associated with chronic diseases. Recent estimates suggest that chronic diseases account for 75% of the total amount spent on health care in the United States (Centers for Disease Control and Prevention, 2005a). Regarding specific conditions, spending is currently approaching $128 billion annually for the combined direct and indirect costs associated with arthritis; the direct and indirect costs associated with smoking exceed $193 billion annually. In 2001, $300 billion was spent on treatment for cardiovascular diseases, and approximately $132 billion was spent on diabetes (Centers for Disease Control and Prevention, 2005a). Therefore, even small reductions in the prevalence of chronic diseases could result in major savings within the U.S. economy.

Future Challenges

In 1900, life expectancy for Americans at birth was 47 years (Kotlikoff & Burns, 2005); today, life expectancy at birth is approximately 76 years and rising. As a result of factors such as better nutrition and advances in health care, Americans are generally living much longer. Data from the U.S. Department of Health and Human Services, the Centers for Disease Control and Prevention, and the National Center for Health Statistics (2006) indicate that men are now expected to live 3 years longer than they did in 1990, and women are now expected to live 1 year longer than they did in 1990. In addition, mortality rates for many conditions are declining, so the population of persons age 65 and over in the United States is expected to increase from 12% in 2000 to nearly 20% by 2030 (Centers for Disease Control and Prevention, 2003).

The dramatic increase in longevity, however, has been occurring at the same time that birth rates in the United States have been declining (Kotlikoff & Burns, 2005). Taken together, these combined trends are resulting in the "graying of America," or the more rapid growth of the percentage of persons over age 65 than the percentage of persons in younger age groups (Kotlikoff & Burns, 2005). Consequently, in the future, an increasingly smaller percentage of working-age U.S. adults will be producing the revenue to fund the social programs that will support an increasingly larger percentage of older Americans.

These demographic trends are worthy of more than casual interest; they have profound implications for the economic future of the United States. In 2008, the oldest baby boomers will be eligible for retirement, and Social Security benefits and Medicare claims will follow not far behind. Indeed, the benefits associated with these federal programs have been promised to future generations, even though they have not been funded in a sustainable manner. Accordingly, the potential funding shortfall for Social Security and Medicare programs is staggering. Currently, the gross official federal debt for the United States is approximately $9 trillion (U.S. Government Accountability Office, 2007). However, the gross official federal debt does not take into account the implicit debt that is inherent in future Social Security and Medicare commitments. The Social Security component of the U.S. implicit debt has been estimated to be $22 trillion; the Medicare component has been estimated to be an additional $50 trillion. These two underfunded programs alone combine for a total implicit U.S. debt of approximately $72 trillion. It has been estimated that to meet debt of this astounding magnitude, today's workers would have to contribute all their earnings to debt retirement for a period of 10 years (Kotlikoff & Burns, 2005). Therefore, the massive debt obligations associated with Social Security and Medicare pose a tremendous challenge to the sustainability of these programs (in their current form) and, indeed, to the economic future of the United States as a whole.

OVERVIEW OF WORLDWIDE HEALTH STATUS

In a figurative sense, the world is becoming "flat" (Friedman, 2005). Specifically, a confluence of forces are operating that, in profound ways, are reducing communication and trade barriers between nations; these forces include the migration toward capitalistic economies in previously communist countries (e.g., the former Soviet Union and China), the emergence of the Internet and related digital technologies, the development of workflow software that facilitates remote participation in commercial activities, and a growing international workforce that is willing to work for relatively low wages (Friedman, 2005). Although possibly less apparent, these trends toward globalization have important implications for worldwide health care. Specifically, the disease profile of the world is undergoing rapid change (World Health Organization, 2005). Although infectious diseases have historically been the major public health concern in developing nations, the total number of people dying of chronic diseases is now twice as high as those dying of the combination of infectious diseases, maternal/perinatal conditions, and nutritional deficiencies (World Health Organization, 2005). More specifically, the emerging epidemics of heart disease, stroke, cancer, and other chronic diseases are beginning to take a tremendous toll in terms of worldwide deaths and disability (World Health Organization, 2005). Without a doubt, there continues to be a tremendous need to address communicable diseases such as HIV/AIDS. There also continues to be a major concern regarding the potential for worldwide pandemics involving infectious conditions such as avian flu. However, trends toward globalization, dietary changes, and migration away from agrarian lifestyles are beginning to introduce a new set of health-related challenges throughout the world.

The health-related impact of globalization is complex, but it involves a dietary transition in low- and middle-income countries toward the consumption of foods that are high in fats, salts, and sugar (World Health Organization, 2005). On the demand side, rising incomes from increased economic productivity have created the ability to purchase processed foods and have reduced the time people have for food production and preparation. On the supply side, a greater percentage of the worldwide population is becoming reachable through marketing and promotional campaigns that encourage consumption of unhealthy foods. Notably, a significant portion of global marketing is now targeted at children (World Health Organization, 2005), which has major implications for the health of future generations. Already, body mass indicators and total cholesterol levels are increasing as national incomes rise in developing countries (World Health Organization, 2005), and approximately 50% of the worldwide population now lives in urban environments, which tend to promote a sedentary lifestyle (World Health Organization, 2005). In addition, as is occurring in the United States, the global population is aging, and the prevalence of persons age 65 and over is projected to reach 973 million worldwide by 2030 (Centers for Disease Control and Prevention, 2003). These trends increase the probability of chronic disease (World Health Organization, 2005). Other risk factors that are known to contribute significantly to global chronic disease include tobacco use, excessive alcohol consumption, and high blood pressure (World Health Organization, 2005).

In spite of the "flattening" world, poverty continues to be a reality for a large segment of the global population, and poverty itself is a risk factor for chronic disease. Poverty occurs in all countries, even the most affluent. Economic deprivation restricts people's access to the essential elements for a healthy life, such as affordable foods, nutrient-rich diets, adequate housing, and access to health care. Poverty also is associated with psychological stress, high-risk behaviors (e.g., tobacco use), and generally unhealthy living conditions. In addition, concerns about physical safety in economically deprived environments often restrict physical activity, and cardiovascular disease has been found to be more prevalent in deprived communities than in affluent ones (Stronks, van de Mheen, & Mackenbach, 1998; Sundquist, Malmstrom, & Johansson, 2004). In poverty-stricken environments, the availability of preventive care, diagnostic services, clinical interventions, and transport to health facilities and access to medications are typically limited (Goddard & Smith, 1998; Lorant, Boland, Humblet, & Deliege, 2002). Persons who live under conditions of economic deprivation also frequently face health care disparities in comparison to persons with greater financial means. Specifically, persons with low incomes are often marginalized within health care systems and do not receive optimally responsive health care services (Goddard & Smith, 1998).

Once chronic disease develops, a downward spiral toward increasing poverty often begins. Persons with chronic diseases are less able to work and hence to generate incomes, so their living conditions tend to deteriorate even further. If a person who becomes ill happens to be the income earner for a family, the living conditions and health status of the entire family, including children and the elderly in multigenerational households, may suffer.

In all nations, there are macroeconomic dimensions to chronic disease. These dimensions include the direct costs of providing health care services, the indirect costs associated with lost productivity, and, in some countries, the loss of national income associated with premature mortality (World Health Organization, 2005). Figure 1.2 shows the projected annual reduction in GDP associated with deaths due to heart disease, stroke, and diabetes in 2005 and as estimated for 2015; the Russian Federation is expected to face an annual reduction in GDP of more than 5% by 2015. Accordingly, for most nations, strong economic incentives exist to reduce chronic disease, and viable strategies are available to improve health-related outcomes; these include laws/regulations (e.g., water fluoridation), taxation to reduce unhealthy behaviors (e.g., cigarette taxes), improvement of public infrastructure (e.g., walking and biking paths), community-based advocacy (e.g., promotion of smoke-free environments), and public education (e.g., programs to improve nutrition and physical activity). In spite of isolated successes, the overall global

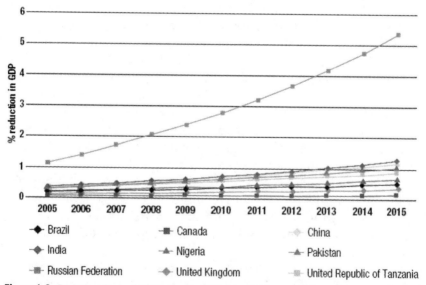

Figure 1.2 Projected Annual Reduction in GDP from Deaths Due to Heart Disease, Stroke, and Diabetes as Proportion of GDP, 2005–2015.

response to chronic disease remains inadequate (Yach, Hawkes, Gould, & Hofman 2004).

MEETING THE HEALTH CARE CHALLENGE

Patient-Centered Health Care

A 2020 vision for health care has been provided by Davis, Schoen, and Schoenbaum (2000) and elaborated by Davis, Schoen, and Audet (2005). Although the vision was conceptualized for U.S. health care, the principles appear to be relevant from a global perspective, even though intermediate achievements likely would be needed in developing countries. Davis, Schoen, Audet, and Schoenbaum describe a vision of affordable health insurance, accessible health care, patient-centered care, information-driven care, and integrated quality improvement systems. They also envision care that is predicated on the latest scientific evidence and supported by robust clinical information systems.

Interestingly, many of these elements of a 2020 vision for health care involve communication systems in one form or another. For example, as described by Davis and associates (2005), patient-centered care involves access to health services that are augmented by digitized communication allowing patients to select their own appointments, to receive timely responses to e-mails, and to obtain electronic prescription refills, among numerous other features. This vision involves active consumer engagement in care, as reflected by well-developed information systems that have the ability to transmit data on health care conditions/problems, treatment options, and treatment plans. Information would be made available to both providers and consumers in the form of reminders and alerts for preventive care or whenever abnormal findings emerge. Consumers would have access to their electronic medical records and be able to receive information that could inform behavior change, patient education, and counseling/guidance.

In addition, Davis et al. (2005) envision access to clinical information systems that would support quality improvement through mechanisms such as patient registries, monitors of adherence, and informed decision making. The patient-centered vision involves effective communication among health care providers and the efficient transfer of clinical information across a virtual provider network; continuous feedback systems would exist in the form of automated patient surveys to facilitate practice improvement. Lastly, Davis and associates envision publicly available information databases that would help consumers select providers and/ or health care facilities on the basis of performance on definable standards of care.

Disruptive Innovations in Health Care

The gap between current health care systems and the idealized vision of patient-centered care is profound. A realistic strategy for bridging this tremendous gap is hard to conceptualize, but Christensen, Bohmer, and Kenagy (2000) describe the possibility of "disruptive innovations" in health care. The key principle is that simpler, less expensive alternatives to costly, inefficient care are possible, but that fundamental disruptions to existing systems and institutions will be required for the necessary changes to occur. Christensen and associates note that prior to 1980, persons with diabetes could only learn their glucose levels through inaccurate urine tests or by visiting a clinic where a blood sample could be drawn and laboratory-based measurements could occur. Today, persons with diabetes are able to carry miniature blood glucose meters wherever they go, which permits them to easily access information that allows self-management of many aspects of a disease that previously required intensive physician management. The advent of miniature blood glucose monitors is an example of a disruptive innovation; endocrinologists experienced less demand for their services, clinic revenues for diabetes care decreased, and the companies that made the large laboratory-based equipment for blood glucose testing were forced to leave the market. More specifically, a technologic innovation that permitted information to be made directly available to people with diabetes at the point of decision making resulted in notably improved (and less expensive) health care.

OPPORTUNITIES IN THE NEW MEDIA LANDSCAPE

In the new media landscape, developments in the fields of information technology and communication systems may enable disruptive innovations and creative solutions that can be brought to bear on many challenging health care problems. The availability of information at the optimal time and place may better inform lifestyle choices, promote preventive health care, improve interdisciplinary coordination of care, and enable more informed selections of health care providers and services. For example,

Woolf, Krist, Johnson, Wilson, Rothemich, Norman, and Devers (2006) found that even a well-designed Web site can promote improvements in stage of change and health behaviors over a short-term follow-up. Several recent studies and editorials also have made a strong case that the basic Google search engine itself will have a substantial impact on clinical decision making and consumer behavior over time (Giustini, 2005, 2006; Tang & Ng, 2006). Through the use of advanced bioinformatics technology, the practice of medicine in the future is expected to personalize health care through access to an individual's unique genetic profile (Giustini, 2007).

Until recently, physicians possessed specialized knowledge to which patients had limited access, but now patients who are willing to invest sufficient time and energy may come to know as much (or more) about a condition than do their providers (Christensen, Anthony, & Roth, 2004). Indeed, the following chapters in this volume explore the various ways that information technology and health communication systems can be used to address challenging health care problems. Although the gap between health systems at the beginning of the 21st century and the ideals of patient-centered care is enormous, there is reason to hope that health communication opportunities in the new media landscape will assist both developed and developing nations to move toward creative, "disruptive" solutions and improved health status for their citizens.

REFERENCES

Centers for Disease Control and Prevention. (2003). Public health and aging: Trends in aging-United States and worldwide. *Morbidity and Mortality Weekly Report, 52*(6), 101–106.

Centers for Disease Control and Prevention. (2004). *The burden of chronic diseases and their risk factors: National and State Perspectives 2004.* Atlanta, GA: U.S. Department of Health and Human Services.

Centers for Disease Control and Prevention. (2005a). *Chronic disease prevention: Chronic disease overview.* Retrieved February 4, 2008, from http://www.cdc.gov/nccdphp/overview.htm

Centers for Disease Control and Prevention. (2005b). Special topic: Obesity. *Chronic Disease Notes & Reports, 17*(2), 1–105.

Centers for Disease Control and Prevention. (2005c). Special topic: Tobacco control. *Chronic Disease Notes & Reports, 18*(1), 1–32.

Centers for Disease Control and Prevention. (2007). Cigarette smoking among adults—United States, 2006. *Morbidity and Mortality Weekly Report, 56*(44), 1157–1161.

Christensen, C., Anthony, S. D., & Roth, E. A. (2004). *Seeing what's next: Using the theories of innovation to predict industry change.* Boston: Harvard Business School Press.

Christensen, C. M., Bohmer, R., & Kenagy, J. (2000). Will disruptive innovations cure health care? *Harvard Business Review, 78*(5), 102–112.

Cohen, R. A., & Martinez, M. E. (2007). *Health insurance coverage: Early release of estimates from the National Health Interview Survey, 2006.* Retrieved March 26, 2008, from http://www.cdc.gov/nchs/data/nhis/earlyrelease/insur200706.pdf

Davis, K., Schoen, C., & Schoenbaum, S. C. (2000). A 2020 vision for American health care. *Archives of Internal Medicine, 160*(22), 3357–3362.

Davis, K., Schoenbaum, S. C., & Audet, A. M. (2005). A 2020 vision of patient-centered primary care. *Journal of General Internal Medicine, 20*(10), 953–957.

Friedman, T. L. (2005). *The world is flat: A brief history of the twenty-first century.* New York: Farrar, Straus and Giroux.

Giustini, D. (2005). How Google is changing medicine. *British Medical Journal, 331*(7531), 1487–1488.

Giustini, D. (2006). How Web 2.0 is changing medicine. *British Medical Journal, 333,* 1283–1284.

Giustini, D. (2007). Web 3.0 and medicine. *British Medical Journal, 335,* 1273–1274.

Goddard, M., & Smith, P. (1998). *Equity of access to health care.* Centre for Health Economics, University of York, York, United Kingdom.

Iglehart, J. K. (2002). Changing health insurance trends. *New England Journal of Medicine, 347*(12), 956–962.

Institute of Medicine & Committee to Design a Strategy for Quality Review and Assurance in Medicare. (1990). *Medicare: A strategy for quality assurance* (Vol. 1.). Washington, DC: National Academy Press.

Jonas, S., Goldsteen, R., & Goldsteen, K. (2007). *An introduction to the U.S. health care system.* New York: Springer Publishing.

Kaiser Family Foundation. (2005). *The USA Today/Kaiser Family Foundation/Harvard School of Public Health, health care costs survey.* Retrieved February 6, 2008, from http://www.kff.org/newsmedia/upload/7371.pdf

Kohn, L. T., Corrigan, J. M., & Donaldson, M. S. (1999). *To err is human: Building a safer health system.* Washington, DC: National Academy Press.

Kotlikoff, L. J., & Burns, S. (2005). *The coming generational storm: What you need to know about America's economic future.* Cambridge, MA: MIT Press.

Lorant, V., Boland, B., Humblet, P., & Deliege, D. (2002). Equity in prevention and health care. *Journal of Epidemiology and Community Health, 56*(7), 510–516.

Martin, J. A., Smith, B. L., Mathews, T. J., & Ventura, S. J. (1999). *Births and deaths: Preliminary data for 1998. National Vital Statistics Report* (Rep. No. Vol. 47, No. 25). Hyattsville, MD: Centers for Disease Control and Prevention, National Center for Health Statistics.

Nolte, E., & McKee, C. M. (2008). Measuring the health of nations: Updating an earlier analysis. *Health Affairs, 27*(1), 58–71.

Ogden, C. L., Flegal, K. M., Carroll, M. D., & Johnson, C. L. (2002). Prevalence and trends in overweight among U.S. children and adolescents, 1999–2000. *Journal of the American Medical Association, 288*(14), 1728–1732.

Phillips, D. P., Christenfeld, N., & Glynn, L. M. (1998). Increase in US medication-error deaths between 1983 and 1993. *Lancet, 351*(9103), 643.

Pleis, J. R., & Lethbridge-Cejku, M. (2007). *Summary health statistics for US adults: National health interview survey, 2006.* National Center for Health Statistics. *Vital Health Stat, 10*(235), 1–105.

Rehabilitation Research and Training Center on Disability Demographics and Statistics. (2007). *2006 disability status report.* Ithaca, NY: Cornell University.

Ross, J. S., Bradley, E. H., & Busch, S. H. (2006). Use of health care services by lower-income and higher-income uninsured adults. *Journal of the American Medical Association, 295*(17), 2027–2036.

Shigaki, C. L., Hagglund, K. J., Clark, M., & Conforti, K. (2002). Access to health care services among people with rehabilitation needs receiving Medicaid. *Rehabilitation Psychology, 47*(2), 204–218.

Shipler, D. K. (2004). *The working poor.* New York: Random House.

Smedley, B. D., Stith, A. Y., & Nelson, A. R. (2002). *Unequal treatment: Confronting racial and ethnic disparities in health care.* Washington, DC: National Academy Press.

Stronks, K., van de Mheen, H. D., & Mackenbach, J. P. (1998). A higher prevalence of health problems in low income groups: Does it reflect relative deprivation? *Journal of Epidemiology and Community Health, 52*(9), 548–557.

Sundquist, K., Malmstrom, M., & Johansson, S. (2004). Neighbourhood deprivation and incidence of coronary heart disease: A multilevel study of 2.6 million women and men in Sweden. *Journal of Epidemiology and Community Health, 58*(1), 71–77.

Tang, H., & Ng, J. H. K. (2006). Googling for a diagnosis—use of Google as a diagnostic aid: Internet based study. *British Medical Journal, 333*, 1143–1145.

U.S. Department of Health and Human Services. (2000). *Healthy people 2010. 2nd ed. With Understanding and Improving Health and Objectives for Improving Health.* (Vol. 1). Washington, DC: Government Printing Office.

U.S. Department of Health and Human Services, Centers for Disease Control and Prevention, & National Center for Health Statistics. (2006). *Health, United States, 2006 with chartbook on trends in the health of Americans.* Washington, DC: Government Printing Office, Retrieved from http://www.cdc.gov/nchs/data/hus/hus06.pdf

U.S. Department of Health and Human Services & National Institutes of Health. (2007). *National Heart Lung and Blood Institute FY 2006 fact book.* Ithaca, NY: National Heart, Lung, and Blood Institute.

U.S. Government Accountability Office. (2007). *Financial audit: Bureau of the Public Debt's fiscal years 2007 and 2006 schedules of federal debt.* Retrieved March 26, 2008, from http://www.treasurydirect.gov/govt/reports/pd/feddebt/feddebt_ann2007.pdf

Woolf, S. H., Krist, A. H., Johnson, R. E., Wilson, D. B., Rothemich, S. F., Norman, G. J., & Devers, K. J. (2006). A practice-sponsored web site to help patients pursue healthy behaviors: An ACORN study. *Annals of Family Medicine, 4*(2), 148–152.

Woolf, S. H., Kuzel, A. J., Dovey, S. M., & Phillips, R. L., Jr. (2004). A string of mistakes: The importance of cascade analysis in describing, counting, and preventing medical errors. *Annals of Family Medicine, 2*, 317–326.

World Health Organization. (1946). *Preamble to the constitution of the World Health Organization as adopted by the International Health Conference, New York, 19–22 June, 1946; signed on 22 July 1946 by the representatives of 61 states (Official Records of the World Health Organization, no. 2, p. 100) and entered into force on 7 April 1948.* Retrieved April 29, 2008, from http://www.who.int/about/definition/en/print.html

World Health Organization. (2005). *Preventing chronic diseases: A vital investment: WHO global report.* Geneva, Switzerland: Author.

Yach, D., Hawkes, C., Gould, C. L., & Hofman, K. J. (2004). The global burden of chronic diseases: Overcoming impediments to prevention and control. *Journal of the American Medical Association, 291*(21), 2616–2622.

2

Emerging Demographics and Health Care Trends

MARY E. NORTHRIDGE, RUBIAHNA L. VAUGHN, AND ALWYN T. COHALL

In this chapter, first an ecological model that traces how health communication tools at various levels (societal/macro, community/meso, and interpersonal/micro) may affect individual and population health and well-being is presented, with examples drawn from ongoing initiatives at the Harlem Health Promotion Center, where the authors are based. Second, the scholarly and scientific public health literature is reviewed in order to explain both emerging demographics and health care trends that are central to the development of health communication approaches and methods in the new media landscape. Next, reflections on the current challenges and possible new strategies for reaching diverse populations with health and health care information are offered for consideration. Finally, a call is issued for needed policy reforms that will abet efforts to improve health and health care through diverse health communication tools, including those envisioned by the other contributors to this volume.

ECOLOGICAL MODEL OF SOCIAL DETERMINANTS OF HEALTH

Table 2.1 presents an ecological model of social determinants of health that was adapted to include health communication tools at various levels of influence.

ECOLOGICAL MODEL OF SOCIAL DETERMINANTS OF HEALTH

Table 2.1

FUNDAMENTAL FACTORS (SOCIAL/MACRO LEVEL)	INTERMEDIATE FACTORS (COMMUNITY/MESO LEVEL)	PROXIMATE FACTORS (INTERPERSONAL/MICRO LEVEL)	HEALTH AND WELL-BEING (INDIVIDUAL AND POPULATION LEVELS)
Health communication tools ■ Web sites ■ Music videos	**Health communication tools** ■ Billboards ■ Ads in subway stations and check cashing establishments	**Health communication tools** ■ Culturally apt DVDs and pamphlets ■ Text messaging	**Health communication tools** ■ Maps of community health indicators and health care facilities ■ Electronic medical records
Natural environment ■ Topography ■ Climate ■ Water supply ■ Air quality	**Built environment** ■ Land use (industrial, residential; mixed use or single use) ■ Transportation systems ■ Services (shopping, banking, health care facilities) ■ Public resources (parks, museums, libraries) ■ Zoning regulations ■ Buildings (housing, schools, workplaces)	**Stressors/buffers** ■ Environmental, neighborhood, workplace, and housing conditions ■ Violent crime and safety ■ Police response ■ Financial insecurity ■ Environmental toxins (lead, particulates) ■ Unfair treatment (stigma, prejudice, discrimination)	**Health outcomes** ■ Mental health ■ Injury/violence ■ HIV/AIDS ■ Obesity/overweight ■ Cardiovascular diseases ■ Diabetes ■ Cancers ■ Infectious diseases ■ Sexually transmitted diseases ■ Respiratory health ■ All-cause mortality

Macrosocial factors

- Historical Conditions
- Political orders
- Economic orders
- Legal codes
- Human rights doctrines
- Social and cultural institutions
- Ideologies (ageism, sexism, racism, social justice, democracy)

Inequalities

- Distribution of material wealth
- Distribution of employment opportunities
- Distribution of educational opportunities
- Distribution of political influence

Social context

- Cultural identity
- Community investment (economic development, maintenance, police services)
- Policies (public, fiscal, environmental, workplace)
- Enforcement of ordinances (public, environmental, workplace)
- Community capacity
- Civic participation and political influence
- Quality of education

Health behaviors

- Health screenings (HIV, cancer, hypertension)
- Physical activity
- Dietary practices
- Substance use (e.g., tobacco, alcohol)

Social integration

- Social participation and integration
- Shape of social networks
- Available resources within networks
- Coping and social support

Well-Being

- Hope/despair
- Life satisfaction
- Psychosocial distress
- Happiness
- Disability
- Concealment of identity
- Expectations of rejection
- Body size and body image

Overview of Model

In its original form (see Northridge, Sclar, & Biswas, 2003), this ecological model introduced a joint urban planning and public health framework that is centrally concerned with the social, political, economic, and historical processes that generate the urban built environment. Specifically, the natural environment, macrosocial factors, and inequalities are fundamental factors operating at the societal/macro level that underlie and influence the health and well-being of individuals and populations via multiple pathways by providing them with differential access to power, information, and resources (Link & Phelan, 1995).

Fundamental factors in turn influence intermediate factors. Table 2.1 presents the intermediate factors consisting of both the built environment and social context. There are two important points worth emphasizing about the community/meso level. First, it is here that interventions may be the most effective in mitigating the more entrenched factors at the societal level (e.g., ageism) to improve the health and well-being of marginalized groups. Second, most of the interventions at the community/meso level necessarily involve organizations and agencies outside the public health sector. Hence, interdisciplinary, participatory collaboration among urban planners, civic organizers, educators, journalists, and public health practitioners may hold the greatest promise for devising effective and sustained community-based interventions.

The more proximate factors influencing health and well-being at the interpersonal level are stressors/buffers, health behaviors, and social integration. This is the more familiar terrain of public health, although Meyer (2003) warns that relying too much on the coping abilities of the oppressed rather than the transgressions of the oppressor could lead to disregard for the need for important political and structural changes.

Finally, the last column in Table 2.1 is labeled health and well-being and lists a wide range of health outcomes, while also identifying various measures of well-being. It is important to emphasize that health and well-being can be measured at both the individual and population levels; that is, societal, community, and interpersonal determinants may affect the health and well-being of individual members of society as well as various populations within it.

To illustrate how Table 2.1 may be used to trace pathways through which health communication tools at various levels may affect individual and population health, case studies from our ongoing work at the Harlem Health Promotion Center are presented next. The hope is that these examples will spur readers to think about ways that new media may be used at diverse levels to reach other communities and populations of interest.

Health Communication Tools by Level of Influence

The examples of health communication tools discussed here cover, in order, fundamental determinants at the societal/macro level, intermediate determinants at the community/meso level, and proximate determinants at the interpersonal/micro level of health and well-being at the individual and population levels. Yet these levels are fluid and changing, and it is important to keep in mind the dynamic nature of the model (Schulz & Northridge, 2004).

Get Healthy Harlem Web Site

To address the need for high-quality, culturally relevant information that does not require a high level of literacy, the Harlem Health Promotion Center (one of the 33 prevention research centers funded by the Centers for Disease Control and Prevention—see www.healthyharlem.org) and Digital Partnerships for Health (an alliance of community and academic partners) are developing an innovative Web-based health portal. Given broad access to Web sites, this project may usefully be considered a health communication tool at the societal/macro level.

When completed, Get Healthy Harlem: Your Door to Health and Wellness in Harlem (see www.GetHealthyHarlem.org) will offer information focusing on obesity written by health professionals as well as community members. Planned features include information about health, nutrition, exercise, and the environment in Harlem; tips from health experts in Harlem; personal stories from people in Harlem who are working to improve their health; tools for learning how healthy the users are and how healthy they could be; links to credible health and wellness information; a listing of Harlem restaurants, fitness centers, gardens, and other community resources; opportunities to meet friends online; and information on how to join online groups and discussions.

Harlem Smoke-Free Home Campaign

In October 2007, the New York City Department of Health and Mental Hygiene (2007), in collaboration with community partners (including the Harlem Children's Zone Asthma Initiative and the Mailman School of Public Health) launched the Harlem Smoke-Free Home campaign to address the issue of secondhand smoke in East and Central Harlem (see www.nyc.gov/html/doh/html/pr2007/pr087-07.shtml). Because it relies on advertisements in subway stations and check cashing establishments, this campaign may be considered a health communication tool at the community/meso level.

The campaign also includes radio promotion and DJ announcements at events throughout Harlem. Produced in English and Spanish, the advertisements feature African American and Latino children suffering from secondhand smoke–related illnesses such as asthma, ear infections, allergies, and chronic cough.

My Life, My Decision

Blending form with function, the DVD titled *My Life, My Decision* developed by the Harlem Health Promotion Center uses realistic plotlines to entertain and educate young adults regarding Plan B, an emergency contraceptive that contains 1.5 milligrams of the hormone levonorgestrel (Allen & Goldberg, 2007). Because the DVD is intended to be utilized in concert with social support from friends, family, and clinical staff as part of Project STAY (Services to Assist Youth), it may be classified as a health communication tool at the interpersonal/micro level. However, the initiative around Plan B also utilizes Web sites and community venues, exemplifying how health communication tools at multiple levels may work in concert to improve individual and population health and well-being.

Filmed in and around Harlem, *My Life, My Decision* features six Black and Latino young adults who are trying to avoid unintended pregnancies. For instance, while Sheila and Victor normally practice safe sex, an unexpected condom break forces them to seek a backup plan. And while Cynthia normally relies on the birth control pill for pregnancy prevention, when her close friend Nia experiences a post-sex dilemma similar to her own, they both need to find a way to prevent pregnancy *after* sex. The aim of this health communication tool is for audience members to feel engaged, informed, and interested in obtaining more information about reproductive health care services, including emergency contraception.

ElderSmile Digital Maps

For the past 5 years, an interdisciplinary team at the Columbia University College of Dental Medicine has been dedicated to improving oral health care access and services for seniors in Harlem and Washington Heights, New York City through an initiative known as ElderSmile. Digital maps created by architectural geographic information system software are effective health communication tools that are used to both document and analyze oral health at the population level (see "ARCgis: Layers and Layers of Data," 2005).

For instance, Borrell, Northridge, Miller, Golembeski, Spielman, Sclar, and Lamster (2006) found that Black racial identity, Hispanic ethnicity, and poverty tend to co-occur spatially in northern Manhattan and the south Bronx. Furthermore, a spatial/transportation barrier may inhibit access to dental care among seniors who live in these areas. The use of multiple layers of local information juxtaposed in digital maps is able to scientifically inform planning as health care workers determine locations for screening and treatment centers to provide oral health care for seniors.

EMERGING DEMOGRAPHICS

From 1990 to 2000, the population center of the United States shifted 12 miles south and 33 miles west, from a location near Steelville, Missouri, to one near Edgar Springs, Missouri (U.S. Census Bureau, 2000). The concomitant population growth of 32.7 million people between 1990 and 2000 represents the largest census-to-census increase in U.S. history (U.S. Census Bureau, 2001a).

The Aging of the U.S. Population

According to the U.S. Census Bureau (2000), the median age of the U.S. population in 2000 was 35.3 years, the highest median age recorded for the United States. Cohort effects are evident within this overall trend. For instance, relatively low birth rates during the late 1920s and early 1930s, the years of the Great Depression, meant that a relatively small number of people celebrated their 65th birthday in time for Census 2000, and for the first time in the history of the U.S. census, the population ages 65 years and older increased at a slower rate than the population as a whole. On the other hand, as the baby boomers (defined as people born in the years after World War II from 1946 to 1964) began passing their 45th birthdays, the population between the ages of 45 and 49 years swelled 49% in just one decade (from 1990 to 2000).

A U.S. Census Bureau report titled "We the People: Aging in the United States" (2004b) provides other useful information from Census 2000 regarding people ages 65 years and older that may be important to the design of targeted health communication strategies. Women outnumber men in this age range (20.6 million women compared with 14.4 million men), and the sex ratio (number of males per 100 females) drops steadily with increasing age. While the sex ratio for people ages 65 to 74 years was 82 in 2000, it declined to 41 for people ages 85 and older in 2000, representing more than two women for every man.

In terms of living arrangements, 28% of people ages 65 years and older lived alone, compared with 10% of the total population (U.S. Census Bureau, 2004b). Close to 7.5 million older women lived alone, as did 2.4 million older men. More than one of four grandparents ages 65 years and older living with their grandchildren under age 18 years were caregivers for their grandchildren.

With regard to the five types of disabilities tracked by the U.S. census (sensory, physical, mental, self-care, and difficulty going outside the home), physical disabilities were the most prevalent, at 28.6% for those ages 65 years and older, compared to only 8.2% for those ages 5 to 64 years (U.S. Census Bureau, 2004b). Almost half (42%) of the population ages 65 years and older reported some type of long-lasting condition or disability in Census 2000. Women are more likely than men to become disabled, and when women experience disability, they are less likely than men to recover (Laditka & Laditka, 2002). As a result, women have both higher disability incidence and higher disability prevalence than men at all ages (Becket et al., 1996; Leveille, Pennix, Melzer, Izmirlian, & Guralnik, 2000).

The growing proportion of the elderly is a direct effect of declining mortality, but also of declining fertility, which results in a greater number of seniors; this also means that they constitute a greater proportion of the population (Albert, 2008). For instance, between 1960 and 2004, overall mortality in the United States declined from about 1,400 to 800 deaths per 100,000 persons per year (Federal Interagency Forum on Aging Related Statistics, 2000). According to Albert (2008), this extraordinary reduction in mortality occurred across the entire life span, resulting in an impressive gain in life expectancy from 70 years to 76 years over the same time period (1960–2004).

Increasing Racial, Ethnic, and Immigrant Diversity

The U.S. federal government considers race and Hispanic origin to be two separate and distinct concepts (U.S. Census Bureau, 2001b). For this reason, race, ethnicity, and immigration status are considered collectively in this subsection. The question on Hispanic origin in Census 2000 asked respondents if they were Spanish, Hispanic, or Latino, while the question on race asked respondents to report the race or races they consider themselves to be: White, Black or African American, American Indian or Alaska Native, Asian, Native Hawaiian or other Pacific Islander, or some other race.

Note that the Census 2000 questions on race and Hispanic origin are based on self-identification, reflecting the social, political, and economic construction of these concepts, rather than disproven "race-as-biology" categories (Goodman, 2000). Furthermore, these categories were revised for Census 2000 to reflect the increasing diversity of the U.S. population and to maintain the ability to monitor compliance with civil rights laws (Wallman, Evinger, & Schechter, 2000); these data from Census 2000 thus are not directly comparable with data from the 1990 census or earlier censuses (U.S. Census Bureau, 2001b).

According to data from Census 2000, 281.4 million people resided in the United States, of whom 35.3 million, or about 13%, self-identified as Latino (U.S. Census Bureau, 2001b). The overwhelming majority (nearly 98%) of respondents reported being only of one race. Of those, 75% reported being White, 12% reported being Black or African American, 5.5% reported being some other race (predominantly people of Hispanic origin), 4% reported being Asian, just under 1% reported being American Indian or Alaska Native, and 0.1% reported being Native Hawaiian or other Pacific Islander.

To further understand the diversity of the U.S. population, it is useful to look at three other Census 2000 measures, namely, foreign born, ancestry, and language use. The U.S. Census Bureau considers anyone who is not born a U.S. citizen to be foreign born (U.S. Census Bureau, 2003a). Of the 281.4 million people measured in Census 2000, 31.1 million, or 11.1%, were foreign born. In the decade between 1990 and 2000, the foreign-born population increased 57%, compared with increases of 9.3% for the native population (i.e., those born in the United States, Puerto Rico, or a U.S. island area, or children born abroad of a U.S. citizen parent) and 13% for the total U.S. population. The majority (52%) of the foreign-born population in Census 2000 were from Latin America (Central America including Mexico, the Caribbean, and South America), and just over half of the foreign-born population lived in three states, namely, California, New York, and Texas.

Ancestry in the U.S. census is a conflated measure, since it has different meanings for different people, including where their ancestors are from, where they or their parents originated, and how they see themselves ethnically (U.S. Census Bureau, 2004a). Notwithstanding this important limitation, it is worth noting that the number of people with the best-represented European ancestries has decreased over the past decade, while the number of individuals with African American, Hispanic, and Asian ancestries has increased.

Finally, both the number and percentage of people in the United States who spoke a language other than English at home increased in the decade from 1990 to 2000 (U.S. Census Bureau, 2003a). In 2000, 18% of the total population ages 5 years and older (47.0 million people) reported that they spoke a language other than English at home, compared with 14% (31.8 million) in 1990 and 11% (23.1 million) in 1980 (U.S. Census Bureau, 2003b). The three major language groups other than English are Spanish (including those who speak Ladino), other Indo-European languages (most languages of Europe and the Indic languages of India), and Asian and Pacific Island languages (including Chinese, Korean, Japanese, and Vietnamese).

The implications of the increasing diversity of the U.S. population for health communication in the new media landscape are enormous. The majority of U.S. households have personal computer and Web access (U.S. Census Bureau, 2005), and as of December 2006, over 18.5 billion text messages were being sent every month—an increase of 250% each year for the previous 2 years (Kaiser Family Foundation, 2007).

HEALTH CARE TRENDS

This section was written at the close of 2007, when health care delivery in the United States was severely stressed. By the time you read this volume, a new U.S. federal administration will likely be in office. While there are a host of health care issues that demand attention, two major concerns will likely dominate upcoming policy debates, namely: how best to care for increasing numbers of seniors and how best to eliminate growing disparities in health care access and treatment between segments of U.S. society.

Caring for Increasing Numbers of Seniors

The increasing numbers of U.S. seniors will require a new world of health care and social service delivery, transportation and housing arrangements, and much more to meet the complex needs of those requiring care (Albert, 2008). According to the National Center for Health Statistics (2006), U.S. men could expect to live 3 years longer and U.S. women could expect to live 1 year longer in 2003 than they did in 1990.

With longer life expectancy comes increasing prevalence of chronic diseases and conditions that are associated with aging (National Center for Health Statistics, 2006). Primary care sensitive conditions such as diabetes, hypertension, and asthma produce cumulative damage if not properly treated, while diseases such as emphysema and certain types of cancers develop slowly or after long periods of exposure to irritants and toxins.

A life course approach to prevention and treatment has proved insightful for a range of chronic diseases and conditions, including oral diseases and conditions (Ben-Shlomo & Kuh, 2002; Northridge & Lamster, 2004). This theory posits that health in later life results from the lifelong accumulation of advantageous and disadvantageous experiences at the personal, interpersonal, community, and societal levels (Northridge et al., 2003). These experiences differ according to a range of factors, including but not limited to gender and sexuality; race, ethnicity, and immigration status; and socioeconomic conditions such as education, income, wealth, and occupation. This is true not only for biological and psychological determinants, but also for social and behavioral determinants, as encompassed in contemporary ecological theories of health and well-being (see, e.g., Krieger, 2001).

A public health model favors directing more societal resources toward the prevention or delayed onset of disabling diseases and conditions rather than toward medically and technologically-intensive care (Crimmins, Saito, & Reynolds, 1997). This view is supported by a growing body of evidence that demonstrates that controlling blood pressure, maintaining appropriate weight, abstaining from smoking, and being physically active lead to lowered prevalence of illness and impairment (Reed, Foley, White, Heimovitz, Burchfiel, & Masaki, 1998; Vita, Terry, Hubert, & Fries, 1998).

According to Laditka and Laditka (2002), "The distinction between 'active' and 'inactive' life disguises a continuum of functional ability" (p. 179). Regardless of the thresholds set for defining disability, long-term care will no doubt exert pressing demands on U.S. society in the coming decades (Laditka & Laditka, 2002). As the large cohort of baby boomers ages, they will require more formal and informal care, in the aggregate, regardless of lifestyle changes, research advances, or morbidity compression (Laditka & Laditka, 2002). Unfortunately, not all segments of U.S. society have equal access to quality health care or treatment for acute and chronic diseases and conditions.

Growing Disparities in Health Care Access and Treatment

For more than a decade, U.S. agencies have documented and confronted inequalities in health care among population groups across a spectrum of diseases and conditions. Perhaps the most influential report published to date is *Unequal Treatment: Confronting Racial and Ethnic Disparities in Health Care* (National Academy of Sciences, 2002). The accumulated evidence underscores the existence of racial and ethnic differences in the quality of health care that are not due to access-related factors or clinical needs, preferences, and appropriateness of intervention (National Academy of Sciences, 2002). In a thoughtful review examining the unequal burden of pain, two sources of disparities were delineated: health care systems and the legal and regulatory climate in which they operate, and discrimination, for example, biases, stereotyping, and uncertainties in clinical communication and decision making (Green et al., 2003).

Together and separately, the authors of this chapter have dedicated their careers to understanding and addressing these two sources of disparities through community-based participatory research and practice initiatives at the Harlem Health Promotion Center. Innovative service delivery models addressing disparities in health care systems and the legal and regulatory climate in which they operate have been designed and evaluated. For instance, Project STAY (Services to Assist Youth) is a haven for young people at risk for or living with HIV/AIDS (see www.projectstay.net). Its comprehensive services fit both the lifestyles and life stages of youths and young adults.

As part of an ongoing project at the Harlem Health Promotion Center, Xavier Ford, a talented health educator who works for a community-based organization, developed a technique that uses computer animation to enable teenagers to communicate with one another via text messaging. In his DVD titled *Cells in the City*, the teenage actors are never shown on screen—we only see their cell phones, accompanied by both the actors' voices and written messages. A series of vignettes around HIV counseling and testing are currently being developed. Youths are involved in developing the messages for the vignettes, while also learning computer animation and storyboarding necessary to create finished media products.

In terms of addressing discrimination in health care service and delivery, struggles experienced at the Harlem Family Asthma Center, especially the difficulties encountered around eligibility for health care coverage by poor men with asthma, have resulted in the provision of advocacy for health care delivery that embraces the diversity of U.S. families (Hutchinson, Northridge, Lebovitz, Northridge, Vaughn, & Vaughan, in press). Other efforts to focus attention on the egregious disparities in health care for men of color have ranged from fundamental causes such as confronting racism and sexism to improve men's health (Treadwell, Northridge, & Bethea, 2007b), to proximate causes such as providing oral health care to prisoners (Treadwell, Northridge, & Bethea, 2007a).

CHALLENGES AND OPPORTUNITIES

The following chapters are devoted to health communication in the new media landscape. A few reflections on the current challenges and possible new strategies are offered here.

First, the aging of the U.S. population means, at the broadest level, that age-friendly health communication strategies ought to be encouraged (Feldman, Oberlink, Simantov, & Gursen, 2004). For instance, inadequate health literacy, as measured by reading fluency, independently predicts all-cause mortality and cardiovascular death among community-dwelling elderly persons (Baker, Wolf, Feinglass, Thompson, Gazmararian, & Huang, 2007). However, limited literacy skills affect all age and population groups in the United States (Davis & Wolf, 2004). In moving beyond describing the problem to devising solutions, it may be advantageous for those developing tailored intervention strategies to ensure that they can be adapted to changing abilities as people age.

Second, for population groups that have been historically oppressed, notably recent immigrants, mainstream approaches to health communication may be ineffective. Elder (2003) advocates using community health advisors to mediate health communication messages for recent immigrants in order to improve comprehension and promote acceptance. A better understanding of who is effective in delivering health messages among different population groups and what approaches work best across settings may help improve public health for those most in need of information and services.

Third, the fragmentation of our health care system has resulted in rising costs, inefficiency, preventable errors, and poor quality of care (Halamka Overhage, Ricciardi, Rishel, Shirky, & Diamond, 2005). A large multi-stakeholder collaborative titled Connecting for Health advocates creating a decentralized and federated model of health information exchange built upon a minimum set of uniform standards and policies, rather than creating a uniform health information infrastructure on a national scale (Halamka et al., 2005). Regardless of the model employed, it is imperative to ensure that medical and dental histories are not lost when people move to new communities or experience other dislocations. Furthermore, improved uniformity of health information will enhance public health tracking, quality evaluation, and health services research in the future. Clearly, policy reforms are needed, including those in the health care, education, transportation, and housing arenas, in order to increase equity in U.S. society.

CALL TO ACTION

In this chapter, the emerging demographics and health care trends to look for in the coming decades have been reviewed in order to lay a foundation for the ensuing chapters in this volume devoted to health communication strategies in the new media landscape. Those of us devoted to improving the health and welfare of the U.S. population need to ensure we move beyond the academy to critically engage with the public sector, the private sector, and community stakeholders, including religious groups (Frodeman & Mitcham, 2007). According to Frodeman and Mitcham (2007), "Our academic research portfolio must include an account of how to effectively integrate knowledge within the decision-making context faced by governments, businesspeople, and citizens" (p. 513).

It is important to remember that, inevitably, any constructive changes in the current health care system will necessarily involve politics and bring up societal values that underlie the debate. As Duane (2007) recently reminded us, "In our democracy, we have the power to implement policies that promote genuine public health. True patriotism demands that we do so" (p. 2123).

REFERENCES

Albert, S. (2008). The aging U.S. population. In I. B. Lamster & M. E. Northridge (Eds.), *Improving oral health for the elderly: An interdisciplinary approach* (pp. 3–13). New York: Springer Publishing.

Allen, R. H., & Goldberg, A. B. (2007). Emergency contraception: A clinical review. *Clinical Obstetrics & Gynecology, 50,* 927–936.

"ARCgis: Layers and layers of data." (2005). *Primus 11.* Retrieved June 13, 2008, from http://dental.columbia.edu/pubs/Primus2005.web.pdf

Baker, D. W., Wolf, M. S., Feinglass, J., Thompson, J. A., Gazmararian, J. A., & Huang, J. (2007). Health literacy and mortality among elderly persons. *Archives of Internal Medicine, 167,* 1503–1509.

Becket, L. A., Brock, D. B., Lemke, J. H., Mendes de leon, C., Guralnik, J. M., Fillenbaum, G. G., et al. (1996). Analysis of change in self-reported physical limitation among older persons in four population studies. *American Journal of Epidemiology, 143,* 766–778.

Ben-Shlomo, Y., & Kuh, D. (2002). A life course approach to chronic disease epidemiology: Conceptual models, empirical challenges and interdisciplinary perspectives. *International Journal of Epidemiology, 31,* 285–293.

Borrell, L. N., Northridge, M. E., Miller, D. B., Golembeski, C. A., Spielman, S. E., Sclar, E. D., & Lamster, I. B. (2006). Oral health and health care for older adults: A spatial approach for addressing disparities and planning services. *Special Care in Dentistry, 26,* 252–256.

Crimmins, E. M., Saito, Y., & Reynolds, S. L. (1997). Further evidence on recent trends in the prevalence and incidence of disability among older Americans from two sources: The LSOA and the NHIS. *Journals of Gerontology Series B: Psychological Sciences and Social Sciences, 52B,* S59–S71.

Davis, T. C., & Wolf, M. S. (2004). Health literacy: implications for family medicine. *Family Medicine Journal, 36,* 595–598.

Duane, J. F. (2007). True patriotism. *American Journal of Public Health, 97,* 2123.

Elder, J. P. (2003). Reaching out to America's immigrants: Community health advisors and health communication. *American Journal of Health Behavior, 27*(Suppl. 3), S197–S205.

Federal Interagency Forum on Aging Related Statistics. (2000). *Older Americans 2000: Key indicators of well-being.* Washington, DC: U.S. Government Printing Office.

Feldman, P. H., Oberlink, M. R., Simantov, E., & Gursen, M. D. (2004). *A tale of two older americas: Community opportunities and challenges. The AdvantAge initiative 2003 national survey of adults aged 65 and older.* New York: Center for Home Care Policy and Research, Visiting Nurse Service of New York.

Frodeman, R., & Mitcham, C. 2007). New directions in interdisciplinarity: Broad, deep, and critical. *Bulletin of Science, Technology, and Society, 27,* 506–514.

Goodman, A. H. (2000). Why genes don't count (for racial differences in health). *American Journal of Public Health, 90,* 1699–1702.

Green, C. R., Anderson, K. O., Baker, T. A., Campbell, L. C., Decker, S., Fillingim, R. B., et al. (2003). The unequal burden of pain: Confronting racial and ethnic disparities in pain. *Pain Medicine, 4,* 277–294.

Halamka, J., Overhage, J. M., Ricciardi, L., Rishel, W., Shirky, C., & Diamond, C. (2005). Exchanging health information: Local distribution, national coordination. *Health Affairs, 24,* 1170–1179.

Hutchinson, V. E., Northridge, M. E., Lebovitz, L. L., Northridge, J. L., Vaughn, R. L., & Vaughan, R. D. (in press). A family-centered approach to providing comprehensive asthma care services: The Harlem Family Asthma Center. *Cardozo Journal of Law and Gender.*

Kaiser Family Foundation. (2007). *HHS and Kaiser Family Foundation team up to promote text messaging in the fight against HIV/AIDS* [Press release]. Retrieved July 2, 2008, from http://www.kff.org/hivaids/phip113007nr.cfm

Krieger, N. (2001). Theories for social epidemiology in the 21st century: An ecosocial perspective. *International Journal of Epidemiology, 30,* 668–677.

Laditka, S. B., & Laditka, J. N. (2002). Recent perspectives on active life expectancy for older women. *Journal of Women and Aging, 14,* 163–184.

Leveille, S. G., Pennix, B. W. J. H., Melzer, D., Izmirlian, G., & Guralnik, J. M. (2000). Sex differences in the prevalence of mobility disability in old age: The dynamics of incidence, recovery, and mortality. *Journals of Gerontology Series B: Psychological Sciences and Social Sciences, 55,* S41–S50.

Link, B. G., & Phelan, J. C. (1995). Social conditions as fundamental causes of disease. *Journal of Health and Social Behavior, 36*(Extra issue), 80–94.

National Academy of Sciences. (2002). *Unequal treatment: Confronting racial and ethnic disparities in health care.* Washington, DC: Institute of Medicine.

National Center for Health Statistics. (2006). *Health, United States, 2006 with chartbook on trends in the health of Americans.* Hyattsville, MD: U.S. Department of Health and Human Services, Centers for Disease Control and Prevention.

New York City Department of Health and Mental Hygiene. (2007). *Health Department Launches Smoke-Free Home Campaign in Harlem* [Press release]. Retrieved June 21, 2008, from http://www.nyc.gov/html/doh/html/pr2007/pr087-07.shtml

Northridge, M. E., Sclar, E. D., & Biswas, P. (2003). Sorting out the connections between the built environment and health: A conceptual framework for navigating pathways and planning healthy cities. *Journal of Urban Health, 80,* 556–568.

Northridge, M. E., & Lamster, I. B. (2004). A lifecourse approach to preventing and treating oral disease. *Sozial- und Präventivmedizin, 49,* 299–300.

Reed, D. M., Foley, D. J., White, L. R., Heimovitz, H., Burchfiel, C. M., & Masaki, K. (1998). Predictors of healthy aging in men with high life expectancies. *American Journal of Public Health, 88,* 1463–1468.

Schulz, A., & Northridge, M. E. (2004). Social determinants of health: Implications for environmental health promotion. *Health Education and Behavior, 31,* 455–471.

Treadwell, H. M., Northridge, M. E., & Bethea, T. N. (2007a). Building the case for oral health care for prisoners: Presenting the evidence and calling for justice. In R. Greifinger (Ed.), *Public health behind bars: From prisons to communities* (pp. 333–346). New York: Springer.

Treadwell, H. M., Northridge, M. E., & Bethea, T. N. (2007b). Confronting racism and sexism to improve men's health. *American Journal of Men's Health, 1,* 81–86.

U.S. Census Bureau. (2000). *All across the U.S.A.: Population distribution and composition, 2000.* Retrieved July 2, 2008, from http://www.census.gov/population/pop-profile/2000/chap02.pdf

U.S. Census Bureau. (2001a). *Population change and distribution: 1990 to 2000.* Retrieved July 2, 2008, from http://www.census.gov/prod/2001pubs/c2kbr01-2.pdf

U.S. Census Bureau. (2001b). *Overview of race and Hispanic origin: 2000.* Retrieved July 2, 2008, from http://www.census.gov/prod/2001pubs/cenbr01-1.pdf

U.S. Census Bureau. (2003a). *The foreign-born population: 2000.* Retrieved July 2, 2008, from http://www.census.gov/prod/2003pubs/c2kbr-34.pdf

U.S. Census Bureau. (2003b). *Language use and English-speaking ability: 2000.* Retrieved July 2, 2008, from http://www.census.gov/prod/2003pubs/c2kbr-29.pdf

U.S. Census Bureau. (2004a). *Ancestry: 2000.* Retrieved July 2, 2008, from http://www.census.gov/prod/2004pubs/c2kbr-35.pdf

U.S. Census Bureau. (2004b). *We the people: Aging in the United States.* Retrieved July 2, 2008, from http://www.census.gov/prod/2004pubs/censr-19.pdf

U.S. Census Bureau. (2005). *Computer and Internet use in the United States: 2003.* Retrieved July 2, 2008, from http://www.census.gov/prod/2005pubs/p23-208.pdf

Vita, A. J., Terry, R. B., Hubert, H. B., & Fries, J. F. (1998). Aging, health risks, and cumulative disability. *New England Journal of Medicine, 338,* 1035–1041.

Wallman, K. K., Evinger, S., & Schechter, S. (2000). Measuring our nation's diversity: Developing a common language for data on race/ethnicity. *American Journal of Public Health, 90,* 1704–1708.

3

Communication Strategies for Reducing Racial and Cultural Disparities

MARÍA E. LEN-RÍOS

Journalists, communication researchers, health professionals, and others have used the mass media to raise public awareness of health problems, to create positive attitudes toward healthful behaviors, and to modify unhealthful behaviors. As health communication researchers have pointed out, "Trying to promote healthy behaviors that offer delayed or uncertain benefits and also entail immediate deprivations makes these efforts even more challenging" (Kar, Alcalay, & Alex, 2001, p. 110). This may be even more challenging for health communication researchers whose mission it is to reach the underserved. Endeavors to reach the underserved may be stymied, as the underserved typically do not have the same economic and community resources as those from higher socioeconomic groups. This sometimes makes it more difficult for people to implement health recommendations. In addition, communication professionals may need to address the underserved through diverse media channels (e.g., radio, television, billboards, transit advertising) using culturally relevant communication, and not all professionals have been trained to be culturally aware.

This chapter summarizes the results of recent mass media health campaigns that have targeted U.S. ethnic audiences and explores what researchers know about media channels and content created for U.S. ethnic audiences. Health disparities[1] are defined "as racial or ethnic differences in the quality of healthcare that are not due to access-related factors or clinical needs, preferences, and appropriateness of intervention" (Smedley, Stith, & Nelson, 2005, pp. 3–4). In other words, many people who belong to U.S. racial and ethnic groups and have access to health care get poorer care. Researchers have identified a variety of reasons why U.S. racial and ethnic groups receive poorer care, including discrimination, prejudice, poor doctor–patient communication, health care system practices, and late detection of disease, as well as the fact that they are provided with fewer treatment options by health care providers (Mayberry, Mili, & Ofili, 2002; Smedley et al., 2005).

The mass media, in particular, can play a role in reducing racial and cultural health disparities by exposing instances of systemic discrimination and prejudice that are responsible for the persistence of unequal health care and by questioning policies that maintain the status quo, by alerting policy makers to health care inequities, and by informing audiences about new prevention recommendations and treatments to affect public attitudes and behaviors. Research from the fields of journalism and mass communication and psychology has demonstrated that there is a connection between what is reported in the mass media and public knowledge about issues (Cho & McLeod, 2007; Gaziano, 2000; Gaziano & Horowitz, 2001; Tichenor, Donohue, & Olien, 1970), attitudes and perceptions of health issues (Jones, Denham, & Springston, 2007; Marcus, Owen, Forsyth, Cavill, & Fridinger, 1998), behavioral intentions (Detweiler, Bedell, Salovey, Pronin, & Rothman, 1999; Len-Ríos & Qiu, 2007), and behaviors (Snyder & Hamilton, 2002). This chapter analyzes the academic literature on mass media health communication campaign efforts to reach underserved U.S. racial and ethnic groups.

DISPARITIES AND INEQUITIES

Early on, the media's role in reporting health disparities focused on exposing institutional prejudice and unequal medical treatment provided to U.S. racial and ethnic minorities, particularly Blacks, and advocating social justice. Journalists put the spotlight on inequities, which led to a major public response. For example, on July 25, 1972, Associated Press reporter Jean Heller (1972) broke the story about the ethically flawed Tuskegee syphilis experiment in which African American men were not told that they had syphilis and were not offered or denied treatment by researchers who wanted to study the natural progression of the disease. The front page headline of the *New York Times* read "Syphilis Victims in U.S. Study Went

Untreated for 40 Years." Its effect of creating mistrust of the health care system in African American communities still reverberates today.

More recently, in 1996, the Centers for Disease Control and Prevention had to explain why it had tested a measles vaccine on 1,500 6- to 9-month-old Black and Hispanic babies ("Vaccine Study Faulted," 1996). The *Los Angeles Times,* the *Washington Post,* and other newspapers carried the story. Observers questioned whether these babies and their parents would have received the same care if they had been upper-middle-class Whites.

On June 13, 2007, Charles Gibson on ABC's *World News Tonight* reported that Edith Isabel Rodriguez died at Martin Luther King Jr.–Harbor Hospital in Los Angeles after waiting more than 45 minutes to be seen in the hospital's emergency room (Associated Press, n.d.). Her death was called an accident—a mistake in an overburdened and mismanaged health system that largely served a poor ethnic community. Again, critics asked whether this would have happened in an upper-middle-class White community.

These types of news stories illustrate to ethnic groups how the system fails to work for them. Cases like these also provide justification for their mistrust of the U.S. health care system.

RESEARCH ON HEALTH COMMUNICATION AND U.S. RACIAL/ETHNIC GROUPS

Several scholars have written reviews of mass media health communication campaigns intended for racial/ethnic populations. This literature focuses on health message design (framing), differences in audience learning from mass media channels (knowledge gaps), media use (media dependency theory, uses and gratifications theory), and media's effects on attitudes and behaviors (diffusion of innovation, social cognitive theory).

A review by Hornik and Ramirez (2006) concluded that no studies have effectively looked at whether racial and ethnic segmentation (i.e., narrowing the target audience of a campaign message to a smaller subset of the general population) in communication campaigns has proved effective. Racial and ethnic segmentation is meant to "increase the relevance and appeal of . . . advertising to specific racial or ethnic groups" (Davis, 1997, p. 448). Hornik and Ramirez argue that the problem is that most studies do not properly design, measure, or carry out evaluation of their interventions. Marcus and associates (1998) reviewed mass media campaigns between 1983 and 1997 on physical activity interventions and reported that the sole study in their sample that included a minority population in its design and made substantial use of mass-mediated messages did not provide an analysis of its effects on that population.

Researchers have paid much more attention to media use and channel preferences of ethnic and racial groups and to the cultural relevance of health messages than they have to implementing and measuring health communication campaign effects. Part of the reason for this is lack of funds, because media campaigns are costly. The following sections review mass media health communication campaigns directed toward U.S. racial and ethnic groups, and the media channels that best serve people belonging to U.S. racial and ethnic groups.

MASS MEDIA HEALTH CAMPAIGNS FOR U.S. ETHNIC/RACIAL GROUPS

Media researchers acknowledge that evaluating health communication campaign effectiveness in general is difficult because there is no common definition for a health campaign and because campaign elements (e.g., time frame, message saturation, levels of analysis) vary from campaign to campaign (Salmon & Atkin, 2003). The assumption that is often made in the health communication literature is that health disparities are caused by a lack of information due to communication inequalities. Viswanath and Emmons (2006) define communication inequalities "as differences in the generation, manipulation, and distribution of information among social groups; and differences in (a) access and use, (b) attention, (c) retention, and (d) capacity to act on relevant information among individuals" (p. S242). The assumption is that if communication and capacity are increased, health outcomes will improve.

Not all researchers agree that ethnic targeting through the mass media is an effective means to deliver health messages to U.S. ethnic and racial groups. For instance, some argue that there is no evidence that racial and ethnic segmentation is more effective than other forms of message targeting and suggest that it may not be worth the expense (Hornik & Ramirez, 2006). In contrast, others argue that general audience targeting fails to reach ethnic groups (Wilkin & Ball-Rokeach, 2006) and that interpersonal channels and ethnic media are most effective. Still other researchers show that the effectiveness of mass media campaigns depends on whom you want to reach. For instance, Salmon and Atkin (2003) argue that community opinion leaders may use general audience media to gather information and then bring those messages back to their communities. It is likely that each of these perspectives has merit, depending on the message and intended audience. Message appropriateness and channel selection are largely dependent on audience characteristics. Important individual-level factors include socioeconomic status, education level, stage of readiness for adopting behavior change, and level of acculturation into mainstream society (Hornik & Ramirez, 2006; Soto, 2006).

Effects Research

This section synthesizes the results of recent mass media health communication campaigns that have sought to affect the knowledge levels, attitudes, and behaviors of members of U.S. racial and ethnic groups. (It should be noted that the size, duration, and conceptualization of the campaigns are not directly comparable.) Some are interventions that have used customized magazines and guides, which do not fit traditional definitions of mass media.[2] There have been few actual mass media campaigns that target ethnic groups and, as Hornik and Ramirez (2006) argue, fewer still that provide a "comparison between segmentation and nonsegmentation by race or ethnicity while comparing progress between racial groups" (p. 874).

Beaudoin, Fernandez, Wall, and Farley (2007) used broadcast and outdoor advertising to reach African American women and motivate them to increase their intake of fruits and vegetables and increase walking. The goal was to reduce the risk of cardiovascular disease among African Americans in New Orleans. The advertising buys were at high saturation levels, meaning the ads appeared frequently to ensure they were seen. Pre- and post-campaign surveys of area residents showed increased positive attitudes toward walking and improved eating habits, but the data indicated that the advertising campaign did not influence actual behavior.

In an effort to reduce children's exposure to harmful lead paint, the Hartford Health Department implemented a campaign that used public relations tactics (e.g., displays at a local hardware store, an art competition) in conjunction with newspaper, outdoor, and transit advertising (McLaughlin, Humphries, Nguyen, Maljanian, & McCormack, 2004). McLaughlin and associates surveyed the campaign's effects on parents of children who attended nine early learning centers in Hartford, Connecticut. Eighty-five percent of respondents were either Black or

Hispanic. Results showed that the best-remembered messages were newspaper advertisements (63%), transit advertising (60%), billboards (60%), and posters on sanitation trucks (40%). In addition, half said that they acted on the information from the newspaper advertisement, and nearly one-third said that a billboard caused them to take some preventative action. The most frequently reported outcome behaviors were talking with a landlord (65%) and asking a doctor about lead testing (58%).

To address cervical cancer health disparities among Vietnamese American women, researchers launched an intervention in California (Mock et al., 2007). Participants either received a combination of education from lay workers about cervical cancer and exposure to a mass media campaign or only had exposure to a mass media campaign. The media campaign used 15 advertisements that ran in Vietnamese newspapers, radio, and television, as well as public relations tactics such as publicity-generated newspaper articles, booklets, and calendars. Results showed that women in the combined intervention group were more knowledgeable about cervical cancer and were more likely to get an updated Pap test than those in the media-only group. Analysis of the mass media components showed that those who had read a newspaper article about Pap tests were also more likely to get a Pap test.

Another study conducted by Wray, Hornik, Gandy, Stryker, Ghez, and Mitchell-Clark (2004) in 1998 and 1999 used 90-second public service announcements to attempt to prevent domestic violence in four African American communities. Results of the study were inconclusive because the local radio stations either did not air the public service announcements or did not air them with sufficient frequency to reliably assess the results. Their study demonstrates that campaign effects may be more difficult to achieve when the saturation and frequency of message exposure cannot be controlled, as is the case with paid advertising or the use of brochures and printed materials.

A campaign that sought to increase the number of older American Indians who get influenza vaccinations used tribal radio in combination with other intervention activities (Traeger, Thompson, Dickson, & Provencio, 2006). However, the unique contributions of radio to the campaign outcomes were not reported.

Several study interventions created printed publications (brochures or magazines) to deliver health information to women of color. Bell and Alcalay (2001) found that White and Black women learned more from the wellness guides they produced than did Hispanic women. In addition, when the level of acculturation was taken into account, acculturated

Hispanic women learned more about and had a better understanding of how to acquire health information they needed than did less acculturated Hispanics. Kreuter and Haughton (2006) created an intervention that delivered magazines that were tailored by culture, behavior, or a combination of culture and behavior to African American women. They found that the combination messages were most strongly associated with getting African American women to eat more fruits and vegetables and get a mammogram. In regard to the latter, the data also revealed that the women most apt to get a mammogram were those who had previously had a mammogram but had fallen behind in scheduling their next one. Thus the media effect was greater for motivating people to repeat a behavior than to exhibit a new one.

The results from these studies show that mainstream and targeted media channels can be used to raise awareness among U.S. racial and ethnic populations about health issues and to encourage preventative behaviors. It appears that advertising (Beaudoin et al., 2007; McLaughlin et al., 2004), printed media such as brochures and magazines (Bell et al., 2001; Kreuter & Haughton, 2006), and a combination of tactics (Mock et al., 2007) may have advantages over efforts that rely solely on non-paid media tactics such as public service announcements (Wray et al., 2004), which rely on the cooperation of media partners. When attitudes were measured, it was found that the media campaigns also appeared to increase positive attitudes (Beaudoin et al., 2007) and perceptions of self-efficacy (Bell et al., 2001). The effects of the campaigns on behavior were mixed, with some campaigns not affecting behavior (Beaudoin et al., 2007), some increasing behavior among those more predisposed (Kreuter & Haughton, 2006; Mock et al., 2007), and some showing multiple behaviors attributed to the campaign (McLaughlin et al., 2004). In considering behavior change and campaign effectiveness, it is important to reflect on the level of change requested of the target audience and the difficulty in implementing that change. For instance, it is easier to talk to one's landlord about lead paint (McLaughlin et al., 2004) or get a Pap test (Mock et al., 2007) than it is to implement a dietary change and exercise program (Beaudoin et al., 2007).

MASS MEDIA CHANNELS

There are several ways to increase cultural message relevance in health communication messages. This can be done through the choice of language (e.g., English versus Spanish), symbolism (e.g., evoking the buffalo or an eagle in communications with certain American Indian tribes), visual representation (e.g., showing members of the ethnic group being targeted), and presentation of values that are closely held by various groups (e.g., religiosity, reverence for elders). But one of the best ways is selection of appropriate media channels (general audience versus ethnic media, or TV versus newspaper).

Studies of media channels and U.S. ethnic and racial minorities address two topics—how racial/ethnic groups access and use mass media and the content of health news consumed by U.S. ethnic and racial group members. The bulk of the existing research addresses African Americans and Hispanics. This is because they are the two largest ethnic minority groups in the United States, each group shares a common language, and each group has well-developed ethnic media (e.g., newspapers, magazines, and television channels). In fact, according to the 2008 *Bacon's Newspaper Directory* (2007) listings, there are 219 U.S. African American newspapers and 401 U.S. Hispanic newspapers. The vast majority are community newspapers. Three of the African American newspapers and 18 of the Hispanic newspapers are published daily. A 2006 report by the Latino Print Network identified 768 Hispanic newspapers, 38 of them dailies, but these include Puerto Rican and Mexican border-town newspapers (Whistler, 2007).

Fewer campaigns target Asian Americans as a monolithic, or panethnic, group because they include a variety of diverse cultural groups that speak many languages. American Indians, although also underserved, are comparatively few in number, are heterogeneous, and do not populate large cities in great numbers, so they continue to be underrepresented in research. In addition, there are few pan-ethnic media channels that reach Asian Americans or American Indians. The following section explores what we know about how racial/ethnic groups use mass media and what is in the media content regarding health information.

Mass Media Use

When it comes to developing health communication campaigns for U.S. racial and ethnic groups, some campaigns approach racial and ethnic minority groups as homogenous, while others look at individual characteristics within a racial or ethnic group (e.g., level of ethnic identity, socioeconomic status). What is clear is that ethnic identity and individual characteristics are more complex than they are often treated. For instance, a White Cuban American in Miami may have a very different cultural orientation than a recent immigrant from Mexico to Los Angeles. Research has also shown that like White populations, less educated ethnic group members are less likely than those with college educations to rely on print media materials (Ribisl, Winkleby, Fortmann, & Flora, 1998).

Since the U.S. census declared Hispanics the fastest-growing U.S. ethnic group, marketers and researchers have begun to research the media habits and behaviors of what has been dubbed the "Hispanic market." Market researcher Isabel Valdés (2000) shows how one commercial research group divides Hispanics into six groups according to their level of proficiency in English and Spanish but points out that "Most Hispanics use both English and Spanish media" (p. 28). Advertising researchers have looked at Hispanic language preferences for ads by asking Hispanics with different levels of language proficiency about their preferences. For instance, Koslow, Shamdasani, and Touchstone (1994) found that bilingual and English-dominant Mexican Americans preferred English-dominant bilingual advertising messages because they felt that the use of Spanish showed the advertiser's cultural sensitivity. Spanish-dominant participants preferred Spanish-only ads.

Mass communication researchers have similarly researched where Hispanics get health information. Data show that Hispanics get a great deal of health information from the media and act on the information they consume (Brodie, Kjellson, Hoff, & Parker, 1999). In surveys of Hispanics, African Americans, and Whites, Brodie and associates found that more than half of Hispanics and Blacks said they were most likely to get health information from television. Their study also showed that both African Americans and Hispanics relied more on general audience media for information than on ethnic media.

While general audience media are used more than ethnic media by African Americans and Hispanics, media use varies by the level of acculturation or assimilation (Brodie et al., 1999). More acculturated Hispanics use general audience media to acquire health news, whereas less acculturated Hispanics prefer ethnic media. For all U.S. ethnic and racial groups, the use of ethnic media offers many benefits—for example, it can help one maintain one's ethnic cultural identity (Lacy, Stephens, & Soffin, 1991; Subervi-Vélez, 1986). Economic research shows that people belonging to ethnic groups consume ethnic media in metropolitan areas where there are large ethnic populations (George & Waldfogel, 2003). Wilkin and Ball-Rokeach (2006) found in surveys of two Hispanic immigrant neighborhoods in Los Angeles that respondents relied first on interpersonal communication for health information (46%), then ethnic television (32%), and last on books or magazines (12%). A Pew Hispanic Center survey (2004) showed that Spanish-dominant Hispanics are more likely to get news from television, while English-dominant Hispanics rely more on newspapers, radio, and the Internet. Likewise, a Kaiser Family Foundation (1998) survey showed that 68% of Spanish-speaking Hispanics preferred getting health information from ethnic media. There have been several studies of Black media consumers (Sylvester, 1993; Vercellotti & Brewer, 2006). One survey by Sylvester (1993) of African American newspaper readers reported that 80% read stories about health risks and 67% said that those stories influenced them to change a health behavior.

There are other individual factors associated with cultural differences in media use. Oetzel, de Vargas and Ginossar (2007) examined Hispanic women's preferences for receiving cancer information and found that a woman's ethnic identity and her "self construal" (whether a person is independent or interdependent on others) influenced whether she relied on mass media for health information. They found that bicultural and interdependent women preferred media channels to interpersonal channels.

Media Content

In that ethnic media are trusted sources of information for members of racial/ethnic groups (Lacy et al., 1991; Sylvester, 1993), it is important to know how well these media present information about health issues.

Studies of African American ethnic media suggest that magazines for women do not do a particularly good job of promoting healthful behaviors. Hoffman-Goetz, Gerlach, Marino, and Mills (1997) found that readers of Black women's magazines in 1994 would have to flip through 55 pages to encounter a tobacco ad but read 748 pages to find an article about cancer. Omonuwa and Bradford (2001) analyzed five Black-oriented magazines and five White-oriented (general audience) magazines and observed that Black magazines dedicated fewer pages to health stories, addressed fewer health topics, and contained more alcohol ads. Duerksen and associates (2005) studied health-related ads in general audience, Black, and Hispanic magazines and found that the general audience magazines had twice the number of advertisements, and that the health ads were more positive. Black and Hispanic magazines had more negative health ads, which they defined as ads for "cigarettes, alcohol, and medical treatments with no apparent value" as well as ads for "candy, ice cream, gelatin desserts," and other foods with little nutritional value. Positive ads promoted good health prevention behaviors, clinical trial participation, nutritional food choices, among other healthful behaviors. Taken together, these findings suggest that any positive messages in the editorial content of ethnic consumer magazines may be overshadowed by the messages conveyed in the advertising.

In contrast, content studies of Black newspapers have found that they do better in some areas than general audience newspapers. For instance, Cohen, Caburnay, Luke, Kreuter, Rodgers, and Cameron (2006) analyzed health news content in Black and general audience newspapers and found that there was more mobilizing information (e.g., telephone numbers, Web site addresses) in Black newspapers. Len-Ríos, Park, Cameron, Luke, and Kreuter (2008) found that Black newspapers reported on the issue of prostate cancer for men in greater proportion than did general audience newspapers. Similarly, Stryker, Emmons, and Viswanath (2007) reported that ethnic newspapers delivered cancer information to readers that was more accessible and prevention-focused than did mainstream newspapers.

Fewer recent studies of Hispanic media content have been conducted. One such study by Vargas and de Pyssler (1999) analyzed 2,386 stories in daily and weekly Hispanic newspapers from six cities. They found that nearly half of their sampled news stories were dedicated to health, but that few stories addressed health policy and the economic and political realities of the health system. For example, only 8% of health stories addressed health care costs, insurance, and health care providers. Vargas and de Pyssler point out that while information about illness is important, it is equally important that media serving immigrant populations help consumers understand how to navigate the health system.

Web-Based Media

Many researchers believe that the Internet and World Wide Web hold promise for reaching members of underserved racial and ethnic groups. Research by Fox (2005) shows that English-speaking Hispanics have closed the Internet access gap, but that African Americans and people older than 65 are still at a disadvantage. A 2007 report showed that 56% of Hispanics, 60% of Blacks, and 71% of White non-Hispanics reported using the Internet (Fox & Livingston, 2007). An academic analysis of Pew data comparing Internet use between 2000 and 2002 showed that there are access inequities between Whites and Blacks and that Whites do more health information seeking than Hispanics (Lorence, Park, & Fox, 2006). Pew Hispanic Center (2004) data also show that while half of English-dominant Hispanics reported getting news from the Internet, only 3% of Spanish-dominant Hispanics said they were likely to do so. Fox and Livingston (2007) suggest that the disparities across all groups are related to not having completed high school. While scholars (Viswanath & Kreuter, 2007) recognize that the Internet and other advances in communication technology can offer new ways to inform and educate the public about health issues, they also caution that steps must be taken to ensure that inequalities are not simply perpetuated in new ways and that it is necessary to ensure access.

Although Web-based mass media may not currently be the best way to convey public health messages to underserved populations, training interventions by telemedicine specialists have shown that computer skills training can have substantial positive effects. Masucci and associates (2006) showed that skills training for participants who had little or no previous Internet access enabled 87% to submit data to a telehealth system. Most participants in the study were more than 64 years old; about half were African American and half were White.

THE FUTURE OF MASS MEDIA CAMPAIGNS

One of the projects of the National Cancer Institute's Centers for Excellence in Cancer Communication Research is Ozioma, which means "good news" or "gospel" in the Nigerian ethnic Igbo language (Chukwuma, 1981). The research project's innovative use of public relations techniques provides Black newspapers with community-level data and culturally relevant cancer news stories at a cost well below that needed for an advertising campaign. The study, which combines expertise in health interventions with mass communication science, is a collaboration between researchers at the Saint Louis University School of Public Health and the Missouri School of Journalism. Data are still being collected for the study, but initial results indicate that the news service has been successful in generating stories in Black newspapers that are culturally relevant and provide resource information (Kreuter, 2006). Audience surveys of Black newspaper readers will determine if the stories are increasing reader knowledge and awareness of cancer prevention and detection behaviors. If this mass media intervention is successful, it could be a meaningful way to reach African American audiences and opinion leaders through a trusted news channel.

CONCLUSIONS

From the studies examined here, application of campaign strategies using the mass media to reach underserved groups appears to achieve some measure of success when controlled media, such as advertising and print media, are used to ensure sufficient levels of message saturation (Beaudoin, 2007; McLaughlin et al., 2004); language preferences and cultural symbols are taken into account (Mock et al., 2007); and the media channels selected are the ones used most and preferred by the audience members (Wilkin & Ball-Rokeach, 2006).

There are also some cautions. For instance, campaigns may only be effective if positive messages, those that advocate healthful behaviors, outnumber or overpower negative ones. Also, there is heterogeneity among ethnic groups (Valdés, 2000), so ethnicity alone may not be the best segmentation technique (Hornik & Ramirez, 2006).

There are critics of a media effects approach to reaching underserved groups. Recent reviews suggest that researchers have focused too much on message characteristics and individual levels of analysis at the expense of exploring social and structural community characteristics (Viswanath & Emmons, 2006). Still others (Kar et al., 2001) argue that communicators often forget to value and reinforce the positive health behaviors that immigrants bring with them (e.g., eating fewer processed foods and sweets). There have been calls from researchers to involve communities in the design of mass media health campaigns (e.g., messaging, outreach) rather than viewing them as target audiences.

The research reviewed here certainly addresses racial and ethnic groups from the perspective that information can help alleviate health disparities. It is true that a person who is unaware of a health problem or how to prevent a health problem will likely not address the health problem. The mass media are effective at the information awareness stage, but we know less about how repeated exposure to messages over time can influence health behavior or how information from the media is spread through social networks throughout a community.

While the research topics addressed in the studies here are pretty straightforward—get a Pap smear, a mammogram, exercise, eat right, check your home for lead—other types of health information may need more specialized understanding. For example, how do people understand their medical benefits, prescription medications, or the public policies that govern the health care system? As some research suggests, this information is not necessarily accessible to those who need it (Vargas & de Pyssler, 1999). Health literacy, or the ability to understand and use health information, is an important component of reducing health care inequities because research shows that those who already suffer health disparities tend to be more likely to have lower levels of health literacy (Davis, Williams, Marin, Parker, & Glass, 2002). As health communication professionals and researchers continue to develop campaigns to improve public health for the underserved, part of the campaign should focus on improving people's understanding of basic health concepts, since nearly half of Americans have medium to low levels of health literacy (Davis et al., 2002).

NOTES

1. Health disparities are not always defined as linked solely to race or ethnicity. It is acknowledged that disparities are influenced by structural factors (e.g., quality of treatment available in communities, environment, educational institutions) and individual-level factors (e.g., mistrust of the medical system, employment, prejudices, communication barriers). Research from various sources shows that health disparities exist for populations that are not privileged: certain racial/ethnic groups; gay, lesbian, bisexual, and transgender group members; people with disabilities, the elderly, and those with a low socioeconomic status. Racial and ethnic minorities can fall within the other groups listed.
2. *Mass media* is defined by *Webster's II New Riverside University Dictionary* as "a means of public communication reaching a large audience" (p. 731). According to a definition elaborated by Severin and Tankard (2001) mass communication reaches "relatively large, heterogeneous, and anonymous audiences," sends messages "timed to reach most audience members simultaneously," and is undertaken by "a complex organization that may involve great expense" (p. 4).

REFERENCES

Associated Press. (n.d.). 911 dispatchers denied dying woman help. *ABC News*. Retrieved June 16, 2007, from http://abcnews.go.com/print?id = 3273647

Bacon's newspaper directory 2008. (2007). Chicago: Cision.

Beaudoin, C. E., Fernandez, C., Wall, J. L., & Farley, T. A. (2007). Promoting healthy eating and physical activity: Short-term effects of a mass media campaign. *Journal of Preventative Medicine, 32*(3), 217–223.

Bell, R. A., & Alcalay, R. (2001). Health communication campaign design: Lessons from the California Wellness Guide distribution project. In S. B. Kar, R. Alcalay, & S. Alex (Eds.), *Health communication: A multicultural perspective* (pp. 281–307). Thousand Oaks, CA: Sage.

Brodie, M., Kjellson, N., Hoff, T., & Parker, M. (1999). Perceptions of Latinos, African Americans, and Whites on media as a health information source. *Howard Journal of Communications, 10,* 147–167.

Cho, J., & McLeod, D. M. (2007). Structural antecedents to knowledge and participation: Extending the knowledge gap concept to participation. *Journal of Communication, 57*(2), 205–228.

Chukwuma, H. (1981). [Review of the book *A dictionary of Igbo names, culture and proverbs*]. *Research in African Literatures, 12,* 121–125.

Cohen, E., Caburnay, C., Luke, D., Kreuter, M., Rodgers, S., & Cameron, G. T. (2006, June). *Evidence of health disparities in cancer coverage of African American communities.* Paper presented at the annual meeting of the International Communication Association, Dresden, Germany.

Davis, J. J. (1997). *Advertising research: Theory and practice.* Upper Saddle River, NJ: Prentice-Hall.

Davis, T. C., Williams, M. V., Marin, E., Parker, R. M., & Glass, J. (2002). Health literacy and cancer communication. *CA: A Cancer Journal for Clinicians, 52*(3), 134–149.

Detweiler, J., B., Bedell, B. T., Salovey, P., Pronin, E., & Rothman, A. J. (1999). Message framing and sunscreen use: Gain-framed messages motivate beach-goers. *Health Psychology, 18*(2), 189–196.

Duerksen, S. C., Mikail, A. M, Tom, L., Patton, A., Lopez, J., Amador, X., et al. (2005). Health disparities and advertising content of women's magazines: A cross-sectional study. *BMC Public Health, 5,* 85. Retrieved September 25, 2007, from http://www.biomedcentral.com/content/pdf/1471-2458-5-85.pdf

Fox, S. (2005, October 5). *Digital divisions.* Washington, DC: Pew Internet & American Life Project.

Fox, S., & Livingston, G. (2007, March 14). *Latinos online.* Washington, DC: Pew Internet & American Life Project.

Gaziano, C. (2000). Forecast 2000: Widening knowledge gaps. *Journalism & Mass Communication Quarterly, 74*(2), 237–264.

Gaziano, C., & Horowitz, A. M. (2001). Knowledge gap on cervical, colorectal cancer exists among U.S. women. *Newspaper Research Journal, 22*(1), 12–27.

George, L., & Waldfogel, J. (2003). Who affects whom in daily newspaper markets? *Journal of Political Economy, 111*(4), 765–784.

Heller, J. (1972, July 26). Syphilis victims in U.S. study went untreated for 40 years. *New York Times,* p. 1. Retrieved June 16, 2007, from ProQuest Historical Newspapers database.

Hoffman-Goetz, L., Gerlach, K. K., Marino, C., & Mills, S. L. (1997). Cancer coverage and tobacco advertising in African-American women's popular magazines. *Journal of Community Health, 22*(4), 261–270.

Hornik, R. C., & Ramirez, A. S. (2006). Racial/ethnic disparities and segmentation in communication campaigns. *American Behavioral Scientist, 49*(6), 868–884.

Jones, K. O., Denham, B. E., & Springston, J. K. (2007). Differing effects of mass and interpersonal communication on breast cancer risk estimates: An exploratory study of college students and their mothers. *Health Communication, 21*(2), 165–175.

Kaiser Family Foundation. (1998). *National and three region survey of Latinos on the media and health.* Menlo Park, CA: Henry J. Kaiser Family Foundation.

Kar, S. B., Alcalay, R., & Alex, S. (2001). Communicating with multicultural populations: A theoretical framework. In S. B. Kar, R. Alcalay, & S. Alex (Eds.), *Health communication: A multicultural perspective* (pp. 109–137). Thousand Oaks, CA: Sage.

Koslow, S., Shamdasani N. P., & Touchstone, E. E. (1994). Exploring language effects in ethnic advertising: A sociolinguistic perspective. *Journal of Consumer Research, 20*(4). 575–585.

Kreuter, M. W. (2006, May 10). *Communication-based strategies to eliminate health disparities.* Presentation to the National Cancer Institute CECCR Symposium. Retrieved June 11, 2007, from http://dccps.nci.nih.gov/hcirb/ceccr/kreuter_5-10b.pdf

Kreuter, M. W., & Haughton, L. T. (2006). Integrating culture into health information for African American women. *American Behavioral Scientist, 49*(6), 794–811.

Lacy, S., Stephens, J., & Soffin, S. (1991). The future of the African-American press: A survey of African-American newspaper managers. *Newspaper Research Journal, 12*(3), 8–19.

Len-Ríos, M. E., Park, S., Cameron, G. T., Luke, D. A., & Kreuter, M. (2008). Study asks if reporter's gender or audience predict paper's cancer coverage. *Newspaper Research Journal, 29*(2), 91–99.

Len-Ríos, M. E., & Qiu, Q. (2007). Newspaper coverage of clinical trials and willingness to participate in medical studies. *Newspaper Research Journal, 28*(1), 24–39.

Lorence, D. P., Park, H., & Fox, S. (2006). Racial disparities in health information access: Resilience of the digital divide. *Journal of Medical Systems, 30*(4), 241–249.

Marcus, B. H., Owen, N., Forsyth, A. H., Cavill, N. A., & Fridinger, F. (1998). Physical activity interventions using mass media, print media, and information technology. *American Journal of Preventative Medicine, 15*(4), 362–378.

Masucci, M. M., Homko, C., Santamore, W. P., Berger, P., McConnell, T. R., Shirk, G., et al. (2006). Cardiovascular disease prevention for underserved patients using the Internet: Bridging the digital divide. *Telemedicine and e-Health, 12*(1), 58–65.

Mayberry, R. M., Mili, F., & Ofili, E. (2002). Racial and ethnic differences in access to medical care. In T. A. LaVeist (Ed.), *Race, ethnicity and health: A public health reader* (pp. 163–197). San Francisco: John Wiley & Sons.

McLaughlin, T., Humphries, Jr., O., Nguyen, T., Maljanian, R., & McCormack, K. (2004). "Getting the lead out" in Hartford, Connecticut: A multifaceted lead-poisoning awareness campaign. *Environmental Health Perspectives, 112*(1), 1–5.

Mock, J., McPhee, S. J., Nguyen, T., Wong, C., Doan, H., Lai, K. Q., et al. (2007). Effective lay health worker outreach and media-based education for promoting cervical cancer screening among Vietnamese American women. *American Journal of Public Health, 97,* 1693–1700.

Oetzel, J., de Vargas, F., & Ginossar, T. (2007). Hispanic women's preferences for breast health information: Subjective cultural influences on source, message, and channel. *Health Communication, 21*(3), 223–233.

Omonuwa, S., & Bradford, D. (2001). How informative on medical conditions and their treatments are black-oriented magazines compared to White-oriented magazines? *American Journal of Health Studies, 17*(2), 75–78.

Pew Hispanic Center. (2004, February/March). *Hispanic media survey.* Retrieved from http://pewhispanic.org/files/reports/27.1.pdf

Ribisl, K. M., Winkleby, M. A., Fortmann, S. P., & Flora, J. A. (1998). The interplay of socioeconomic status and ethnicity on Hispanic and White men's cardiovascular disease risk and health communication patterns. *Health Education Research, 13*(3), 407–417.

Salmon, C. T., & Atkin, C. (2003). Using media campaigns for health promotion. In T. L. Thompson, A. M. Dorsey, K. I. Miller, & R. Parrott (Eds.), *Handbook of health communication* (pp. 449–472). Mahwah, NJ: Erlbaum.

Severin, W. J., & Tankard, J. W., Jr. (2001). *Communication theories: Origins, methods, and uses in the mass media* (5th ed.). New York: Longman.

Smedley, B. D., Stith, A. Y., & Nelson, A. R. (Eds.). (2005). *Unequal treatment: Confronting racial and ethnic disparities in health.* Washington, DC: National Academies Press.

Snyder, L. B., & Hamilton, M. A. (2002). A meta-analysis of U.S. health campaign effects on behavior: Emphasize enforcement, exposure, and new information and beware the secular trend. In R. C. Hornik (Ed.), *Public health communication: Evidence for behavior change* (pp. 357–383). Mahwah, NJ: Erlbaum.

Soto, T. J. (2006). *Marketing to Hispanics: A strategic approach to assessing and planning your initiative.* Chicago: Kaplan.

Stryker, J. E., Emmons, K. M., & Viswanath, K. (2007). Uncovering differences across the cancer control continuum: A comparison of ethnic and mainstream cancer newspaper stories. *Preventive Medicine, 44,* 20–25.

Subervi-Vélez, F. (1986). The mass media and ethnic assimilation and pluralism: A review and research proposal with special focus on Hispanics. *Communication Research, 13*(1), 71–96.

Sylvester, J. (1993). Media research bureau Black newspaper readership report. In F. Black (Ed.), *Milestones in Black newspaper research* (pp. 11–13, 56–81). Washington, DC: National Newspaper Publishers Association.

Tichenor, P. J., Donohue, G. A., & Olien, C. N. (1970). Mass media flow and differential growth in knowledge. *Public Opinion Quarterly, 34*(2), 159–170.

Traeger, M., Thompson, A., Dickson, E., & Provencio, A. (2006). Bridging disparity: A multidisciplinary approach for influenza vaccination in an American Indian community. *American Journal of Public Health, 95*(5), 921–925.

Vaccine study faulted. (1996, June 17). *Tampa Tribune,* p. 5. Retrieved June 16, 2007, from LexisNexis Academic database.

Valdés, M. I. (2000). *Marketing to American Latinos: A guide to the in-culture approach.* Ithaca, NY: Paramount.

Vargas, L. C., & de Pyssler, B. J. (1999). U.S. Latino newspapers as health communication resource: A content analysis. *Howard Journal of Communication, 10,* 189–205.

Vercellotti, T., & Brewer, P. R. (2006). "To plead our own cause" public opinion toward Black and mainstream news media among African Americans. *Journal of Black Studies, 37*(2), 231–250.

Viswanath, K., & Emmons, K. M. (2006). Message effects and social determinants of health: Its application to cancer disparities. *Journal of Communication, 56*(S1), S238–264.

Viswanath, K., & Kreuter, M. W. (2007). Health disparities, communication inequalities and eHealth. *American Journal of Preventative Medicine, 32*(5S), S131–133.

Webster's II New Riverside University Dictionary. (1988). Boston: Houghton Mifflin.

Whistler, K. (2007). *The state of Hispanic print 2006.* (2007). Carlsbad, CA: Latino Print Network.

Wilkin, H. A., & Ball-Rokeach, S. J. (2006). Reaching at risk groups: The importance of health storytelling in Los Angeles Latino media. *Journalism, 7*(3), 299–320.

Wray, R. J., Hornik, R. M., Gandy, O. H., Stryker, J., Ghez, M., & Mitchell-Clark, K. (2004). Preventing domestic violence in the African American community: Assessing the impact of a dramatic radio serial. *Journal of Health Communication, 9*, 31–52.

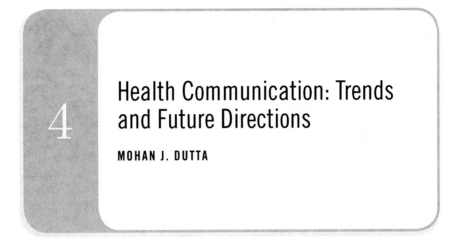

Health Communication: Trends and Future Directions

MOHAN J. DUTTA

Health communication scholars have increasingly called for the development and synthesis of theoretical insights in understanding, interpreting, explaining, predicting, analyzing, and critiquing communication processes, strategies, tactics, and messages in health care settings (Thompson, Dorsey, Miller, & Parrott, 2005). The theoretical emphasis in health communication demonstrates the relevance of theory in the development of meaningful and effective applications and is an exemplar of the ways in which theory and practice can inform each other in the context of communication problems. As Thompson (2005) points out, the field has been increasingly sensitized to the importance of theoretically driven insights that can equip scholarly understanding of communication processes in health care and thus inform the development of health care solutions both in the United States and around the global. Theorizing in health communication has by its very nature been driven by practice and, in turn, has contributed to the ways in which the delivery of health care has been practiced.

The goal of this chapter is to review the state of the field in health communication; examine the micro (small), meso (medium), and macro (large) levels of health communication; examine key trends in health care and their impact on health communication; and finally summarize the grand challenges facing health communication, including those of health care access, culture, health care quality, and technology.

CONTEXTS OF HEALTH COMMUNICATION

As a discipline, health communication may be defined as the study of communication principles, processes, and messages directed toward the development of micro-, meso-, and macro-scale health solutions (Du pre, 2005; Dutta, 2007a). Whereas the process-based perspective suggests that communication is an ongoing human effort to create and share ways of interpreting the world around us (Du pre, 2005), the message-based perspective emphasizes the ways in which effective communication materials may be created to have desired effects on the audience (Murray-Johnson & Witte, 2005). The different scales of the solutions in health care are dictated by the nature of the problem being studied and the level of emphasis that guides the identification of the problem (Dutta-Bergman, 2004a).

Furthermore, the levels at which health communication solutions are articulated are embedded within the contexts in which we construct the health care problem to be studied. For instance, the study of physician–patient communication typically focuses on the locally situated context of the physician's office or examination room, where the interaction between the physician and patient takes place (Dutta, 2007b). In contrast, the study of radio-based health promotion messages focuses on the context of the communities (local, state, and/or national) in which the radio programming is broadcasted (Dutta, 2007b).

The scale and context of the health care problem are central to the ways in which health communicators go about developing and utilizing theories to address the problem. This emphasis on the broader context of health care is increasingly evident in health communication research that underscores the importance of an ecological perspective that locates health communication within the broader environment in which health care structures, institutions, and processes are situated (Airhihenbuwa, 1995; Airhihenbuwa & Obregon, 2000; Dutta, 2007a, 2007b; Dutta-Bergman, 2003, 2004a, 2004f, 2004h; Street, 2005). In other words, health communication theorists as well as practitioners are becoming increasingly sensitized to the complexities and interrelated webs of communicative processes within which health care is situated and health meanings are continuously negotiated.

Figure 4.1 depicts the different levels and contexts for health communication research from an ecological perspective. Health communication here may be conceptualized in the realm of health organizations and the principles of organizing of health care systems, communities, and cultures. Health care is typically delivered by health organizations such as clinics and

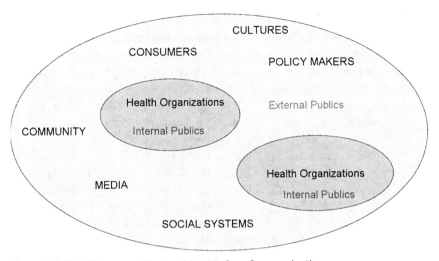

Figure 4.1 The Nature and Scope of Health Care Communication

hospitals that communicate with a variety of stakeholders such as patients, relatives, media, communities, and policy makers in order to provide health solutions. Depending upon the lens that is applied to investigate a health problem, the study of health communication in the context of the health organizations can be categorized as micro, meso, or macro level.

The micro-level emphasis in health communication typically focuses on the interpersonal relationships that play out in the context of health organizations, families, friendship networks, and various forms of organizing. Studies of physician–patient interactions and social support in health communication typically fall within this domain. Scholars studying physician–patient interactions typically focus on describing and explaining the nature of physician–patient relationships and the characteristics of competent health communication skills and then create skills training programs that are directed at providers and patients. The micro-level perspective in health communication is also evident in the diffusion of health interventions through the use of peer networks and opinion leaders to communicate health information. In such instances, one-on-one interactions among individuals diffuse the information in the community and create opportunities for diffusing the information into the broader community, thus demonstrating the possibilities of linking the micro- with the macro-level elements of health communication (Dutta, 2007b).

The meso-level emphasis in health communication examines the nature of communication processes, infrastructures, and messages in health organizations and in the relationships between health organizations and their multiple publics (Lammers, Barbour, & Duggan, 2005). Whereas traditional health organizations include those organizations that are directly involved in the delivery of health care, such as physicians' offices, medical groups, hospitals, nursing homes, hospices, and departments of public health, it is important to widen the scope of our definition to include workplaces, because a significant proportion of health care is delivered through workplaces. Organizational studies in health communication investigate the nature of communication in health care teams, occupational identification, management of organizational change, the role of leadership in health organizations, the nature of health care in organizations, the points of delivery of health care, and the like. The relationship between health organizations and their publics falls within the purview of strategic communications, and health communicators working on organization–public relationships focus on the various strategies that might be utilized by organizations to build effective and meaningful relationships with various stakeholder groups. Strategic communicators investigate the various messaging techniques that might be deployed to accomplish persuasive tasks, to achieve organizational objectives, to prevent crises, and to respond to crises.

The macro-level perspective in health communication studies the community- and societal-level aspects of health care processes and systems (Airhihenbuwa, 1995; Dutta, 2007a, 2007b; Dutta-Bergman, 2003, 2004a). Health communicators, for instance, often engage in community-based interventions that utilize communities as channels to diffuse health information, health beliefs, health attitudes, and health behaviors. The community serves as a point of entry for reaching out to the target audience of health promotion campaigns (Murray-Johnson & Witte, 2005). A significant proportion of community-based health communication programs harness the high reach of mass media to reach out to large audiences. The macro perspective is further evident in studies of health communication that investigate social patterns in the distributions of disease and health and suggest strategies for developing societal-level interventions to address health problems. Health communicators studying health care policies also adopt a macro-level perspective to understand the ways in which health policies are discursively constructed and the ways in which such policies limit possibilities for health and suggest transformative communication strategies that open up opportunities for changing unhealthy structures in social systems (Dutta, 2007b).

Although the micro-, meso-, and macro-level perspectives provide different entry points for understanding, describing, interpreting, explaining, and ultimately transforming health care systems, much of current health communication work exists at the intersections of these levels. For instance, workplace health promotion programs utilize one-on-one peer networks and mass-mediated channels to diffuse health behaviors in the organization. What we see here is the interpenetration of the micro (one-on-one), meso (organizational), and macro (mass-mediated) dimensions of health communication.

In the next section, I will review some of the key areas of health communication research in recent years. In identifying these key areas, I have particularly paid attention to the major thrusts of scholarly research evident in the two mainstream health communication journals: *Health Communication* and *Journal of Health Communication*. I have also supplemented my observations with the key areas identified in the *Handbook of Health Communication*. The areas reviewed briefly in the next section include physician–patient communication, community-based health communication, media-based health communication, and health policy. This discussion will provide the backdrop for looking at the trends in health care, and connecting these trends in health care to the trends in health communication research.

AREAS OF HEALTH COMMUNICATION

The areas of health communication included in this section range from the micro to the meso to the macro levels. At each of these levels, I will draw attention to the theoretical impetus, followed by a discussion of the methodological and pragmatic elements of health communication research. Furthermore, as I discuss the research in these key areas of health communication, I will attempt to build linkages among the areas and demonstrate the possible domains of overlap where health communication research brings together various levels of health communication processes and messages, suggesting the complexities of intertwined relationships that define health communication processes. Ultimately, my goal would be to suggest the importance of a polymorphic approach to the scholarship of health communication that generates and builds on dialogue across the various levels and paradigms of health communication research (Dutta, 2007a, 2007b; Dutta-Bergman, 2004f, 2004h).

Physician–Patient Communication

The area of physician–patient communication was one of the first areas in which communication scholars contributed to the study of health care processes. Much of the immediate experience of health care happens in the context of providers of health. Under the dominant model of health care that circulates in the United States, much of this immediate health care delivery happens in the office of the physician. Therefore, studies of the domain of physician–patient interaction explore the communication strategies and messages used by physicians and patients during medical encounters.

This research on provider–patient communication suggests that provider–patient communication styles influence a variety of patient behaviors and outcomes, including patient satisfaction with care (Street, 2005). Beyond patient satisfaction, studies of provider–patient interactions point out that the nature of these interactions influences physiological outcomes, adherence to treatment, and the likelihood of malpractice complaints (Duggan, 2006). Satisfaction measures have typically tapped into overall satisfaction and aspects related to the provider such as humanity and competence, as well as aspects related to the system such as costs and physical infrastructures (Street, 2005).

Researchers studying communication styles of physicians have looked at the ways in which patient-centered and doctor-centered styles influence outcomes (Street, 2005). The patient-centered style is characterized by communicative strategies that invite the patient's perspective in the consultation such as open-ended questions, requests for opinions and concerns, and offers of support and counseling. In contrast, the doctor-centered style primarily emphasizes clinician control; doctors practicing in this style tend to ask closed-ended questions, interrupt the patient, give directions. After controlling for the demographic characteristics and degree of participation of patients, Street (2005) observed that individual physicians demonstrated variances in communication styles in the extent to which they provided information, used partnership-building strategies, and utilized positive socioemotional strategies such as reassuring and encouraging the patient. In addition to observing variances in individual physician communication styles, health communication researchers have also observed that physicians vary in the ways in which they communicate to different patients, and thus the ways in which they adjust their styles. Such variances in physician communication styles have been observed in the extent and nature of the patient's health care status, age, gender, and ethnicity.

In addition to investigating the role of provider communication styles, scholars have also investigated the influence of patient communication styles on a variety of outcomes. Patients vary in their communication styles; they range from being expressive and communicative to being submissive and passive during the physician–patient interaction. Scholars studying patient communication styles suggest variance in patient styles in terms of age, gender, education, income, race, and other characteristics. For instance, patients with more formal education are more likely to be expressive than their less educated counterparts (Street, 2005). Studies report that patients who have a large repertoire of linguistic and informational resources for communication are more likely to actively participate in the medical encounter (Street, 2005). Patients with internal locus of control, high levels of self-efficacy, and high skill levels are also more likely to provide more information, ask more questions, and speak longer in general in their consultation with physicians (Duggan, 2006).

The research on communication styles and communication skills has provided impetus for the development of training programs that are directed at training physicians and patients in communication skills. Programs that emphasize training providers teach a variety of skills such as data gathering, interviewing, rapport building, facilitation, checking and clarifying comments, asking open-ended questions, establishing eye contact, seeking patients' views, making empathic statements, eliciting patients' concerns, listening, engaging in psychosocial discussion, and probing for patients' understanding (Cegala & Broz, 2005). Such training programs utilize a variety of strategies, such as modeling through the use of instructional videos, role playing with feedback, lectures, live demonstrations, and discussions. Interventions directed at patients have mostly focused on patient information exchange skills—primarily information seeking, information provision, and information verifying (Cegala & Broz, 2005). Strategies for patient training have included modeling of question asking, videotaped training, booklets, handouts, leaflets, and practice sessions (Cegala & Broz, 2005).

Communication skills and the ways in which we conceptualize effective communication skills vary according to local, cultural, economic, and social contexts. The provider–patient relationship and the communication skills and strategies deployed in the relationship have also evolved with the changing trends in health care today. The increasing emphasis on patient participation (to be discussed later in this chapter), coupled with increasing attention to the sociocultural environment that constitutes provider–patient relationships, has provided the foundation for Street's (2005) ecological model of provider–patient interactions, which draws attention to the social contexts within which health care relationships are situated. He suggests that in addition to looking at the interpersonal context of provider–patient consultation that is embedded in the immediate setting of the medical encounter, we also pay attention to the mediated context (e.g., Internet, telemedicine, mass media), cultural context (e.g., issues of race/ethnicity, culture, socioeconomic status, religion), political legal context (e.g., patient bill of rights, malpractice litigation, Medicaid/Medicare coverage), and the organizational context (e.g., managed care, services offered, standards of care) of health care interactions.

The ecological model points out that the interpersonal communication between physicians and patients is embedded within a broader environment and this environment plays a crucial role in the ways in which physicians and patients communicate with each other, the communication styles and strategies that are used, and the outcomes associated with these styles and strategies. This model particularly highlights the changes in technology that have occurred, the role of culture, and the level and type of access available to patients (Dutta, 2007b). We will look at some of the current trends in health communication research on provider–patient interactions when discussing the response of health communicators to the changing landscape of health care in the last section of this chapter.

Community-Based Health Communication

Health communicators have increasingly focused on the community context of health care as they have attempted to address the locally situated nature of health issues (Dorsey, 2005). A community is defined as an "informally organized set of loose associations among residents"(Dearing, 2003, p. 209). There has been an emerging acknowledgement that community participatory processes can provide important avenues for disseminating health interventions, particularly in the context of underserved communities in the United States and across the globe. Furthermore, there is an increasing awareness that local communities ought to be at the heart of health promotion efforts (Scherer & Juanillo, 2003). Community-based health communication projects have taken a wide variety of forms, ranging from top-down campaigns that utilize community platforms as channels to diffuse health information to health communication programs that utilize grassroots mobilization strategies and community coalitions to seek out resources for the community and to bring about structural changes (Dearing, 2003; Dutta-Bergman, 2004a, 2004c, 2004g).

At the heart of community-based health communication is the idea that communities can serve as channels of communication about health issues. The formal and informal networks that are present within a community offer avenues for creating and sustaining healthful beliefs, attitudes, and behaviors within communities (Beaudoin, Thorson, & Hong, 2006). The importance and usefulness of community participation have been underlined by a variety of health campaigns for causes like heart disease prevention, smoking prevention and cessation, HIV prevention, healthy eating, and road safety (Kawachi, Kennedy, & Glass, 1999). Stephens, Rimal, and Flora (2004) point out that since participation and membership in community organizations are voluntary, health messages that come out of community organizations are likely to be considered with greater trust. Scholars like Rappaport (1987) and Repucci, Woolard, and Fried (1999) note that individual-level preventive efforts should be complemented by community-based approaches.

According to Merzel and D'Afflitti (2003), the rationale for the community-based approach to health promotion stems from the notion that individuals cannot be considered separate from their social milieu, and that context is interdependent with the health and lives of individuals in the community, and hence the community as a whole. Campbell and Jovchelovitch (2000) state that participation allows community members to formulate strategies that are based on the barriers they face and their perceived health needs. As a result, health program messages and program implementation procedures are created within the community; this enhances their chances of eliciting desired results. Related to this is the notion of empowering the community. Communities with actively participating members are likely to perceive that they are more in charge of their lives. Hence they are also more likely to take control of their health, engage in health-enhancing behaviors, and actively seek out health resources (Campbell & Jovchelovitch, 2000). A conglomeration of individuals with such high loci of control will result in a community that ranks high in terms of being healthy and engaging in health promotion practices. In other words, situating a health communication model within a participatory community–based framework empowers members of the community to articulate their needs, map available resources, mobilize in the production of positive health outcomes, and engage in health sustenance behaviors (Dutta-Bergman, 2003).

This community-based health communication work has been complemented by health communication projects that underscore the role of communities in fostering healthful contexts. This line of work is captured under the broader umbrella of social capital and health. Social capital refers to the formal and informal ties in a community that bring a community together and create community cohesiveness (Dutta-Bergman, 2004e, 2004g). It is also reflective of the resources available in the social structure that can be accessed and mobilized for strategic actions (Dutta, 2007b). Health communication research examining the role of social capital in health points out that community participation is positively associated with a variety of positive health behaviors (Dutta-Bergman, 2004e, 2004g). In other words, those individuals who are more likely to participate in their communities are also more likely to engage in a variety of health-related behaviors.

Social capital generates positive health outcomes by creating a supportive environment, by mitigating the stress and loneliness experienced by individual community members, and by fostering high levels of self-efficacy (Kawachi et al., 1999). People with higher levels of social capital and trust also report lower mortality rates and better health status than other people (Kawachi & Berkman, 2000).

Communicating in community contexts nurtures, sustains, and fortifies health behaviors. Community social networks serve as points through which health information can be accessed and disseminated, resources for health information, resources for community mobilizing and organizing around key health issues, resources for mobilizing to secure additional structural resources, and points of access for bringing about changes in unhealthy local, national, and global structures. The literature reports that not only are communities with high social capital more likely to serve as conduits for health promotion efforts, but they are also likely to provide the needed resources for community mobilization around structural issues (Dutta, 2007b). In other words, communities with high social capital have community capacity for mobilizing network resources to address questions of policy and to go about seeking to change unhealthy policies.

This community capacity-building aspect of health communication provides impetus for the next generation of research that explores the role of community participation in promoting infrastructural change, examines the participatory mechanisms for engaging with community members, and suggests ways of building community capacity for developing community-based solutions. In addition, the role of technology in community-based health organizing is yet another area that has started receiving increasing attention in communication research.

Media and Health Communication

The role of the media in health as an influencer and shaper of health beliefs, health attitudes, and health behaviors is well documented in the health communication literature (Parrott, 2004). In fact, one of the earliest strands of health communication research explored the ways in which mass media could be utilized for disseminating health information to the public, informing health beliefs, shaping health attitudes, and ultimately influencing health behaviors (Salmon & Atkin, 2003). As articulated by Rogers and Storey (1987) in their seminal piece on campaigns, campaigns are purposive in their desire to generate certain outcomes in a relatively large number of individuals within a specified time period through the use of an organized set of communication activities. This area of health communication campaigns has historically focused on the mass media as the mass media have provided large-scale reach to the intended audiences of campaign messages (see Salmon & Atkin, 2003, for a review). Theories of mass media and persuasion have provided valuable guidelines regarding the strategic choice of media vehicles, sources to be used in campaign messages, the content of campaign messages, the appeals to be presented through campaigns messages, and the like (Salmon & Atkin, 2003; Slater, 1999; Snyder, 2001).

Particularly in the domain of campaigns, health communication scholars have examined the role of the information- and entertainment-based media in promoting both healthy and unhealthy behaviors. What are the types of health beliefs, health attitudes, and health behaviors promoted through programming such as news programming? Traditionally the promotion of health through the mass media has been conceptualized in terms of the diffusion of health information. The diffusion-of-innovations framework widely circulated in the health communication literature has been built on the assumption that the mass media can serve as conduits for diffusing health interventions by informing the public about health issues. Outlets such as radio and television news have been widely used to diffuse health information to at-risk communities. Specific news segments have been developed that are directed at serving the health information needs of particular target audiences. Radio programming was particularly crucial in early campaign research and practice, as radio provided a large reach for campaigns, particularly among otherwise-hard-to-reach segments of the population. Analysis of media usage patterns suggests that the information-based approach to mediated campaigns often contributes to the gaps between the haves and have-nots by serving as a resource for members of the health-oriented segments, who are more likely to follow news-based programming than are members of the low health–oriented segments, who are more likely to consume entertainment programming (Dutta-Bergman, 2004c, 2004d, 2004g, 2005b).

Starting with this early emphasis on communication as information, health communication scholars moved on to articulate the role of entertainment programming as a source of health information for target audiences (Dutta-Bergman, 2004d). The term "entertainment-education" describes the embedding of information in entertainment contexts. Since the early entertainment-education programs that were carried out in the realm of development communication programs, health communication scholars have investigated the ways in which health messages might be strategically placed in entertainment programs and the content strategies that might be deployed in such programs. Dutta-Bergman (2004c, 2005b) argues that entertainment-education programs serve as channels for reaching out to the less health–oriented segments of the population, as such segments of the population often acquire health information serendipitously through exposure to health content within the context of entertainment programming.

The notion that entertainment programs provide role models, information resources, and decision-making cues for the performance of a variety of health-related behaviors led health communication scholars to examine the role of entertainment programming in the realm of a variety of health behaviors. Scholars have conducted content analyses to examine the nature of health-related content in entertainment programming. Assessments of such portrayals have provided the impetus for health advocacy that is directed at improving or shifting the type of coverage of a specific health issue in the media (Morgan, Harrison, Chewning, Davis, & Dicorcia, 2007).

Finally, media-based health communication scholars have increasingly started adopting a strategic approach to the utilization of the mass media for health-related purposes. One of the core components driving the strategic approach is the awareness that health care consumers use the mass media to gratify a wide range of felt needs. Uses and means of gratification and selective exposure theories draw our attention to the various ways in which media audiences utilize the mass media for a wide variety of purposes. From a selective exposure standpoint, health communication scholars have empirically demonstrated that within-population differences in involvement in health-related issues significantly influence the processing of health content in the media.

For instance, individuals who are already highly motivated regarding their health are the ones who are likely to seek out health-related news from a variety of channels (print, television, radio, Internet etc.) and process health information received from mediated channels (Dutta-Bergman, 2004a, 2004b, 2004d, 2004e, 2004f, 2004h). As a consequence, mediated messages are less likely to reach those segments of the population that are less likely to be interested in issues of health. This leads to the increasing gaps between the health haves and have-nots as mediated messages continue to serve as resources for health information for the health-oriented segments of the population.

Applications of uses and gratifications theory in health contexts also emphasize the motivation-based perspective and suggest that there exists within-population variance in people's motivations for using health-based media content. Understanding these within-population differences allows health communicators to formulate strategies for reaching out to different segments of the population, specifically the underserved segments of the population that are less likely to have access to health care resources. Similar patterns are observed in the research that examines the relationship between access to new media technologies and health care disparities, suggesting that underserved segments of the population are also less likely to have access to new media technologies such as the Internet that serve as health information resources (Dutta-Bergman, 2004c, 2005b, 2005e).

Furthermore, there are within-population differences in people's motivation to use such technologies and the knowledge of ways to use new media technologies for health-related purposes. Summarizing these differences in patterns in access to, motivation and knowledge to use, and efficacy of health-related media uses, health communication scholars suggest the importance of a strategic approach to health communication that utilizes formative research on media usage patterns to develop campaign strategies. Recent years have witnessed a dramatic increase in health communication studies and applications that apply new media technologies for disseminating health information.

Policy and Health Communication

Health communicators are increasingly underscoring the roles of health care policies in shaping the landscape of health, based upon the realization that health communicators have been rather slow in examining the role of communication in shaping health care policies and practices (Kreps, Bonaguro, & Query, 1998; Wallack & Dorfman, 2001). They have drawn attention to the notion that it is ultimately in the realm of policies that decisions are made about health care and the ways in which health care is distributed in the population. Policies also determine the ways in which health initiatives consider the role of communication and the emphasis on communicative strategies in the realm of public health problems (Kreps, 2003). Such policies cover a wide gamut ranging from the local levels to the state levels to the national and international levels. Ultimately, policies determine the ambit of health communication practice, defining the scope of the problems we work with and the solutions we develop in order to address these problems (Dutta, 2007a, 2007b). Health care policies, in other words, dictate the terrain on which communicative practices are defined, enacted, and evaluated (Wallack & Dorfman, 2001; Zoller, 2005).

Health communicators working at the level of policy explore the ways in which policies construct discourses of health care, drawing attention to the health-promoting and health-damaging aspects of such policies (Dutta, 2007a, 2007b; Wallack & Dorfman, 2001; Zoller, 2005). The emphasis here is on understanding the ways in which such policies promote or threaten health, and the communicative processes through which these policies are articulated, discussed, implemented, and evaluated.

Similarly, health communication provides an entry point for examining the relationship between the rhetoric of health care policies and the practices of these health care policies. It is worthwhile to examine the match or mismatch between the rhetoric and practice of health care policies because it is by examining these gaps that problems may be identified in the health care system. The gaps in health care policy discourses and the practice of such policies provide tools for evaluating the real impact of the policies that are circulated and supported in mainstream health care. Furthermore, a discursive approach to health care policies provides invaluable entry points for interrogating the communicative processes through which health care discourses marginalize and silence certain sectors of society. By raising questions such as "Who gets to speak in the discursive space?" "Who has voice and who does not?" and "How are agendas and issues discursively constituted by dominant social actors?" health communication scholars can draw our attention to the processes through which certain policy articulations are normalized.

For instance, critical health communication scholars examining the discursive spaces constituted by campaign policies question the individual-level focus of health campaigns and suggest the need for policy discourse to examine the unhealthy structures of health that are supported, reified, and recirculated by mainstream agendas in health care. The emphasis on the individual as the subject of health care interventions draws attention away from the need to address the structural inequities and resource deprivation faced in certain communities.

The examination of the rhetoric of health care policies and the positioning of these policies in the backdrop of health outcomes provides the basis for examining communication strategies for changing those health care policies that limit access to basic health care, support health care disparities, and sustain unhealthy social structures. The emphasis is on developing communication processes and messages that are directed toward shifting public opinion around key policies and influencing policy makers. The emphasis is on advocacy and activism directed at bringing about large-scale changes, instead of individual health behaviors. The communication interventions developed in this realm ultimately seek to create healthy communities by bringing about changes in the structures constituting these communities. Theories such as agenda setting, priming, and framing provide important entry points for looking at ways of shifting health care policies.

Now that we have reviewed the major strands of health communication research in the areas of physician–patient communication, community-based health communication, health communication and media, and health communication in the realm of policy, we will consider these discussions within the context of key trends in health care today. This discussion will serve as the basis for our exploration of new directions in the next generation of health communication research.

KEY TRENDS IN HEALTH CARE

What are the key trends in health care, and what are the effects of these trends on the ways in which we conceptualize health communication, design health communication research, and develop health communication solutions? In this section, we will look at these trends and review the ways in which health communicators might go about addressing these trends in their work. In other words, an awareness of the trends presented in this section is based on the premise that they might provide ways for thinking about communication solutions and the processes through which these solutions might be deployed to address the grand challenges in the health care industry. The knowledge of the trends provides ways of conceptualizing and developing communication solutions in health care. Ultimately, knowledge of the trends allows health communicators to take stock of the existing research in health communication and find new avenues that might provide the impetus for the next generation of health communication research.

Increasing Consumer Participation

One trend is increasing consumer participation in health care processes (see Chapter 6). The increasing participation of the public in health care processes has opened up avenues for questioning the expertise-driven model of health care that has traditionally dominated the health care industry (Sharf, 2005). This shift from an expert-driven model to a more participatory model has been brought about by changes in technology as well as broader changes in the delivery of health care. The reconfiguration in health care delivery processes has also brought about opportunities for addressing the ways in which consumer participation might open up opportunities for addressing health care issues in democratic ways.

The emphasis on a consumer-driven model, however, has also introduced questions on topics such as the construction of health care as a commodity in a capitalist economy, the role of the state and nongovernmental organizations in delivering health care, and the relationship between health care access and the ability to participate in the consumer economy. Whereas certain segments of the population have increasing access to health care services, preventive resources, and communicative platforms promoting health, other segments of the population are increasingly marginalized through their lack of access to health services, preventive resources, health information, and those communication channels that serve as resources for health (Dutta-Bergman, 2004b, 2004c, 2004d, 2004e, 2004f, 2004g, 2005b, 2005e, 2005f).

For instance, the research on health orientation demonstrates that the health-motivated segments of the population are also more likely to participate actively in physician–patient relationships, seek out health information from a variety of communication channels, process health information actively, and participate in communication-based health-enhancing platforms than are the segments of the population that are not health oriented. This situation regarding participation in health-based communication channels, coupled with people's lack of access to participatory platforms, introduces questions regarding ways to introduce communicative resources to underserved segments of the population in developing communicative capacities for utilizing these resources, as well as in addressing the broader structures that create and sustain the conditions that foster people's lack of access.

Increasing Diversity

The United States has become increasingly diverse over the last few decades, and there has also been increasing acknowledgement that culture plays an important role in health care interactions, health care delivery, reception of health information, and the like (Huff & Kline, 1999). Health organizations have become increasingly sensitized to the need for the development and delivery of culturally sensitive messages that take the nature of a population's culture into account in conceptualizing health communication interventions. What are the ways in which culture influences the communication needs of communities in health care settings? How can health care organizations be responsive to the communicative needs that are presented in differing cultural contexts? What are the ways in which culturally responsive messages can be developed in health communication campaigns that are sensitive to the various needs of local cultural communities and therefore more likely to be influential in multicultural contexts?

Furthermore, looking at health communication within the context of globalization processes has also brought about fundamental questions about the nature and characteristics of health and illness (Dutta, 2007a, 2007b). The flow of health communication across the globe called into question the universal languages of health care and brought us face-to-face with the multiple and often contradictory frames in which health and illness might be defined and understood.

While globalization is an increasingly important factor in health communication, researchers must still be sensitive to the local contexts within which health meanings are narrated, interpreted, and communicated. What is the role of the local context in the various meanings of health that circulate in local communities? What processes and strategies might health communicators develop in order to centralize the role of the context in health care interactions and experiences?

For health communicators, new challenges have evolved in terms of defining the very nature of health, articulating health problems, and configuring health solutions through participatory strategies that engage local communities. What are the ways in which health communication theorists, researchers, and practitioners can contribute to the creation of spaces for dialogue and conversation that invite the participation of local community members? The emphasis on dialogue and conversation has provided impetus for participatory health communication research that explores the ways in which participatory spaces might be created and sustained in local communities and in the interactions of the local communities with key stakeholder groups.

Increasing Use of Technology

As discussed throughout this chapter, technology has emerged as a key player in the delivery of health care information and services (Murero & Rice, 2006). An increasing percentage of Internet users use the Internet to receive, process, and share health information in their decision-making processes. Health information technologies have facilitated the flow of health information, preventive resources, and health care services. The increasingly visible role of health information technologies in health care decision-making processes has also fundamentally shifted the landscape of health care services delivery in the United States and in other parts of the globe. With the widespread access to health information facilitated by new media technologies, health care providers have become increasingly concerned about the quality of health information received by patients and the role of such health information in patient decision-making processes. Furthermore, the differential patterns of distributions of technologies in communities and societies have triggered interest in the linkages between the digital divide and health care disparities.

Increasing Health Care Disparities

Finally, and perhaps most importantly, a survey of the landscape of health services, U.S. age patterns, and health care access demonstrates increasing national and global disparities in people's access to and usage of health care services. Whereas the health-rich continue to have better access to health care choices, the underserved segments of the population continue to lack access to basic health care. Disparities in health care in the United States are affected by characteristics such as race, socioeconomic status, gender, and geographic location (Dutta, 2007a; 2007b). What are the communicative avenues for addressing these disparities? In examining the role of communication, health communication scholars observe that individuals, groups, and communities that have poor access to a wide range of health care services also have poor access to communicative infrastructures (Dutta, 2007b; Dutta, Bodie, & Basu, 2007). In other words, structural disparities in communication infrastructures mirror structural disparities in health care infrastructures and reflect deep-seated disparities within social systems (Dutta, 2007b). (See Chapter 3 for more on disparities in health care.)

Socioeconomic Disparities

Low socioeconomic status (SES) is one of the critical indicators of structural violence and plays out its role in the realm of health care by limiting people's access to a variety of health care resources that are considered necessary for human survival. Individuals living in poor communities are directly exposed to violence through the absence of basic infrastructures and opportunities, and through the presence of a variety of threats to their health. Social class is a critical indicator of health capacity in underserved communities, with poorer communities having lower health capacity than communities that have higher levels of income.

The basic health infrastructure in such communities is either absent or minimal, with a limited number of providers, limited medical supplies, limited health care technologies, limited transportation, and limited access to preventive resources. In addition to affecting the distribution of resources at a community level, SES fundamentally affects individual health by determining the amount and types of health care services that are available to individuals. Class contributes to a culture of poverty that is built around narratives of pain, struggle, and resistance. It is through these narratives of suffering and survival that we gain insight into the agency of marginalized communities and the ways in which such communities make sense of their limited structural resources.

The SES of an individual directly determines the types of preventive services, health care services, and communication infrastructures he or she has access to. Higher-SES groups are more likely than lower socioeconomic groups to have better access to a variety of health-related services. For instance, individuals from higher-SES groups have greater access to providers than do individuals from lower-SES groups. Similarly, higher-SES individuals have greater access than individuals who belong to lower-SES groups to cancer screening resources. An increasing number of studies document the disparity in access to basic health care services among higher- and lower-SES groups in the United States.

Furthermore, disparities exist between higher- and lower-SES groups in the realms of access to policy platforms, civil society forums, health delivery organizations, and organizations that evaluate the ways in which policy gets implemented by health care organizations. In other words, lack of access to basic health care is supplemented by lack of access to basic means of communication such that lower-SES individuals also have minimal access to fundamental communication infrastructures. Also, the quality of communication experienced by individuals varies by SES such that low-SES individuals are more likely to experience unpleasant interactions with their providers.

Whereas higher-socioeconomic groups typically can afford a plethora of preventive services, lower-socioeconomic groups are limited in the ways in which they can access preventive services in terms of the costs of these resources, the effort needed to access them, and the time consumed by individual efforts to take preventive steps. In addition, higher-SES groups typically live in resource-rich communities that have greater levels of access to preventive resources of various types, including parks and walkways for physical exercise, screening facilities, and food resources. In addition, higher-SES groups also have greater access to hospitals and medical centers, physicians, nurses, and a variety of treatment options (medicines and surgical options) than individuals from lower-SES groups. Of particular concern in the realm of SES is the health of those who are not covered by health insurance, the health of the working classes, the health of homeless populations, and the health of individuals who live in rural communities. Each of these segments of the population is marked by its lack of access to basic health care resources.

Racial Disparities

Historically, race-based differences in U.S. society have resulted in differential access to socioeconomic resources like educational and employment opportunities. This situation has meant lower levels of income in racial minority families, and lower socioeconomic status. Unhealthy living conditions and limited access to structural resources like transportation, food, medicine, and insurance are all products of this race-based social differential, and in turn they exert a considerable impact on the health and well-being of minorities. Low socioeconomic status, adverse health behaviors, and lack of health insurance serve as the primary pathways through which racial disparities are played out in the realm of health (Black, Ray, and Markides, 1999; Brodie, Flournoy, Altman, Blendon, Benson, & Rosenbaum, 2000; Williams & Collins, 2001).

Several studies have demonstrated just how race-based differences cause disparities in access to medical care. Even after adjustment for socioeconomic status, health insurance, and clinical status, these studies show that Whites are more likely than Blacks to receive a broad range of specific medical procedures (Williams, 1999). Among Medicare inpatients, Williams notes, Blacks are less likely than Whites to receive all 16 of the most common procedures. This demonstrates the prevalence of prejudiced treatments in health care within the United States, even when social class is controlled for.

Gender Disparities

In their day-to-day experiences of health, women regularly experience limited access to a health care system that is dominated by men, funded and supported by a health care industry that is run by men, and regulated by policy makers who are mostly men (Tong, 2002). Women's limited access is the result of such factors as lack of financial resources, lack of time because of household commitments, the epistemological construction of a medical system that is unresponsive to women's personal experiences, and fundamental differences in communication expectations and goals of patients and their providers. Limited access also is a key issue regarding women's access to adequate and healthy food, spaces for exercising, and screening programs. Worth noting are the ways in which race and class interact with gender to further marginalize women.

The many issues surrounding disparities in health care services, access, and delivery raise numerous questions for health communication researchers. What is the role of health communicators in addressing these disparities? Given the complementary patterns of disparities in distributions of health care resources and the unequal distribution of communication infrastructures and resources, what are the ways in which health communicators can reach out to the underserved segments of the population? What communication processes and strategies might prove meaningful in addressing the structural disparities in health care? How might current and future research in health communications develop strategies for challenging and transforming unhealthy structures in health care? What are the ways in which participatory processes in health communication might be organized in order to bring about changes in the unhealthy structures that lie at the root of health care disparities? What are the communication processes through which cultures can be theorized and understood as entry points for communicating about issues of health and for creating accessible health care? What communication processes and strategies might be deployed in order to create and sustain community capacities, particularly in those communities that are most likely to be underserved and have minimal access to basic health capacities?

GRAND CHALLENGES IN HEALTH CARE COMMUNICATION

What are the grand challenges in health communication, and what are the ways in which the next generation of health communicators might respond to these grand challenges? The trends reviewed in the previous section underscore the importance of addressing issues of access, culture, quality, and technology in health communication theorization, research, and practice (more on each of these to follow). My goal in this section is to outline some central questions for the next generation of health communication research and suggest ways in which these questions might be addressed through the theorization, research, and practice of health communication. Ultimately, my hope is that this section will open up new opportunities for dialogue in health communication about the ways in which health communication scholars can go about providing communicative entry points for responding to the major trends in the health care industry.

Culture-Centered Approach

The culture-centered approach to health communication provides a theoretical entry point for addressing the major challenges facing health communicators today (Airhihenbuwa, 1995; Dutta, 2007a, 2007b; Dutta-Bergman, 2004d, 2004e). Challenging the top-down processes reflected in much of the existing health communication theory and research, the culture-centered approach suggests that health communication is embedded within local contexts and is itself a culturally situated process that is continuously negotiated.

In the culture-centered approach, the emphasis is on communicative meanings and the ways in which these meanings are constituted by members of a culture as they negotiate cultural contexts and social structures in their day-to-day health experiences. It further suggests that a culturally centered understanding of health communication processes leads us to new ways of thinking about health that have otherwise been disregarded. Therefore, the approach highlights the importance of listening to local communities and creating dialogic spaces for local participation through which locally narrated issues might be voiced and that might serve as axes for structural transformations. The creation of participatory spaces in local communities and of spaces for dialogues between local communities and external stakeholders serves as the basis for developing health communication applications that are directed toward addressing the needs of local communities. In the culture-centered approach, the emphasis of health communicators is on creating and sustaining participatory infrastructures that facilitate the development of health solutions driven by the articulations of local communities.

The culture-centered approach foregrounds the elements of culture, structure, and agency in the construction of health meanings (Dutta, 2007b). Figure 4.2 outlines the basic tenets of the culture-centered approach. Structure is one of the core components of the culture-centered approach and refers to the institutions, policies, codes, rules, and processes that determine and constrain the health choices that are available to community members. The emphasis of the culture-centered approach, therefore, is on addressing health care disparities and on issues related to the lack of access discussed in the previous section. That many of the health experiences of individuals, groups, and communities are structured is an invaluable realization in health communication research, as it shifts the emphasis from the traditional individual-level approach of health communication to emphasizing the role of health care structures in health experiences.

Culture reflects the dynamic and complex web of contexts within which health meanings are negotiated. Cultures provide the scripts for understanding and interpreting structures.

Agency reflects the capacity of local community members to make choices and to participate in processes that negotiate and seek to transform the structures of health.

The rest of the chapter will explore the ways in which the culture-centered approach provides a meaningful theoretical, methodological, and pragmatic lens for envisioning a health care communication system that suggests insights about responding to these grand challenges. The culture-centered approach to health communication is built on the

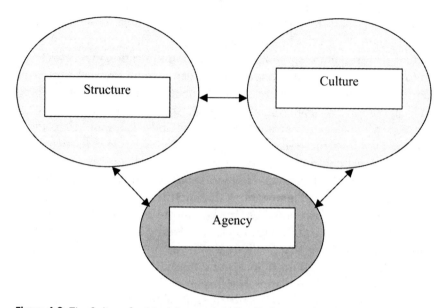

Figure 4.2 The Culture-Centered Approach to Health Communication

central notion that the voices of local communities ought to be the centerpiece of health communication research. Furthermore, it stresses that the voices of these local communities have been systematically silenced by the top-down health communication programs that have often taken for granted problem and solution configurations in local communities. Although formative research is often done in the early stages of health communication programs, such formative research almost always predetermines the nature of the problem and takes for granted the characteristics of the solutions that are to be diffused in the communities.

Health Care Access

As reiterated throughout the chapter, access is one of the important issues in health care. That certain segments of the population do not have access to some of the basic capacities of health care is a key realization that ought to provide the guiding vision for the next generation of health communication research. The basic necessities of health care need to be brought to the forefront, and health communication scholars ought to play a pivotal role in understanding the ways in which communication strategies might be used to build basic health care capacities in local communities. Furthermore, although much of the existing health communication work has taken issues of access for granted, the next generation of health communication research can begin by starting to interrogate the accessibility of communicative spaces, particularly in the realm of those communities that have traditionally been marginalized. In a nutshell then, the emphasis of future health communication ought to be on:

- Examining the ways in which communicative processes, strategies and tactics might go about developing access to health care infrastructures in underserved communities. Note the emphasis here on the mobilization and community organizing aspects of communication in order to build basic health capacities in underserved communities.
- Examining the ways in which communication scholars and practitioners might create points of access to communication infrastructures (e.g., communication technologies, communication platforms). Future research ought to examine the roles of communication theorizing, research, and practice to create points of access to community participatory platforms for setting health care agendas.
- Examining the processes and strategies through which communication skills might be developed among health care experts for listening to the voices of underserved communities locally, nationally, and globally. The thought process is complete.

Culture

That culture is central to the communication of health meanings is a key tenet in an increasing body of health communication work. The importance of the role ascribed to culture in health communication processes has grown with the realization that health care professionals ought to be sensitized to the changing cultural landscape of the United States, coupled with the rapid demographic shifts within the United States. Furthermore, the concept of culture has become particularly relevant in the context of health communication processes as an increasing number of scholars have questioned the "universal" logic of health that runs through much of health communication scholarship and application. On one hand, health communicators have started articulating the value of developing culturally sensitive interventions that take into account the cultural characteristics of local communities; on the other hand, a growing body of work on the culture-centered approach has discussed the importance of local participation in the articulation of problems and in the development of solutions. The understanding that culture is important serves as the foundation for:

- Examining the role of culture in the realm of health care decision making. What role does culture play in the ways in which individuals, groups, and communities construct meanings of health? How does culture constitute identities of individuals, groups, and communities, and how do these identities interact with meanings of health, health beliefs, health care decisions, and the ways in which the decisions are practiced in local communities?

- Examining the role of culture in developing health-related messages. What are the ways in which culture shapes the ways in which individuals, groups, and communities perceive health and construct the various barriers to health? What are the strategies for taking culture into account in the development of health communication messages? How can health communication be responsive to the variances in cultures? Understanding the influence of culture in health communication shapes the framework for cultural sensitivity programs.

- Examining the role of culture in the development of communication strategies for addressing unhealthy structures. What are the ways in which unhealthy structures play out in the local cultural contexts of underserved communities? What are the health ramifications of such structures? What are the processes through which structural features marginalize certain cultural communities? What are the mainstream communication strategies that are utilized in order to marginalize local communities? How can transformative communication processes and strategies that are directed at addressing the underlying structures that manifest in health care disparities be developed?

- Developing culture-centered approaches to health communication that underscore the relevance of cultural context and community agency in articulating health communication problems and health solutions in local communities. Ultimately, the goal of the culture-centered approach is to develop communicative solutions that emerge from within the community through the involvement of community members. The emphasis is on creating participatory spaces for the discursive co-constructions of health issues and the communication of these issues to external stakeholders who influence policies of health. The articulation of local cultural contexts in the health communication process lies at the core of culture-centered health communication.

Health Care Quality

An Institute of Medicine report on health care in the United States suggests the importance of addressing the quality of health care that is being delivered within the United States. Questions of quality not only are salient in the United States but are quintessential in the delivery of health care across the globe. What is the quality of the health information, health resources, health services, and preventive services that are available to the different segments of the population? What are the within-population differences in the ways in which the quality of health information resources, preventive services, and health care services are delivered? What are the relationships between differentials in these patterns and differentials in the quality of health communication resources? More specifically, the emphasis on quality plays out in the following realms:

- Quality of provider–patient communication. This line of research examines the differences in communicative patterns in different cultural communities, and the ways in which these communicative patterns in physician–patient interactions vary by race, gender, socioeconomic status, and other characteristics. What are the ways in which culture influences the constructions of health and relationships with health care providers? What are the influences of social structures in the quality of experiences that patients have with providers? How do patients enact their agency in the context of the physician–patient relationship, and how does this enactment influence the quality of the physician–patient interaction?
- Quality of organizational (e.g., hospital, agency) communication. What are the ways in which health care infrastructures influence the quality of communication in hospitals and other health care agencies? What are the cultural features that play out in the realm of the quality of communication in such organizations?

- Quality of health information (trust, completeness, comprehensibility, etc.). What are the indicators of the quality of health information? What are the strategies consumers use to evaluate the quality of health information that they receive? How do these quality evaluations vary in different sectors of the population? What strategies might be utilized to develop communication programs that are directed toward training patients in strategies for evaluating the quality of health information?
- Quality of communication technologies. In addition to the emphasis on health information, an increasing number of health communication projects emphasize the importance of evaluating the quality of health communication technologies. This emphasis on technologies is particularly relevant in the delivery of health care, given the growing use of communication technologies as avenues for delivering health services, particularly to the underserved sectors of the global population. What are the ways in which measures of quality might be developed for evaluating health care technologies? How can these measures of quality be responsive to the cultural contexts within which the technologies are constituted? What are the ways in which the quality of health care technologies can be located and discussed within the context of the social structures within which the technologies are deployed?
- Quality of health infrastructures. Finally, an increasing number of health communication scholars have drawn attention to the quality of health care infrastructures and the ways in which infrastructure quality is distributed within the population.

Technology

As discussed in the section on the trends in health care, technology has emerged as a key player in the delivery of health information, preventive resources as well as health care resources. The culture-centered approach suggests that technology exists at the intersections of structure, culture, and agency. On one hand, access to technology (and lack thereof) creates and constrains the possibilities for health care in local communities, and on the other hand, it is through the use of technologies that individuals, groups, and communities create spaces for communicating about social structures and transforming these structures. The meanings of technologies become culturally localized as technologies take on local meanings for local community members and they use these technologies to participate in their health care decision making. The intersections of technologies and participatory spaces provide new ways of thinking about the ways in which health communication technologies might be harnessed toward the goal of creating and sustaining equitable, accessible, and democratic health care processes. This chapter's review of the interdisciplinary connections around technology suggests that the next generation of health communication research ought to focus on:

- Examining uses of technology for health-related purposes such that technologies can be utilized in order to deliver need-specific solutions. In this sense, the technology serves as a resource for solving community-specific problems and is conceptualized as an element of community capacity. The applications developing from this line of work focus on creating technology-based infrastructures in underserved communities and developing programs that teach the skill sets needed to utilize the technologies. Furthermore, a use-based perspective also informs the ways in which technology-based platforms might be developed in order to serve the needs of users.

- Examining consumer access to health care technologies in order to be able to create sustainable technology access points for individuals, groups, and communities. This line of research provides the impetus for studying the correlations between digital divides and other kinds of disparities within the population. For instance, the differential patterns of access in broadband technologies are often correlated with socioeconomic disparities, thus suggesting the importance of locating technologies in the realm of broader structures. Applications developing from this line of work provide the basis for the development of technology infrastructures in underserved communities such that the technologies might be utilized by community members for transformative politics.

- Examining consumer knowledge about using technology for health-related purposes. Health communication researchers are increasingly pointing out that people's knowledge of ways to use technology makes a great deal of difference in consumer uses of technologies for health-related purposes. Health communication research exploring the knowledge of technology uses locates these differential knowledge patterns in the context of broader population-level characteristics. Health communicators have the opportunity for suggesting the ways in which differences in knowledge play out in the realm of health care usage patterns, health experiences, and a variety of outcomes, including morbidity and mortality patterns.

- Developing e-health literacy programs to train patients in gathering, evaluating, and using health information. It is through these literacy programs that individuals, groups, and communities in the underserved sectors of the population can be equipped with skills that enable them to access health care resources. E-health literacy programs need to be developed in a manner that takes cultural characteristics into account.
- Examining the ways in which technology-based platforms might be mobilized to address and transform unhealthy structures. In this realm, community-based activism projects have started looking at ways in which technologically mediated platforms serve as communities for individuals to mobilize around issues of health and communicate their concerns about these issues to key policy makers.

CONCLUSION

Health communication scholars have significant opportunities for influencing the landscape of health care in the United States and globally. That communication is central to the realization of health is an important understanding that has shaped the practice of health care today (Kreps, 2003). The ways in which individuals, groups, and communities develop meanings of health and the processes through which they communicate about health are central to practices of health care. Furthermore, experiences of health care are situated within broader structural contexts that determine the communicative resources available to individuals, groups, and communities as they participate in their day-to-day health practices. It is in the realm of the broader structures that health experiences get defined. Furthermore, structures become meaningful to cultural members through the local cultural contexts that provide scripts for interpreting structures and for negotiating them. Therefore, in addition to looking at individual behaviors, there is an increasing need for the next generation of health communication scholarship to start exploring more macro-level features such as infrastructures. Furthermore, there is an increasing need to understand the culturally constituted and contested nature of health communication processes.

The complex interplay of structure and culture also draws our attention to the ways in which local meanings of health are continuously defined in the terrain of broader structures. In summary, communication about health is socially constituted in the realm of broader structures and is embedded within local cultural contexts. The next generation of health communication research is charged with the broader agenda of taking this ecological approach to understand the roles that health communicators might play in the delivery of accessible and high-quality health care. Such an ecological approach calls for polymorphic theorizing that brings together multiple theoretical approaches in order to develop a more meaningful understanding of the complex processes in health care today. Furthermore, the next generation of health communication scholarship ought to engage in multi-level approaches that are sensitized to incorporating the micro-, meso-, and macro- level contexts of health communication. Also, more scholarship is needed in multi-method approaches that tap into various methodological approaches for studying health care problems and developing communication solutions to these problems. In summary, there is need for greater dialogue across disciplinary and paradigmatic emphases in order to develop fruitful spaces of conversation for challenging the grand health care challenges of tomorrow.

REFERENCES

Airhihenbuwa, C. (1995). *Health and culture: Beyond the Western paradigm.* Thousand Oaks, CA: Sage.

Airhihenbuwa, C., & Obregon, R. (2000). A critical assessment of theories/models used in health communication for AIDS. *Journal of Health Communication, 5*(Suppl.), 101–111.

Bandura, A. (2002). Social cognitive theory of mass communication. In J. Bryant & D. Zillman (Eds.), *Media effects: Advances in theory and research* (pp. 121–154). Mahwah, NJ: Erlbaum.

Beaudoin, C. E., Thorson, E., & Hong, T. (2006). Promoting youth health by social empowerment: A media campaign targeting social capital. *Health Communication, 19,* 175–182.

Black, S. A., Ray, L. A., & Markides, K. S. (1999). The prevalence and health burden of self-reported diabetes in older Mexican Americans: Findings from the Hispanic established populations for epidemiologic studies of the elderly. *American Journal of Public Health, 89,* 546–552.

Brodie, M., Flournoy, R. E., Altman, D. E., Blendon, R. J., Benson, J. M., & Rosenbaum, M. D. (2000). Health information, the Internet, and the digital divide. *Health Affairs, 19,* 255–265.

Campbell, C., & Jovchelovitch, S. (2000). Health, community, and development: Towards a social psychology of participation. *Journal of Community & Applied Social Psychology, 10*, 255–270.

Cegala, D. J., & Broz, S. L. (2005). Physician communication skills training: A review of theoretical backgrounds, objectives and skills. *Medical Education, 36*, 1004–1016.

Dearing, J. W. (2003). The state of the art and the state of the science of community organizing. In T. L. Thompson, A. M. Dorsey, K. I. Miller, & R. Parrott (Eds.), *Handbook of health communication* (pp. 207–220). Mahwah, NJ: Lawrence Erlbaum.

Dorsey, A. (2005). Lessons and challenges from the field. In T. L. Thompson, A. M. Dorsey, K. I. Miller, & R. Parrott (Eds.), *Handbook of health communication* (pp. 607–608). Mahwah, NJ: Erlbaum.

Duggan, A. (2006). Understanding interpersonal communication processes across health contexts: Advances in the last decade and challenges for the next decade. *Journal of Health Communication, 11*, 93–108.

Du pre, A. (2005). *Communicating about health: Current issues and perspectives.* Boston: McGraw Hill.

Dutta, M. (2007a). Communicating about culture and health: Theorizing culture-centered and cultural-sensitivity approaches. *Communication Theory, 17*, 304–328.

Dutta, M. (2007b). *Communicating health: A culture-centered approach.* London: Polity Press.

Dutta, M., Bodie, G. D., & Basu, A. (2007). Health disparity and the racial divide among the nation's youth: Internet as an equalizer? In A. Everett (Ed.), *Learning race and ethnicity: Youth and digital media* (pp. 175–197). Cambridge, MA: MIT Press.

Dutta-Bergman, M. (2003). Demographic and psychographic antecedents of community participation: Applying a social marketing model. *Social Marketing Quarterly, 9*, 17–31.

Dutta-Bergman, M. (2004a). An alternative approach to social capital: Exploring the linkage between health consciousness and community participation. *Health Communication, 16*, 393–409.

Dutta-Bergman, M. (2004b). A descriptive narrative of healthy eating: A social marketing approach using psychographics. *Health Marketing Quarterly, 20*, 81–101.

Dutta-Bergman, M. (2004c). Developing a profile of consumer intention to seek out additional health information beyond the doctor: Demographic, communicative, and psychographic factors. *Health Communication, 17*, 1–16.

Dutta-Bergman, M. (2004d). Health attitudes, health cognitions and health behaviors among Internet health information seekers: Population-based survey. *Journal of Medical Internet Research, 6*, e15. Retrieved June 2, 2004, from http://www.jmir.org/2004/2/e15/index.htm

Dutta-Bergman, M. (2004e). The impact of completeness and Web use motivation on the credibility of e-Health information. *Journal of Communication, 54*, 253–269.

Dutta-Bergman, M. (2004f). Poverty, structural barriers and health: A Santali narrative of health communication. *Qualitative Health Research, 14*, 1–16.

Dutta-Bergman, M. (2004g). Primary sources of health information: Comparison in the domain of health attitudes, health cognitions, and health behaviors. *Health Communication, 16*, 273–288.

Dutta-Bergman, M. (2004h). The unheard voices of Santalis: Communicating about health from the margins of India. *Communication Theory, 14*, 237–263.

Dutta-Bergman, M. (2005a). Access to the Internet in the context of community participation and community satisfaction. *New Media and Society, 7,* 89–109.

Dutta-Bergman, M. (2005b). A formative approach to strategic message targeting through soap operas: Using selective processing theory. *Health Communication, 19,* 11–18.

Dutta-Bergman, M. (2005c). Idiocentrism, involvement, and health appeals: A social-psychological framework. *Southern Communication Journal, 70,* 46–55.

Dutta-Bergman, M. (2005d). Psychographic profiling of fruit and vegetable consumption: The role of health orientation. *Social Marketing Quarterly, 11,* 1–20.

Dutta-Bergman, M. (2005e). The readership of health magazines: The role of health orientation. *Health Marketing Quarterly, 22,* 27–49.

Dutta-Bergman, M. (2005f). The relationship among health orientation, provider–patient communication, and satisfaction: An individual difference approach. *Health Communication, 18,* 291–303.

Dutta-Bergman, M. (2006). Media use theory and Internet use for health care. In M. Murero & R. E. Rice (Eds.), *The Internet and health care: Theory, research, and practice* (pp. 83–103). Mahwah, NJ: Lawrence Erlbaum.

Huff, R., & Kline, M. (Eds.) (1999). *Promoting health in multicultural populations: A handbook for practitioners.* Thousand Oaks, CA: Sage.

Institute of Medicine. (2002). *Unequal treatment: Confronting racial and ethnic disparities in healthcare.* Washington, DC: National Academy Press.

Kawachi, I., & Berkman, L. F. (2000). Social cohesion, social capital and health. In L. F. Berkman & I. Kawachi (Eds.), *Social epidemiology* (pp. 99–108). New York: Oxford University Press.

Kawachi, I., Kennedy, B. P., & Glass, R. (1999). Social capital and self-rated health: A contextual analysis. *American Journal of Public Health, 89,* 1187–1193.

Kreps, G. L., Bonaguro, E. W., & Query, J. L. (1998). The history and development of the field of health communication. In L. D. Jackson & B. K. Duffy (Eds.), *Health communication research: A guide to developments and directions* (pp. 1–15), Westport, CT: Greenwood Press.

Kreps, G. L. (2003). Opportunities for health communication scholarship to shape public health policy and practice: Examples from the National Cancer Institute. In T. L. Thompson, A. M. Dorsey, K. I. Miller, & R. Parrott (Eds.), *Handbook of health communication* (pp. 609–624). Mahwah, NJ: Lawrence Erlbaum.

Lammers, J., Barbour, J., & Duggan, A. (2005). Organizational forms and the provision of health care. In T. L. Thompson, A. M. Dorsey, K. I. Miller, & R. Parrott (Eds.), *Handbook of health communication* (pp. 319–346). Mahwah, NJ: Erlbaum.

Merzel, C., & D'Afflitti, J. (2003). Reconsidering community-based health promotion: Promise, performance and potential. *American Journal of Public Health, 93*(4), 557–574.

Morgan, S., Harrison, T., Chewning, L., Davis, L., & Dicorcia, M. (2007). Entertainment (mis)education: The framing of organ donation in entertainment television. *Health Communication, 22,* 143–151.

Murero, M., & Rice, R. E. (2006), *The Internet and health care: Theory, research, and practice.* Mahwah, NJ: Erlbaum.

Murray-Johnson, L., & Witte, K. (2005). Looking toward the future: Health message design strategies. In T. L. Thompson, A. M. Dorsey, K. I. Miller, & R. Parrott (Eds.), *Handbook of health communication* (pp. 473–496). Mahwah, NJ: Erlbaum.

Parrott, R. (2004) Emphasizing "communication" in health communication. *Journal of Communication, 54,* 751–787.

Rappaport, J. (1987). Terms of empowerment/exemplars of prevention: Toward a theory for community psychology. *American Journal of Community Psychology, 15,* 121–148.

Repucci, N. D., Woolard, J. L., & Fried, C. S. (1999). Social, community, and preventive interventions. *Annual Review of Psychology, 50,* 347–418.

Rogers, E. M., & Storey, J. D. (1987). Communication campaigns. In C. R. Berger & S. H. Chaffee (Eds.), *Handbook of communication science* (pp. 817–46). Beverly Hills, CA: Sage.

Salmon, C. T., & Atkin, C. (2003). Using media campaigns for health promotion. In T. L. Thompson, A. M. Dorsey, K. I. Miller, & R. Parrott (Eds.), *Handbook of health communication* (pp. 449–472). Mahwah, NJ: Erlbaum.

Scherer, C. W., & Juanillo Jr., N. K. (2003). The continuing challenge of community health risk management and communication. In T. L. Thompson, A. M. Dorsey, K. I. Miller, & R. Parrott (Eds.), *Handbook of health communication* (pp. 221–240). Mahwah, NJ: Lawrence Erlbaum.

Sharf, B. (2005). How I fired my surgeon and embraced an alternative narrative. In L. Harter, P. Japp, & C. Beck (Eds.), *Narratives, health and healing: Communication theory, research, and practice* (pp. 325–342). Mahwah, NJ: Lawrence Erlbaum.

Slater, M. (1999). Integrating application of media effects, persuasion and behavior change theories to communication campaigns: A stages-of-change framework. *Health Communication, 11,* 335–354.

Snyder, L. (2001). How effective are mediated health campaigns? In R.E. Rice & C. K. Atkin (Eds.), *Public communication campaigns* (3rd ed., pp. 181–190). Thousand Oaks, CA: Sage.

Street, R. (2005). Communication in medical encounters: An ecological perspective. In T. L. Thompson, A. M. Dorsey, K. I. Miller, & R. Parrott (Eds.), *Handbook of health communication* (pp. 63–89). Mahwah, NJ: Erlbaum.

Thompson, T. L. (2005). Introduction. In T. L. Thompson, A. M. Dorsey, K. I. Miller, & R. Parrott (Eds.), *Handbook of health communication* (pp. 1–5). Mahwah, NJ: Erlbaum.

Thompson, T. L., Dorsey, A. M., Miller, K. I., & Parrott, R. (Eds.). (2005). *Handbook of health communication.* Mahwah, NJ: Erlbaum.

Tong, R. (2002). Love's labor in the health care system: Working toward gender equity. *Hypatia, 17*(3), 200–213.

Wallack, L. M., & Dorfman, L. (2001). Putting policy into health communication: The role of media advocacy. In R. E. Rice & C. K. Atkin (Eds.), *Public communication campaigns* (3rd ed., pp. 389–401). Thousand Oaks, CA: Sage.

Williams, D. R. (1999). Race, socioeconomic status, and health: The added effects of racism and discrimination. *Annals of the New York Academy of Sciences, 896,* 173–188.

Williams, D. R., & Collins, C. (2001). U.S. socioeconomic and racial differences in health: Patterns and explanations. *Annual Review of Sociology, 21,* 349–386.

Zoller, H. M. (2005). Health activism: Communication theory and action for social change. *Communication Theory, 15,* 341–64.

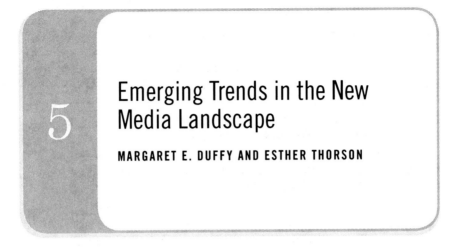

Emerging Trends in the New Media Landscape

MARGARET E. DUFFY AND ESTHER THORSON

Physicians, medical researchers, health policy specialists, and health communicators have crucial information that citizens and consumers need so they can make better decisions about their health. Indeed, health communication of a variety of types is crucial for informing and persuading people to make better lifestyle choices, as well as aiding them in managing their own and others' medical conditions.

Twenty years ago health communication was mainly accomplished through interpersonal interactions between patients and health care providers, or through mass media vehicles like news stories, television/radio public service announcements and commercials, and printed materials that were picked up or mailed. But in the last few years, the digital revolution has completely changed the nature of both interpersonal and mass communication. Much of interpersonal communication is now actually mediated by cell phone, text messaging, e-mail, and social networking vehicles like Facebook and MySpace. Correspondingly, much of mass communication has become "personalized" with options like RSS feeds, targeted e-mail, cell phone–delivered messages, and customized advertising that can be delivered by mail or through some digital device. Indeed, as the number of choices for communication modes and devices has grown, the distinctions between interpersonal and mass communication are blurring.

Along with these effects of the digital revolution have come sea changes in how people choose to communicate with each other and how they are reached by professional communicators with news, information, and persuasive messages. It is crucial that health communicators understand this new media landscape and people's behavior in that landscape. This understanding will enable them to change their approach to doing health communication, allowing them to take advantage of the opportunities for greater reach and effectiveness.

People today are perceiving, remembering, and engaging with information in ways that are revolutionizing communication systems. The Project for Excellence in Journalism's most recent *State of the News Media Report* (2008) provides some startling statistics. People spend an average of 22% of their day online. The news media are in a state of crisis, with television and newspaper news audience eroding faster each year. There is a growing divide between advertising and news/entertainment content. In the past, advertisers needed news and entertainment shows to get into the consumer's home by riding in with newspapers, news magazines, and radio and television programming; this is no longer the case. More and more advertisers are reaching people with Web sites, drawing them with use of search engines, and entering the fray of social network activity like that on YouTube, Facebook, and MySpace. Of course, without advertising, many forms of news and entertainment companies are losing their main source of revenues and indeed, the advertising-dependent business model for news appears to be expiring.

As new technologies and massive behavioral changes in the public roil mainstream media businesses and outlets, traditional dissemination practices are becoming less and less effective. Moreover, in the new digital communication world, much of the health information available is riddled with omissions, factual errors, and undisclosed commercial interests (Hoffman-Goetz, 2000; Slater, 2003; Walji, Sagaram, Sagaram, Meric-Bernstam, Johnson, Mirza, & Bernstam, 2004). In fact, while the amount of authoritative health and medical knowledge has grown exponentially, abilities to effectively disseminate that information have become obsolete.

Given these changes, it is crucial that health communicators realize and understand the difficult challenges presented by a new and bewildering media landscape. In this chapter, we suggest these challenges can be successfully countered with sophisticated research-based strategies focusing on individuals' media choices and behaviors.

THE HEALTH COMMUNICATION MEDIA CHOICE MODEL

This chapter introduces the health communication media choice model, a research-based strategy that shows how health communicators can develop effective information programs in the new media landscape. First, we sketch the primary features of today's media world, describing how consumers are using media and technology to fulfill their needs and desires. Second, we briefly review some of the most salient health communication research offering insights into how individuals are seeking and accessing health information in the current environment. Third, we offer a theory and an organizing framework that suggests a communication needs and features-based segmented audience strategy. We link these communication needs and features with the notion of aperture, a window of enhanced opportunity for sending a persuasive and/or informative message at the optimal time. Finally, we outline a research strategy that describes how health communicators can design effective evidence-based campaigns.

In developing our model, we drew on a number of important resources. First, in work with the Newspaper Association of America (2006) we utilized the Life Styles database, a highly respected survey conducted yearly by the advertising agency DDB. Using that database, we were able to examine the trend of consumer media choices across the years 1995, 2000, and 2005. Further, we gathered and continue to compile extensive research from a wide variety of secondary sources to gain additional insights into media changes and apply them to health communication questions.

WHAT'S HAPPENING IN TODAY'S MEDIA?

As consumers abandon traditional media channels, news organizations, advertisers, and media companies have scrambled for explanations and solutions. Health communicators are seeking new approaches as past tactics using print and broadcast media have become increasingly ineffective. Expanding choices have shifted power from authoritative sources as consumers take control in searching for information and entertainment and even in creating content.

The ever-expanding array of technology-enabled media features allows people to select among those they find most desirable in fulfilling their communication needs. They may choose the power of search in their shopping activities. Those who want to express themselves may be drawn to health communication models that allow them to create or contribute health messages, comment on products or services, or communicate with companies.

Evidence clearly shows that the digital environment has changed media behaviors for almost everyone. As mentioned above, the array of media choices available has exploded since 1975. Viewers may now watch news, sports, and entertainment videos online and on their mobile devices. Advertising.com reports that 62% of consumers, a significant percentage of whom are 35 and older, are watching videos online (Loechner, 2007). The most youthful of adults might be called "screen-agers" in light of the amount of time they spend watching the screens of their phones, their iPods, their video games, and of course television. Figures 5.1 and 5.2 illustrate the enormous changes that have occurred in media choice.

Consumers are embracing the options available to them, clearly recognizing the opportunity to construct their media, information, and advertising worlds through personalized content, time shifting, and other media features. This is seen in growth of daily RSS feeds, TiVo, and pod and vodcasts.

Migration to the Web

It is no surprise that consumers are fulfilling many of their news and entertainment needs via the Internet and spending less time with traditional

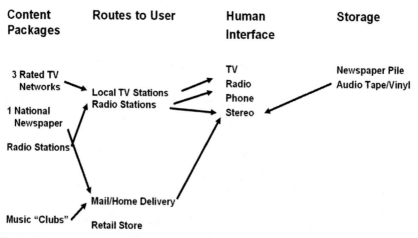

Figure 5.1 Content/Delivery Options 1976
Copyright 2006 wolzein l.l.c.

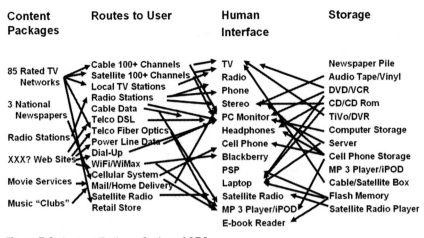

| Content Packages | Routes to User | Human Interface | Storage |

Figure 5.2 Content/Delivery Options 1976
Copyright 2006 wolzein l.l.c.

media. A 2007 Pew survey revealed that 71% of U.S. adults are online (Pew Internet & American Life Project, 2007). A Harris poll reported that the number of U.S. adults who have ever gone online seeking health or medical information increased from 136 million in 2006 to 162 million in 2007. The poll refers to health seekers as "cyberchondriacs," and the results suggest that online information significantly affects doctor–patient interactions (Harris, 2007).

Demographic differences in Internet and technology use do exist, but they are not as significant as one might expect. The same percentage of women and men use the Internet, though there are age differences: 85% of those between the ages of 18 and 29, 78% between the ages of 30 and 49, 69% between the ages of 50 and 64, and 31% 65 and older are online. Indeed, baby boomers (those born between 1946 and 1964) are adopting technology much faster than the next older generation, and they are expected to continue their technologically advanced behaviors as they age. Boomer behaviors are important to health professionals as this large cohort ages and encounters age-related health challenges. According to the most recent U.S. census data, by 2010 there will be 84 million adults between the ages of 43 and 61 in the United States. Mediabuyerplanner.com reports that this cohort is spending less time and money on television and newspapers, and more on Internet-related technologies and cell phones ("Boomer Media Consumption," 2007).

News organizations, advertisers, and information dissemination specialists of all kinds are finding that approaches that were successful in the past are no longer effective. Advertisers are responding to changing consumer habits, and Internet ad spending grew 34% in 2006 to $16.8 billion, a record high (Peterson, 2007).

Further, our research shows decreased reliance on traditional media sources for information. Key indicators are changing responses to the survey question "I need to get the news (national, international, local) every day." Across all ages, agreement was down 6% from 1995 to 2005, agreement among baby boomers was down 5% from 1995 to 2005, and agreement among those 60+ down 8% from 1995 to 2005. In addition, the mean of the youngest group's expressed need for news is 29% lower than oldest group's. Clearly, approaches that rely on print and broadcast news media will be increasingly less effective in health campaign and dissemination initiatives.

Our research also reveals that people desire personalized input and customized content. As mentioned above, this is seen in the growth of RSS feeds, personalized home pages, TiVo, personalized cell phone ring tones, and a growing preference for news with a viewpoint that is in concert with the beliefs of the viewer. For example, personalized ring tone sales are estimated at more than $5 billion worldwide (Pogue, 2007).

Another aspect of the trend toward customized and personally relevant media is the impulse to create content. Many observers have commented about the growth of blogs, podcasting, and other consumer-generated content. Acccording to Technorati, users create about 120,000 new blogs each day, or 4 new blogs every second (Sifry, 2007).

Brands are now using blogs as part of their strategic planning, recognizing that some bloggers and their fans are extremely influential as they comment upon and review products, services, and advertising campaigns. In addition, market researchers are using blogs and social networks as guides for analyzing online consumer behavior (Havenstein, 2007). The *Wall Street Journal*, in its "Blog Watch," reports that among the range of health-related blogs are those devoted to dealing with allergies and inability to digest gluten (Bright, 2007).

HEALTH COMMUNICATION RESEARCH IN THE NEW MEDIA LANDSCAPE

Health communication researchers are responding to consumers' changing media behaviors. A bibliography compiled by Petya Stoeva (2006) reviewed 95 studies on new media and health communication. One key finding of that review was that individuals seeking health information rely on search engines (Peterson, 2003). Moreover, consumers' search habits are cursory, as most people access Web sites only from the first page of the search results (Peterson, 2003).

A related concern is the quality of the information found through Internet searches. Some studies identified significant gaps and omissions (Fahey et al., 2003; Walji et al., 2004) and even harmful information (Walji et al., 2004). Researchers also uncovered concerns about commercial sourcing and sponsorship of health-related sites (Slater & Zimmerman, 2003). According to a Pew survey, only 15% of searchers always verified their search findings, and Fox (2006) extrapolated that some 85 million people are searching without investigating whether the information is reliable. A number of organizations are providing specific instructions to people on how to access quality information about health from the Internet (e.g., Schnall, n.d.).

Doctor–patient interactions are affected by patients' access to health information. The fact that individuals are more informed has led to the creation of a phenomenon Akerkar and Bichile (2004) calls the "e-patient," a patient who "lobbies" for certain types of treatment, who often has less trust in the physician's authority, and who may access online support groups.

Other research shows that online channels that offer support mechanisms for individuals with various conditions can improve outcomes (Gustafson et al., 2001, 2005; Lieberman et al., 2003; Reeves, 2000; Shaw, McTavish, Hawkins, Gustafson, & Pingree, 2000). Some researchers are expressing concern that the digital divide limits the access of disadvantaged groups, who may not have the resources to use digital technologies (Fogel, Albert, Schnabel, Ditkoff, & Neugut, 2002; Gustafson et al., 2005; Kittler, Hobbs, Volk, Kreps, & Bates, 2004; Rideout, Neuman, Kitchman, & Brodie, 2005). These studies suggest, as will be discussed, that health communication initiatives must be "media agnostic" and begin with the preferred communication channels of the target audience.

THE HEALTH COMMUNICATION MEDIA CHOICE MODEL

As mentioned above, creation of the model began with extensive and ongoing review of the academic and professional literature related to consumer media behaviors. Examination of advertising, newspaper, and broadcast trends showed that media professionals have an abundance of facts and information about the changes but have few mechanisms with which to respond strategically to changing consumer preferences. For example, newspapers tried ongoing experiments with a variety of ideas, such as youth-oriented print products, social networking, and page redesigns in hopes of winning back readers and advertisers (Angwin & Hagan, 2006). As fewer people continued to consume traditional media, advertisers sought other venues through which to present their persuasive messages.

Advertisers once could expect that their messages would enter people's homes attached to newspaper or broadcast content. Similarly, health messages, PSAs, and other public relations efforts such as news stories and press releases were delivered packaged in traditional media vehicles. Traditional health communication techniques and campaigns were usually premised on people's reliance on old media and the assumption that the old media, particularly news content, were authoritative and credible to target audiences. Effective health communication today must acknowledge the emergence of the powerful and technologically connected consumer. Unlike the one-to-many model of old media, the new media world is best imagined as a dynamic network of human beings and technology. It is a world in which people have access to vast stores of data and often trust the recommendations of their online friends more than authoritative sources.

The evidence reveals active consumers who are taking charge of their communication needs and desires and rejecting passive acceptance of information. In developing a theoretical model, we began with a venerable and highly researched theory known as uses and gratifications (Katz, 1950). This theory moves the discussion away from the notion that media "do" things to people, and toward the idea the people use media to fulfill various needs. Imagine, for example, the daily tasks and activities you and your family must perform to meet various needs. Of course, basic human physiological needs must be met first with food, shelter, and so on. Similarly, as psychologists have pointed out, humans have needs beyond the physiological for connections with other people, including safety, self-esteem, and entertainment.

Our model posits that people have communication needs that drive them to select communication media and adopt communication behaviors that best gratify those needs at a given time. It is important to note that human beings may choose to fulfill needs in interpersonal and face-to-face interactions or they may select what we call "mediated" channels.

For example, the need to gather information about a health condition may be filled by a visit to a physician, a call to a knowledgeable friend, or an Internet search. As more and more media alternatives emerge, people will choose the sources that best gratify a given communication need. Another key factor is that different media sources offer different features such as participation, immediacy, and customization that play into consumer's decision making.

A brief review of the evolving literature in the uses and gratifications tradition will provide better context for the media choice model. Early on, researchers distilled several important concepts (Katz, Blumler, & Gurevitch, 1974):

1. The social and psychological origins of *needs* that;
2. generate consumer expectations;
3. of the mass media or other communication options leading to;
4. different media choices, resulting in;
5. fulfillment of needs (p. 20).

Rosengren (1974) pointed out that individual differences, such as demographics and lifestyles as well as the different needs individuals want to fill in differing situations, are critical aspects of choice.

Uses and gratifications research has been usefully summarized by Rubin (1983, 1994) and by Ruggiero (2000). In addition, researchers have deployed the theory in a wide range of media, including television (Babrow, 1987; Conway & Rubin, 1991; Heeter & Greenberg, 1985), newspapers (Elliott & Rosenberg, 1987), and the Internet (Beaudoin & Thorson, 2004; Kaye & Johnson, 2002; Rodgers & Thorson, 2000). Lacy (2000) argued that five communication needs—surveillance, diversion, social-cultural interaction, decision making, and self-understanding—interact with variables such a cost, quality, and features in determining amounts of time people allocate to different media.

In Figure 5.3, the elements of the health communication media choice model are shown. We next describe each of the elements and how they work together to form audience choices.

In our research with the news and advertising industries, it became clear to us that focusing on the four major communication needs self-identified by individuals in our research provided a powerful yet simple model on which to base strategic decision making. In our work in health communication focusing on media choices, this schema seemed most appropriate as well. Following are the communication needs:

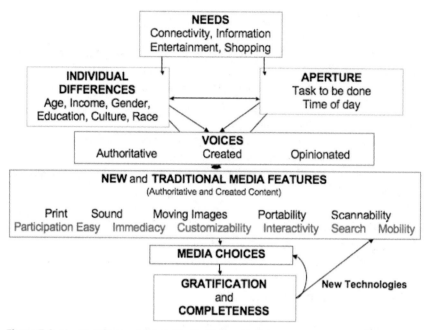

Figure 5.3 Health Communication Media Choice Model

1. Connectivity (need to relate, support, engage with and communicate with others face-to-face or through media)
2. Information (surveillance or the need to gain knowledge important for accomplishing goals both large and small)
3. Entertainment (need to be amused, relaxed, and diverted)
4. Shopping (need to acquire goods and services)

Of course, people's needs can overlap and be important in different ways to different people. Searching for health information may be a diversion to certain individuals, for example. However, it is important to note that the needs were self-identified by individuals in our research, rather than imposed by us, so we believe the categories represent individuals' psychological realities.

Connectivity

Every instance of media use is motivated by a communication need. Connectivity is extremely important and can be seen in friendships, religious affiliations, clubs, and community ties. For example, logging into

Revolutionhealth.com communities and belonging to a support group for a particular condition are connectivity behaviors. Hundreds of YouTube videos are related to health and medical procedures. It is common to see people sharing highly personal information regarding surgeries, medical experiences, and even the experiences of their children. This sharing and connecting behavior often involves interactions with unknown respondents who vicariously share and comment on the posted data. Social networking sites such as Facebook have hundreds of sites related to various conditions. For example, a search for juvenile arthritis produced 22 different groups. A study by Wilkin and Ball-Rokeach (2006) regarding health communication strategies for Latino neighborhoods suggests that effective dissemination strategies involve "storytelling networks" that utilize media, interpersonal, and digital venues.

Information

Informational behavior might involve searching WebMD or going to see a health professional with specific questions. Usually, however, the consumer turns first to a major search engine. We cannot overstate the importance of search and search engine optimization for health communication. Eighty percent of Internet users, or 93 million Americans, have searched online for one of 16 major health topics. One in five has researched mental health information, and 13% have researched vaccination data. Most important for health communicators to consider is that fact that people expect search engines to provide them with reliable health information, an assumption that is questionable at best (Fox, 2006).

Other data show how consumers are increasingly satisfying their information needs online:

- Thirty-six percent of e-caregivers say the Internet helped them find advice or support from other people.
- Thirty-four percent of e-caregivers say the Internet helped them find professional or expert services.
- Twenty-six percent of e-caregivers say the Internet helped them find information or compare options (Fox, 2006).

Entertainment

Entertainment as a communication need might be seen as frivolous to some. However, to be psychologically healthy, human beings must play and be diverted. When seeking entertainment, consumers have a wide range of sources with which to fulfill that need, including physical activities and mediated amusements. For certain applications, it is important that some health-related messages be presented in an entertaining fashion similar to the strategies using humor, sexual appeal, and other attention-getting devices that advertisers use to "cut through the clutter."

In a related area, the growth of celebrity culture is becoming a more significant part of day-to-day life for many people. For example, celebrity is the only magazine category to maintain circulation and advertising sales (Project for Excellence in Journalism, 2008). Digital sites including popular Web sites such as TMZ.com, Perez Hilton, and Jossip are also growing (Gossip Websites, 2007). We hypothesize that technology has enhanced people's abilities to access celebrity information and has reduced the informational and psychological distance between consumers and celebrities and this is an important area for future study, especially in health communication.

Psychologists have long observed that audiences are affected by celebrities' comments, behaviors, and health issues. Brown and Basil (1995) studied the impact of the revelation of Magic Johnson's HIV diagnosis and found that because of parasocial factors—factors concerning relations that occur between people and either real or fictional people represented in the media (Horton & Wohl, 1956)—celebrities can be an important mediating variable in health communication. Similarly, Brown, Basil, and Bocarnea (2003) studied attitudes toward a celebrity athlete, and their results suggested a parasocial relationship with the athlete leading to identification with the celebrity and promotion of his attitudes and beliefs. Cram, Vijan, Inadomi, Cowen, Carpenter, and Fendrick (2000) found that significantly improved colon screening behaviors resulted when Katie Couric publicized her own procedure. Boon and Lomore (2001) found that celebrities' behaviors may affect young adult's identities and self-esteem.

Other research revealed some intriguing trends: 45% of adults surveyed said that celebrity opinions make a large difference on issues and causes the celebrities promote (Harris, 2008). Non-celebrity business owners say they see celebrities as role models (Sherman, 2004).

Of course, there are negative and unintended health-related consequences that can result from celebrity obsession. Randerson (2007) reported on a range of unsubstantiated health and prevention claims from celebrities such as Madonna that may be not only misleading, but dangerous. For example, a British celebrity suggested that certain types of vaccinations thought to be sound by the medical community are dangerous.

Shopping

Shopping behavior might involve accessing canadadrugs.com, going to the local drugstore, or ordering vitamins online. This is another area that might seem trivial, though for virtually every economy in the world, consumer behaviors are major drivers of economic success. Increasingly, health consumers are moving away from dependence on sources from which they have traditionally bought health-related goods and services, and they are using searches to inform their purchase decisions. Consumers now have expanded, and even global, resources from which to choose.

Individual Differences in Communication Needs

Individuals' communication needs vary based on their demographic, cultural, and personal variables and are then expressed in different ways when they are interested in health matters. There is not sufficient space to fully discuss this here, but marketers and media scholars have long known that age, education, gender, and other individual characteristics are among the variables that affect media choice (Also see the more detailed review of demographic patterns in chapter 2.)

Someone who is twenty has different media and health priorities than someone who is 50. The generation to which one belongs is an important differentiator of how communication needs are activated. Millions of young people are spending hours on social networks, and older people in the United States are accessing online dating in increasing numbers with mainstream sites such as eHarmony showing significant growth among Baby Boomers (Marsan, 2008). While these demographic data are valuable, they offer only a limited picture of how people are behaving in this new media landscape. As mentioned above, members of older generations should not be stereotyped as technophobes based only on age.

The Concept of Aperture

Introduced by advertising executive William Wells, the concept of aperture refers to the optimal time when people are most receptive to a persuasive message (Wells, Moriarty, & Burnett, 2006). Apertures can be defined in terms of dayparts (e.g., readiness for vitamin messages in the morning) or in terms of times of life or types of human connections with a particular health issue. For example, when a celebrity is diagnosed with an illness, audience members who care about that person or identify with her or him might be more receptive to promotions for health screening for the illness.

There is an important need for more research in this area, but as Cohen and Kaczorowski (2005) report, there are differences between different life stage groups that are important to all media, health communicators in particular. For example, they found that older people seek information on Sunday mornings, while younger adults search for entertainment on Sunday mornings. Thus health information in terms of news features in Sunday newspapers can be very valuable to one demographic but unseen by others.

Whether health communicators are using digital or traditional media, aperture is important. Beyers (2004) showed that the Internet and television show clear daypart patterns. As Thorson and Thorson (2006) found, differences in different types of news—local versus national, for example—can be aperture sensitive in different ways with different segments of the population. It seems clear that health communicators must be highly sensitive to variations in media use by different segments of the population.

Media Features

Another key element of the media choice model involves media features. Consider the popularity of mobile telephones. They have increasingly sophisticated features that make them more than just a simple phone. People use them to text message, send and receive e-mail, watch videos, listen to music, check sports scores, and other activities. What is important for the health communicator is the recognition that different media have features that make them attractive to different target audiences who fulfill their communication needs at different times of the day. A broadcast public service announcement offers visuals and rich media that are attractive to audiences viewing certain types of news or entertainment programming. Newspapers are appealing to audiences who value portability, exposure to unexpected content, or the ritual of the reading experience. Digital media offer instant updates, the capability to personalize and customize content, and the chance to share with like-minded others. Specifically, new media offer at least these seven features:

1. Immediacy: the ability to access information on demand
2. Mobility: the ability not only to transport the product/service but to get updated content wherever one is
3. Rich media: video and audio delivered online
4. Participation: the ability to create and publish (personal authorship)
5. Search: the ability to quickly and easily find accurate information on topics of interest
6. Customization: the ability to tailor the types and frequency of messages to personal interests
7. Time shifting: The ability to download digital content and replay it at the consumer's convenience

Our research shows that features of customization, personalization, and participation are important to many key target audiences who are abandoning media that do not offer such capabilities.

Table 5.1 shows how these features are distributed across the major news media.

As the uses and gratifications theory suggests, after individuals choose a medium and use it, they decide whether the use satisfied the need. If they are satisfied, they continue using that medium. If not, they search for a better or more effective media.

Voice in Health Communication

The model emphasizes the concept of voice, a way to describe changing expectations and desires regarding what sources are credible, engaging, and trustworthy. In years past, the model of the trusted anchorman was that of Walter Cronkite, who told audiences, "And that's the way it is." Audiences believed that quality newspapers were credible and had a belief that the news did not express opinions, but facts. However, we are seeing a society-wide change in that acceptance of the authoritative voice of the news (e.g., Gillmor, 2006). As audiences depend more and more on nontraditional sources of information, they are saying they have less confidence that mainstream media are trustworthy or objective. A Pew study (2002) found that:

1. From 1985 to 2002 the number of Americans who thought news organizations were highly professional declined from 72% to 49%.

Table 5.1

USABILITY FEATURES OF EACH MEDIUM

MEDIA FEATURES	MEDIA				
	NEWSPAPERS	RADIO	TV	CABLE NEWS	INTERNET
Participation easy					X
Customizability					X
Time shifting	X				X
Time flexibility (24/7)				X	X
Mobility	X				X
Interactivity					X
Search capacity					X
Immediacy		X	X	X	X
Images			X	X	X
Sound		X	X	X	X
Doesn't require high level of attention		X	X	X	X
Doesn't require reading skills		X	X	X	X

2. The number of those who felt news organizations tried to cover up their mistakes rose from 13% to 67%.
3. The number who thought news organizations were biased politically rose from 45% to 59%.
4. The number of those who thought news organizations got facts straight fell from 55% to 35%.

Other research confirms this. Research by MTV suggests that young people define news and news values differently, saying they want facts only if they are offered in the context of their own lives (Catapano, 2006).

Jarvis, quoted in a Carnegie study, remarked that young people like *The Daily Show* because it is "bringing news down off its pedestal and presenting it at eye-level" (Brown, 2005, p. 9). The popularity of talk shows and Fox News is an example of how "news with an attitude" (a very different voice from the authoritative one) is becoming more popular and more trusted.

News and advertising created by nonprofessionals are becoming increasingly visible. The notion of "citizen journalism," or reporting and blogging by those who are not journalists, is growing in power and audience (Gillmor, 2006). Changes in the perceived credibility of new voices is a key aspect of the media choice model. In creating content and selecting media, health communicators must use the preferred voice of the target audience to convey information. According to the model, some audiences prefer health information that comes from a long-established source and find it most credible. We call this the *authoritative voice*. Others find that health information that seems to share their own viewpoints and attitudes is most trustworthy; we refer to this as the *opinionated voice*. Others prefer getting health information from the perspective of people who are experiencing it; we call this the *created voice*.

IMPLICATIONS FOR HEALTH COMMUNICATION

As we suggested earlier in this chapter, uses and gratifications theory and the health communication media choice model offer insights into why health consumers behave as they do and how health communicators can create research-based campaigns that have a better likelihood of success. The gratification people receive from the media has led to a redistribution of time spent on media and to the sources people trust, enjoy, or act upon.

Following is a brief discussion of how the health communication media choice model offers a research protocol.

Measure the Communication Needs and Preferences of the Target Audience

First, crucial questions concerning the level of importance of various factors to people's choices to get health information from one form of media over another must be answered by the target audience.

Specifically, the researcher seeks responses for each of the communication needs. The following are examples of variables that the researcher might investigate.

Health Information Related to Connectivity Needs:
- Getting health information I can share with my friends.
- Getting health information that makes me feel smarter.
- Knowing who wrote or compiled the health information.
- Being able to see who is reporting the health information.

Health Information Related to Information Needs:
- Alerting me to damaging or harmful situations.
- Providing me with information I can use to improve my condition or that of a friend or family member.
- Identifying new research in nutrition or exercise or research that offers information on disease prevention.

Health Information Related to Entertainment:
- Entertains me, makes me feel relaxed, is supportive of my point of view.
- Diverts me with health-related stories about celebrities.
- Provides me with important ideas in a way that is amusing or diverting.

Measure Target Audience Preference for Media Features

The second step in the research design involves measuring what features different audiences prefer in message delivery. This relates to those issues of immediacy, customizability, and participation discussed previously.

How important are each of the following in your choice to get health information from one form of media over another?

- Getting health information when I want it.
- Getting only the health information I want.
- Getting health information as soon as it becomes available.
- Getting health information that's easy to understand.
- Getting health information that's rich with images.
- Getting health information that I can share with my friends.

Measure Aperture for the Health Messages You Intend to Convey

The issue of aperture is similarly critical and must be measured for each target audience.

> What media do you use in the ___ time of day to get health information, stay connected with others, be entertained, purchase health-related products?

Just as the businesses of news, advertising, and promotion have become more complex and fragmented, health communication faces important challenges. As the mass media become ever more fragmented and increasingly personalized, health communicators must constantly adjust their strategic and creative approaches so that they align with changing audience needs. Although the media world has become more complex, it also offers unprecedented opportunities to bring health consumers the information they need in the most effective ways possible. The United States faces daunting challenges in the areas of prevention and treatment of conditions, which are complicated by an aging population, millions of uninsured or underinsured citizens, and a growing divide in income and access to health resources. In the developing world, even greater challenges face health policy makers, medical providers, researchers, and dissemination professionals.

The findings from our research suggest these guidelines:

- Begin with a theoretical approach that will guide your decision making and utilize a strategic rather than a tactical approach. This means that rather than starting with a tactic such as developing a blog or a social networking site, communicators will want to begin with goals and objectives for each targeted audience.
- Conduct needs, features, and aperture research for each target audience and narrow the segments as precisely as possible. Communicators should seek an approach that approximates one-to-one or interpersonal communication for highest-priority goals and audiences.
- Be willing to abandon past practices and so-called best practices. Each campaign goal for each audience will require distinct research-based strategies. What worked in the past will not necessarily work for the current problem or opportunity.

- Be medium agnostic. By that, we mean that communicators should draw on the variety of tools available to them to create the most effective and persuasive message and deliver it at the right time to the right person. These tools could include direct mail, social networks and Web sites, blogs, mobile devices, television, outdoor media interpersonal approaches such as meetings and gatherings, and word-of-mouth, viral, and experiential marketing.
- Test and refine approaches for each target audience. The media world today is constantly shifting as people use new options and new technologies to meet their communication needs.

Just as a skilled physician draws on research and uses sophisticated tests to accurately diagnose an individual's condition, the health communicator must "diagnose" the needs, habits, behaviors, and preferences of her target audiences. He or she then continues to monitor the effectiveness of the campaign or program and make the appropriate adjustments to achieve an optimum result. Through research, testing, strategic thinking, and evidence-based approaches, health communicators can achieve the results they seek.

REFERENCES

Akerkar S. M., & Bichile, L. S. (2004). Doctor patient relationship: Changing dynamics in the information age. *E-Medicine.* Retrieved August 5, 2008, from https://tspace.library.utoronto.ca/bitstream/1807/2635/2/jp04038.pdf

Angwin, J., & Hagan, J. (2006, March 22). As market shifts, newspapers try to lure new, young readers. *Wall Street Journal,* p. 1.

Babrow, A. S. (1987). Student motives for watching soap operas. *Journal of Broadcasting and Electronic Media, 31*(3), 309–321.

Beyers, H. (2004). Dayparting online: Living up to its potential? *International Journal on Media Management, 6*(1/2), 67–73.

Beaudoin, C. E., & Thorson, E. (2004). Testing the cognitive mediation model: The roles of news reliance and three gratifications sought. *Communication Research, 31*(4), 446–471.

Boon, S. D., & Lomore, C. D. (2001). Admirer-celebrity relationships among young adults: Explaining perceptions of celebrity influence on identity. *Human Communication Research, 27*(3), 432–465.

Bright, B. (2007, September 24). Baby boomers embracing mobile technology. *Consumer Technology Blog Watch,* p. R9.

Brown, M. (2005). Abandoning the news. *Carnegie Reporter, 3*(2). Retrieved August 5, 2008, from http://www.carnegie.org/reporter/10/news/index.html

Brown, W. J., & Basil, M. D. (1995). Media celebrities and public health: Responses to "Magic" Johnson's HIV disclosure and its impact on AIDS risk and high-risk behaviors. *Health Communication, 7*(4), 345–370.

Brown, W. J., Basil, M. D., & Bocarnea, M. C. (2003). The influence of famous athletes on health beliefs and practices: Mark McGwire, child abuse prevention, and androstenedione? *Health Communication, 8*(1), 41–57.

"Boomer media consumption: Less TV, newspaper; more PC, cell phone." (2007, September 17). Retrieved August 5, 2008, from Mediabuyerplanner.com

Catapano, M. (2006, March 22). *Growing audience: New thinking for a new media age.* NAA Marketing Conference, Orlando, FL.

Cohen, B., & Kazcorowski, C. (2005). Life-stage segmentation: An effective tool for audience growth strategies. Retrieved August 5, 2008, from http://www.growingaudience.com/downloads/ga_lifestage.pdf

Conway, J. C., & Rubin, A. M. (1991). Psychological predictors of television viewing motivation. *Communication Research, 18*(4): 443–464.

Cram, S., Vijan, J., Inadomi, V. J., Cowen, M. E., Carpenter, D., & Fendrick, A. M. (2000). *The impact of a celebrity spokesperson on preventive health behavior: The Katie Couric effect.* Division of General Medicine, Department of Internal Medicine, School of Medicine.

Elliott, W. R., & Rosenberg, W. L. (1987). The 1985 Philadelphia newspaper strike: A uses and gratifications study. *Journalism Quarterly, 64*(4), 679–687.

Fogel, J., Albert, S. M., Schnabel, F., Ditkoff, B. A., & Neugut, A. I. (2002). Use of the Internet by women with breast cancer. *Journal of Medical Internet Research, 4*(2): e9.

Fox, S. (2006). *Online health search 2006.* Retrieved August 5, 2008, from http://www.pewinternet.org/pdfs/PIP_Online_Health_2006.pdf

Gillmor, D. (2006). *We the media.* Sebastopol, CA: O'Reilly Media.

Gossip websites: Talk is cheap, but celebrity gossip can be priceless. (2007, October 15). *The Independent.* Retrieved August 13, 2008, from http://www.independent.co.uk/news/media/gossip-websites-talk-is-cheap-but-celebrity-gossip-can-be-priceless-396881.html

Gustafson, D. H., McTavish, F. M., Stengle, W., Ballard, D., Hawkins, R., Shaw, B., et al. (2001). Use and impact of eHealth System by low-income women with breast cancer. *Journal of Health Communication, 10,* 195–218.

Gustafson, D. H., McTavish, F. M., Stengle, W., Ballard, D., Jones, E., Julesberg, K., et al. (2005). Reducing the digital divide for low-income women with breast cancer: A feasibility study of a population-based intervention. *Journal of Health Communication, 10,* 173–193.

Harris Poll. (2007). Harris Poll shows number of "cyberchondriacs"—Adults who have ever gone online for health information—Increases to an estimated 160 million nationwide. Retrieved August 5, 2008, from http://findarticles.com/p/articles/mi_m0EIN/is_2007_July_31/ai_n27326409

Harris Poll. (2008, April 17). Half of Americans believe celebrities make little or no positive difference on issues and causes they promote. *The Harris Poll®* #43. Retrieved August 5, 2008, from http://www.harrisinteractive.com/harris_poll/index.asp?PID=897

Havenstein, H. (2007, March 6). Tool uses blogs, social networks for market research. *Computerworld.* Retrieved August 5, 2008, from http://www.computerworld.com/action/article.do?command=viewArticleBasic&articleId=9012362

Heeter, C., & Greenberg, B. S. (1985). Cable and program choice. In D. Zillmann & J. Bryant (Eds.), *Selective exposure to communication* (pp. 203–224). Hillsdale, NJ: Lawrence Erlbaum.

Hoffman-Goetz, L., & Clarke, J. N. (2000). Quality of breast cancer sites on the World Wide Web. *Canadian Journal of Public Health, 91*(4), 281–284.

Horton, D. R., & Wohl, R. (1956). Mass communication and para-social interaction: Observations on intimacy at a distance. *Psychiatry, 19*(3), 215–229.

Katz, E. (1959). Mass communication research and the study of popular culture. *Public Communication, 2,* 1–6.

Katz, E., Blumler, J. G., & Gurevitch, M. (1974). Utilization of mass communication by the individual. In J. G. Blumler & E. Katz (Eds.), *The uses of mass communications: Current perspectives on gratifications research* (pp. 19–32). Beverly Hills, CA: Sage.

Kaye, B. K., & Johnson, T. J. (2002). Online and in the know: Uses and gratifications of the Web for political information. *Journal of Broadcasting & Electronic Media, 46*(1), 54–71.

Kittler, A. F., Hobbs, J., Volk, L. A., Kreps, G. L., & Bates, D. W. (2004). The Internet as a vehicle to communicate health information during a public health emergency: A survey analysis involving the Anthrax scare of 2001. *Journal of Medical Internet Research, 6*(1), e8.

Lacy, S. (2000). Commitment of financial resources as a measure of quality. In R. G. Picard (Ed.), *Measuring media content, quality, and diversity: Approaches and issues in content research* (pp. 25–50). Turku, Finland: Suomen Akatemia.

Lieberman, M. A., Golant, M., Giese-Davis, J., Winzlenberg, A., Benjamin, H., Humphreys, K., et al. (2003). Electronic support groups for breast carcinoma. *Cancer, 97,* 920–925.

Loechner, J. (2007). *Mobile video popularity suggests significant advertising potential.* Retrieved August 5, 2008, from http://publications.mediapost.com/index.cfm?fuseaction = Articles.showArticle&art_aid = 63397

Marsan, C. D. (2007). The hottest trends in online dating. Network world, February 7. Retrieved August 5, 2008, from http://www/networkworld.com/news/2008/020708-valentines-online-dating.html

Newspaper Association of America. (2006). *Better ideas for journalism.* Retrieved August 5, 2008, from http://www.naa.org/docs/Events-Marketing-Conference-Presentations-2006/tuesday-growingaudience-newthinking-thornson.pdf

Peterson, G., Aslani, P., & Williams, K. A. (2003). How do consumers search for and appraise information on medicines on the Internet? A qualitative study using focus groups. *Journal of Medical Internet Research, 5*(4): e33.

Pew Center for the People and the Press Report (2002). *News media's improved image proves short-lived.* Retrieved August 5, 2008, from http://people-press.org/report/?pageid=629

Pew Internet & American Life Project. (2007, June). *Home broadband adoption 2007* [Data memo]. Retrieved August 5, 2008, from http://www.pewinternet.org/pdfs/PIP_Broadband%202007.pdf

Pogue, D. (2007, September 13). A baffling new phenomenon: Personalized ring-tones. *New York Times.* Retrieved August 6, 2008, from http://www.nytimes.com/2007/09/13/technology/circuits/13pogue-email.html?_r=1&oref=slogin

Project for Excellence in Journalism. (2008). *State of the news media 2008.* Retrieved August 5, 2008, form http://www.stateofthenewsmedia.com

Randerson, J. (2007, January 3). Neutralise radiation and stay off milk: The truth about celebrity health claims. *The Guardian.* Retrieved July 9, 2008, from http://www.guardian.co.uk/science/2007/jan/03/health.research

Reeves, P. M. (2000). Coping in cyberspace: The impact of Internet use on the ability of HIV positive individuals to deal with their illness. *Journal of Health Communication,* 5(Suppl.), 47–59.

Rideout, V., Neuman, T., Kitchman, M., & Brodie, M. (2005). *E-Health and the elderly: How seniors use the Internet for health information.* Menlo Park, CA: Henry J. Kaiser Family Foundation.

Rodgers, S., & Thorson, E. (2000). The interactive advertising model: How users perceive and process online ads. *Journal of Interactive Advertising.* Retrieved August 5, 2008, from http://www.jiad.org/vol1/no1/rodgers/index.htm

Rosengren, K. E. (1974). Uses and gratifications: A paradigm outlined. In J. G. Blumler & E. Katz (Eds.), *The uses of mass communications: Current perspective on gratifications research* (pp. 269–286). Beverly Hills, CA: Sage.

Rubin, A. M. (1983). Television uses and gratification: The connections of viewing patterns and motivations. *Journal of Broadcasting & Electronic Media,* 27, 37–51.

Rubin, A. M. (1994). Media uses and effects: A uses-and-gratifications perspective. In J. Bryant & D. Zillmann (eds.), *Media effects: Advances in theory and research* (pp. 417–436). Hillsdale, NJ: Erlbaum.

Ruggiero, T. E. (2000). Uses and gratifications theory in the 21st century. *Mass Communication & Society,* 3(1), 3–37.

Schnall, J. (n.d.). *Untangling the Web: How to find quality health information.* Retrieved June 24, 2008, from http://healthlinks.washington.edu/hsl/liaisons/schnall/UntanglingTheWeb.pdf

Shaw, B. R., McTavish, F., Hawkins, R., Gustafson, D. H., & Pingree, S. (2000). Experiences of women with breast cancer: Exchanging social support over the CHESS computer network. *Health Communication,* 5(2), 135–159.

Sherman, A. P. (2004, May). Star qualities: How celebrity role models have inspired us. *Entrepreneur.* Retrieved August 6, 2008, from http://findarticles.com/p/articles/mi_m0DTI/is_5_32/ai_n6023844

Sifry, D. (2007). *The state of the live Web, April 2007.* Retrieved August 6, 2008, from http://www.sifry.com/alerts/archives/000493.html

Slater, M. D., & Zimmerman, D. E. (2003). Descriptions of Web sites in search listings: A potential obstacle to informed choice of health information. *American Journal of Public Health,* 93(8), 1281–1282.

Stoeva, P. (2006). Unpublished health communication annotated bibliography, Missouri School of Journalism, University of Missouri, Columbia, MO.

Thorson, E., & Thorson, K. (2006). *Choice of news media sources in the new media landscape: The crucial 18–34 demographic.* Technical paper. Missouri School of Journalism.

Walji, M., Sagaram, S., Sagaram, D., Meric-Bernstam, F., Johnson, C., Mirza, N. Q. & Bernstam, E. V. (2004). Efficacy of quality criteria to identify and alternative medicine Web sites. *Journal of Medical Internet Research*, 6(2), e21.

Wells, W., Moriarty, S., & Burnett, S. (2006). *Advertising principles and practice* (7th ed.). New Jersey: Pearson International.

Wilkin, H. A., & Ball-Rokeach, S. J. (2006). Reaching at risk groups: The importance of health storytelling in Los Angeles Latino media. *Journalism, 7*(3), 299–320.

Health Communication in the New Media Landscape

PART
II

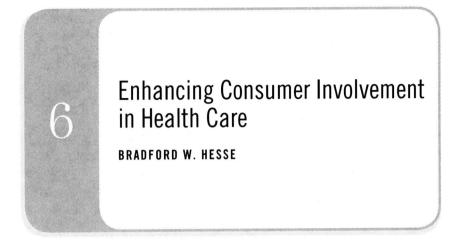

Enhancing Consumer Involvement in Health Care

BRADFORD W. HESSE

THE DAY THE WORLD CHANGED

On May 24, 2001, the Public Broadcasting System aired a featured report titled "Health on the Web" on its popular news show *NewsHour with Jim Lehrer*. The feature began with a statistic, surprising to many at the time, suggesting that in the previous year some 60 million Americans had gone online looking for health information. In the feature, breast cancer patient Pat Hodges summarized what her experience had been when she looked on the Internet for information about her breast cancer treatment.

> The Internet gives you so much more. You can be as inquisitive [as you want] as long as you're awake. And there's no one that judges you on the questions that you ask or the searches that you do. I just went on to a regular search engine and typed the words "breast cancer drug," and I knew the name of the drug, Femara. And I actually got 1,060 references. (Dentzer, 2001)

A New Turn in Health Care

Hodges's experience captured the essence of a new turn in health care, a turn that we are just beginning to understand but that will continue to play out—for better or worse—in coming decades. Her statements are telling, as they are emblematic of larger changes occurring in health care that are worth noting. For example, Hodge expressed a sense of hope at the abundance of medical information immediately available to consumers. In the past, medical knowledge was seen primarily as the purview of highly trained medical care providers. Because of the protected nature of the knowledge, patients often had no choice but to assume a passive role regarding their own health, usually waiting until a problem emerged before submitting themselves to the will and expertise of highly paid professionals (Taylor, Aspinwall, Costa, & VandenBos, 1996). In the new media world, information about health—as well as almost any other topic—has been made freely available to anyone with an Internet connection and a desire to search. The Internet has brought about an atmosphere of "disintermediation," or an opportunity for consumers to bypass the middleman and go directly to the source for information and services delivered on demand (Crowston, Sawyer, Wigand, & Allbritton, 2000).

This shift in the availability of health information has precipitated a change in the ways in which patients are approaching their own health and health care (Hesse et al., 2005). As Hodges put it, when patients go online, "there is no one that judges you on the questions you ask." Patients can be as proactive in seeking new knowledge in this new world as they wish. Quite simply the barriers are down. With just a few key strokes entered into a computer at any time of day or night, people can enter into the conversation about their own health. They can be selective in their choice of treatments or can seek help on such pernicious habits as smoking (Saul et al., 2007) at the exact moment at which they reach a stage of readiness to change (Prochaska, Teherani, & Hauer, 2007; Weinstein, Lyon, Sandman, & Cuite, 1998).

This change from passivity to a proactive approach implies a significant alteration in the way that researchers and policy makers should think about health communication. Health communication, like all types of service communication, is no longer a matter of "push" through one-way media; it is increasingly becoming a matter of "pull" as consumers go online in search of their own research for products and services (Beckjord et al., 2007; Johnson, 1997; Napolli, 2001; Nelson et al., 2004). The chief executive officer of Proctor & Gamble put it this way when speaking about the new media era in 2006: "Consumers are more participative and selective [than they have ever been before] and the trend from push to pull is accelerating" (Creamer, 2006).

Finally, as Hodges's experience in looking up the drug Femara illustrates, the information revolution is not without its challenges. In 2001, Hodges's search for information on the drug produced just over 1,000 hits—a daunting number, to be sure. In 2007, just 6 years later, the same search would produce approximately two million hits, according to indices posted on the popular search engine Google. The information revolution is producing an information glut, what journalist David Shenk (1997) called "data smog," as consumers are inundated with more information than they are able to process (Arora, Hesse, Rimer, Viswanath, Clayman, & Croyle, 2007). Biomedical scientists often add to the problem inadvertently by releasing early, and often contradictory, findings to the popular press prematurely (Woloshin & Schwartz, 2006). Staying fully abreast of the scientific literature in medicine means keeping track of the more than 12,000 newly referenced articles added to the National Library of Medicine's online bibliographic retrieval system weekly (U.S. National Library of Medicine, 2007). It is no wonder that in a survey conducted in 2003, an estimated 71.5% of the U.S. public felt that "there are so many recommendations about preventing skin cancer that it's hard to know which ones to follow" (Niederdeppe & Levy, 2007).

PURPOSE OF THE CHAPTER

The purpose of this chapter will be to explore the potential for enhancing consumer involvement in health care within the context of a rapidly changing new media environment. The focus will unabashedly be on behavior—that is, on understanding how healthy behaviors can be supported in a way that will extend life and improve quality of living. In the previous century, the greatest threats to public and personal health were often associated with malnourishment and infectious disease. In this century, the greatest threats in the United States are posed by an aging population and the onset of avoidable chronic conditions (Bhattacharya, Choudhry, & Lakdawalla, 2008). Understanding how to support preventive behavior in this new environment, it can be argued, will be as important to the problem of extending longevity and improving quality of life in the next century as was the development of safe water treatments and vaccines in the last (Quam, Smith, & Yach, 2006; Strong, Mathers, Epping-Jordan, & Beaglehole, 2006; World Health Organization, 2006).

CONSUMER BEHAVIOR IN THE NEW MEDIA ENVIRONMENT

To understand how the new media environment can be optimized to support changes in consumer behavior, it is worthwhile to examine how and under what conditions the environment has evolved over the past several decades. One of the seminal articulations of the power that computer media can have in changing behavior can be found in a white paper written by computer scientist Douglas Engelbart (1962) and his colleagues in 1961. Titled "Augmenting Human Intellect: A Conceptual Framework," the paper borrowed heavily from multiple fields, including communication theory, cognitive science, mathematics, human factors, and computer engineering. Its main premise was borrowed from the linguistic notion that human thought has co-evolved with the development and sophistication of language (Whorf, 1956); that is, the more sophisticated the system of symbolic interaction became, the greater the capacity for intellectual advancement. Engelbart and his colleagues believed that information systems represent a type of structured system for symbolic interaction. Engineered appropriately, these systems had the potential to augment human thought and empower human behavior.

HUMAN FACTORS

For Engelbart (1962), the problem of designing a truly augmentative environment for human thought was a human factors issue; that is, it was a matter of optimizing the interface between the underlying systems architecture and the user's own intellectual predilections through evidence-based iterations of the system's design. Perhaps best known for his contributions to the design of the computer mouse, Engelbart championed the cause of creating better and more productive interfaces between developing computer systems and their human users (Bardini, 2000)—an area of research that came to be known as the field of human–computer interaction. In his mind and in the minds of other computer pioneers, the computer should not replace human thought or action; rather it should augment it.

Shoshana Zuboff (1988), a social psychologist studying the ways in which computer systems enhanced business productivity, put it this way. The information revolution, she explained, was not about automating human performance as machines did during the industrial revolution; it was about informating human performance, using computing machines to augment or add to human intellectual capacity. The distinction may seem subtle, but it has had a big impact on the ways in which informatics applications can be designed to support health. Early medical informatics pioneers often asked "the wrong question" in system design (Hesse & Shneiderman, 2007; Shneiderman, 2002). They tried to automate physician performance and knowledge through expert systems and artificial intelligence. The more effective designers recognized that the patient's health was central; all designs should be brought to bear in improving the experience that all patients have (Brailer, 2005).

Engelbart and his colleagues also recognized that the true power of the new emerging information systems should not be limited to the capacity of any one single computer but should expand to include the broader view of collective capacity as users interacted with new knowledge and with each other over computer-based communication networks. Thirty years later, in 1991, computer scientist Tim Berners-Lee proposed a project that would bring the early computer pioneers' ideas to fruition. By combining the usability of a graphical user interface environment with the connectivity offered by the Internet, Berners-Lee was able to propose a truly collaborative environment for interaction: an environment that would be easy to join and simple to navigate (Berners-Lee & Fischetti, 1999). He referred to his proposed project as the "World Wide Web."

AN ERA OF UNFETTERED ACCESS TO INFORMATION

Undoubtedly, the World Wide Web has put a global wealth of human knowledge and information within reach for contemporary consumers. The growth of information on Web-based servers has literally exploded from the mere megabytes (10^6) of data available when the Web was first made available to the petabytes (10^{15}) of data accessible through the millions of servers accessible in 2007 and beyond (National Science Foundation, 2007). Penetration of the Web as a new communication technology was rapid; while a small percentage of American citizens were online in 1993, almost 75% of adults were estimated to be online in 2006 (Pew Charitable Trust, 2007). The information revolution ushered in by the World Wide Web heralded a new era in communication research, one in which the information stores of a global community can be made available on demand to consumers (Viswanath, 2005).

It created a tectonic shift in the ways in which health communication researchers consider supporting the health of the public (Hesse, 2005; Hesse et al., 2005).

Moreover, the communication revolution precipitated by the Web did not just bring the power of information to individuals; it expanded the reach and capacity of social networks. Computer-mediated communications allowed individuals to interact with each other dyadically (one-to-one) and with whole groups (one-to-many), it let preexisting groups communicate with each other (many-to-many), and it let new relationships emerge in virtual rather than physical space (Kiesler, 1997; Kiesler & Sproull, 1987; Sproull & Kiesler, 1991). The medium provided newer, quicker ways for people to find answers to questions (either through search engines or by querying online discussion groups), it connected people to services and information about services, it offered support for decision making and self-management, and it gave people remote access to powerful new computer systems. In general, virtual environments allowed users to overcome boundaries traditionally imposed by place (Stokols, Montero, Bechtel, & Churchman, 2002) and temporality (Hesse, Werner, & Altman, 1988). It allowed users to benefit by interacting with data, resources, and people locally and globally, and it bridged the gap between real-time (synchronous) and delayed-time (asynchronous) communication.

Transformed Context for Consumer Behavior

These early historical roots of new media environments lie at the foundation of some of the most significant economic transformations in both local and global economies over the past two decades (T. L. Friedman, 2007). They have altered the very context in which work, health, and consumer behavior should be considered (Hesse & Grantham, 1991).

One of the first broad sectors of the economy to grapple with change from the new computing technologies was the financial sector. Because the exchange of monetary information is so vital to what financial institutions do, the financial sector pioneered some of the first real accomplishments in enabling standards for electronic data interchange. Once data could be transferred in reliable ways, it did not take long for business managers to consider ways of adapting the electronic data interchange infrastructures for direct use by the public. The automatic teller machine was the first consumer adaptation designed to put the ability to manipulate personal funds directly into the hands of customers. Rather than having to wait in line for small deposits, transfers, and withdrawals, consumers could manage many of these transactions at their own pace and in their own time. The bank would win by attracting more customers and reserving personnel time for more challenging financial problems (Grantham & Nichols, 1993).

Other industries have undergone similar transformations. For example, in the airline industry, American Airlines debuted its Semi-Automated Business Research Environment (SABRE) system as an experimental technology for coordinating seat assignments, reservations, and price offerings in 1960. Although the pioneering computer system was originally developed to serve reservations specialists at American Airlines, the company began selling access to independent travel agents in 1976. In 1996, at the beginning of the dot-com boom, a subsidiary of SABRE Holdings called Travelocity was created with the express purpose of opening access to consumers. Today, the ubiquity of Travelocity and other online travel services has provoked an industry-wide change in airline business practice to cope with the influx of price-conscious consumers going online for best value (Grantham & Carr, 2002).

Transformations in Health Care

So, the question remains: if we can achieve such monumental change in empowering consumers in *wealth care,* why can't we achieve the same successes in *health care*? The health care industry has been notoriously slow to adapt the kinds of broad-scale changes in its use of information technology that would improve its quality of direct service to patients. Reasons for the disconnect are multifaceted, ranging from the complex set of incentives and disincentives woven into the fabric of insurance-provider relationships to an "illness care" system that has been historically oriented toward reacting to symptoms once they emerge (Brailer, 2005). Nevertheless, conditions are changing. With aging populations in many large developed countries, it is untenable to think of an illness-oriented and disconnected health system as being economically viable in the decades to come (Cayton, 2006). National health directors in the United States and Europe are urging their governments to adopt a new approach to health care, one that would take preemptive action to stave off these health care costs by encouraging the public to be proactive in its choice of healthy lifestyles and participative in its management of personal care.

In testimony to Congress, the director of the U.S. National Institutes of Health suggested that medical research must undergo a transformation to enable substantive progress against the complex, multifaceted health problems confronting the nation at the beginning of the 21st century. The science must move from being reactive, imprecise, and ultimately expensive in terms of lives and money to being predictive, personalized, preemptive, and ultimately cost effective by intervening in people's lives early before tissue damage occurs and function is lost (Culliton, 2006). Health information technology must play a key role in harnessing the power of a more personalized, preemptive health care system for consumers (Hesse, 2005). To this end, the secretary for the U.S. Department of Health and Human Services declared that it will be necessary to create an electronic infrastructure based on transportable, interoperable electronic medical records in order to achieve progress against chronic disease in the 21st century. The president of the United States echoed the secretary's sense of priority in two State of the Union addresses and upped the ante by declaring a national goal of connecting the majority of Americans to electronic medical records by 2014 (Brailer, 2005).

All these changes are creating a new environment for consumer involvement in health care. As will be explained in this chapter, the time is ripe to sculpt this environment in ways that will improve health and extend life. It is time to think proactively about how to embed the benefits this new technology can offer into the fabric of daily living.

THE ACTIVATED PATIENT

In an article published in the journal *Patient Education and Counselling*, Harry Cayton (2006), national director for patients and the public in the United Kingdom, mentioned some of the changes that will be occurring in the United Kingdom and other countries in the area of health care. As he explained, economic analyses show that current trajectories in health care expenditures are not sustainable in the long term. The only way to stave off financial crisis is to reduce demand while improving supply. The way for that to happen, he suggested, is to create an environment in which patients and physicians create good health together.

In this new environment, the use of new technologies to answer day-to-day questions and to reduce administrative workload would be high. Members of the public would become engaged in managing their own health in proactive ways, taking prevention seriously, and staying on track for suggested checkups and routine screenings. When they do need the assistance of the health care system, they would demand high-quality care and insist that components of the system work together to support positive health outcomes. The result would be longer life expectancies, with more rewarding and productive years per person, and significant cost savings for delivery of care (Cayton, 2006).

Is the Public Ready for Active Involvement?

Future predictions notwithstanding, a big question remains as to whether the public is ready to make such a significant transition. To monitor changes in the ways in which Americans utilize health information, the U.S. National Cancer Institute launched the Health Information National Trends Survey (HINTS) in 2001. HINTS is a biennial survey that uses a nationally representative sample of adults ages 18 and older. Random digit dial telephone interviews were used for the first HINTS data collection in 2003, a second administration used random digit dial plus Web surveys in 2005; and a third administration used random digit dial plus mail surveys (to account for the increase in cell phone–only households) in 2007 (Rutten, Moser, Beckjord, Hesse, & Croyle, 2007).

In 2003, the survey asked respondents to imagine they had a strong need to get information about cancer and then to indicate where they would go first to obtain information. An estimated 49% of the U.S. population said they would go to their health care providers, while an estimated 33.2% said they would go to the Internet (percentages for other options were negligible). In the same survey, interviewers asked respondents if they had ever had an occasion to look for information about cancer from any source. An estimated 45% of the population said they had. Interviewers asked respondents who answered in the affirmative to recall the most recent time they had looked for information about cancer from any source, and to indicate what source they had gone to first. In this case, the order of responses was reversed. An estimated 47% of the information-seeking group indicated that they had gone to the Internet first, and only 23% indicated that they had gone to their health care providers (Hesse et al., 2005).

To understand further how Americans were using the Internet for health information, the survey asked respondents if they had ever gone online to access the Internet or World Wide Web or to send and receive e-mail. For those who reported being online, the survey then asked respondents whether or not they had engaged in a number of health-related activities in the previous 12 months. Figure 6.1 shows a comparison from 2003 to 2005 of these health-related activities for the online populations identified through each survey. The first two sets of bars show general increases in the percentages of online Americans looking for health information either for themselves or for others. The third and fifth sets show small increases in the percentages purchasing medicine online and in e-mailing their physicians, respectively. The fourth set, showing the percentage using online support services, remained stable (Beckjord et al., 2007; Rutten et al., 2007).

Health communication is not just about exposure to information; it is about attention and trust (Hesse et al., 2005; Institute of Medicine, 2001; Kreps & Thornton, 1992). To understand how the new mix of media channels was influencing the public's confidence in health information sources, HINTS interviewers asked respondents to indicate how much they would trust information about cancer that they received from their doctors, families, newspapers, radio, television, and the Internet. Figure 6.2 offers population estimates for the percentage of adult Americans who feel a lot of trust for sources in each of these categories. For health information, the public had the greatest trust in

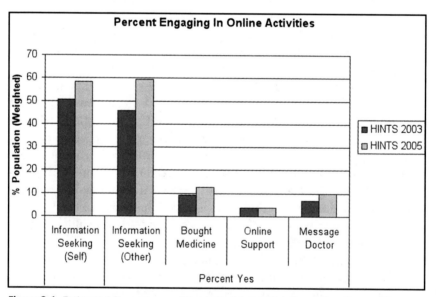

Figure 6.1 Estimated Percentages of the U.S. Adult (18+) Population Engaged in Health-Related Activities Online From the 2003–2005. Administrations of the Health Information National Trends Survey.

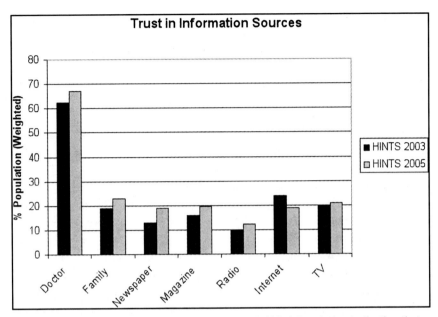

Figure 6.2 Estimated Percentages of the U.S. Adult (18+) Population Indicating that they would Trust Health Information from Each of Seven Sources "a Lot."

physicians, a trend that grew from 2005 to 2006. Trust in other sources, at least for health or medical information, was significantly lower. There appeared to be a slight erosion of trust for the Internet as a source (Rutten et al., 2007).

Collectively, these data suggest that the majority of users are going online to look for health-related information either for themselves or others. Involvement in other online health-related activities, such as buying medication or communicating with physicians, currently lags behind general information seeking, but those areas are continuing to grow. Support for these other online activities will likely evolve as the infrastructure matures. In spite of the profusion of health information on the Web, these data suggest that the need for qualified medical personnel will not go away. If anything, consumers' reliance on the training and experience of qualified medical teams to answer questions from materials otherwise found online will become greater (Beckjord et al., 2007; Mazur, 2003). Enhancing consumer involvement means focusing first on the perceptions and needs of the user, and then supplying consumers with integrated solutions that augment the physician–patient relationship.

Focus on Users

The HINTS data suggest that people are indeed taking advantage of this dramatic shift in the media environment to improve their own health care experiences. The question this chapter asks is: How can new media planners catch up to people's needs? How can this connective, augmentative information environment be leveraged in ways that will enhance, not detract from, consumers' desires to lead optimally healthy lives and to protect the health of their loved ones (Fox, 2007; Fox & Rainie, 2002)? To find an answer to that question, it is worthwhile to look into the psychological literature on the role of motivation in human performance.

The study of human motivation has a long history in the psychological sciences, from early quantification of drive or tissue need to studies of reinforcement in behavior and contemporary theories on social influence and cognition. After years of studying motivational issues among students and employees, social psychologists Edward Deci and Richard Ryan (2002) observed that most people are driven by a need to influence the outcomes that affect their lives. That is, humans seek self-determination in thought and action. When the environment reinforces self-determination, people become effective and thrive. When the environment takes away that goal, they can become listless and depressed (Deci & Vansteenkiste, 2004; Seligman, Rashid, & Parks, 2006).

Using factor analytic and structural equation modeling approaches, Deci and Ryan (2000) identified three universal needs that appear to influence the cultivation of self-determined behavior. The first was a need for autonomy, or the need to perceive actions as stemming from internal motivations, not from external sources. The second motivational need they observed was a need for competency, or the desire we all have to learn from the environment and gain mastery over skills and talents. The third was a need for relatedness, of the social need to gain a sense of respect and belonging from valued others.

Supporting these universal needs, Deci and Ryan argued, lies at the heart of creating an environment that will lead to personal empowerment. It is instructive to take each of these needs and examine the contributions that the new media can offer each in supporting a shift toward consumer involvement.

A Need for Autonomy

In many respects, the ethos of the information revolution has emerged from a collective desire to achieve autonomy in behavior and thought

(Markoff, 2005). At its heart, the personal computer revolution has been a movement aimed at wresting power away from centralized gatekeepers, and then putting that power back into the hands of individuals for personal action (Toffler, 1990; Toffler & Toffler, 1993). It is easy to see why individuals are flocking to the Internet as a way of regaining personal autonomy in their own personal health issues. Consider what happens under the traditional medical model of health care.

In the traditional model, patients are typically inclined to wait until they got sick—that is, when symptoms appear late in the disease cycle and function is at threat or lost—before contacting their health care provider. Once they have a need, they call an overburdened office staff to put themselves on a waiting list to see a physician. The first appointment could not be for days or weeks, during which time the underlying disease pathology might very well progress. To enter the system, the patient must provide proof of coverage, fill out medical history forms, describe medications from memory, and then wait in a waiting room filled with other patients while reading popular news or gossip magazines to pass the time. In the examination room, a nurse might take routine—but nonspecific—measurements (weight, blood pressure), after which the physician and patient must condense weeks' worth of pathology and review into a short 15-minute exchange. The patient is given a diagnosis or put on a treatment plan that may require visits to other components of the health care system or referrals to specialists, or is given a prescription for a pharmaceutical product with three- or four-word instructions on the pill bottle's label, and perhaps accompanied by an indecipherable insert designed to meet legal requirements rather than to instruct.

Each of these interactions appears to be focused on requirements exogenous to the patient's interest and is part of the "thousand little assaults" on personal autonomy that plagues the modern consumer on a daily basis (Zuboff & Maxmin, 2002). What is worse is that the first generation of information technology applications did not solve the problem but in many ways made it worse. Early dot-com companies myopically looked to the single Web visit (much as the traditional health care system looked only to the single office visit) as the sole point of interaction. Designers then set out to extract as much value from that single transaction as possible. A consumer visiting a site would be forced down the same rigid set of marketing paths, with little support for self-determined needs, while pop-up ads took time away from the consumer's goal. Often no other way of contacting the organization (telephone numbers, mailing addresses) was provided, and when a telephone number was given, a set of complex telephonic menus ("Press '1' if you have a question about billing") took even more time away from the time devoted to meeting the customer's needs.

Today, with greater business acumen, the more successful companies are changing that (O'Reilly, 2005). These companies look to developing long-term relationships with and a sense of loyalty among their customers. When technology is used, it is used in a way that is transparent and that reinforces the organization's core commitment to providing customers with responsive, ongoing support (Collins, 2001). Consider companies such as UPS or FedEx. These are some of the most advanced users of information technology in the current global market, yet customers do not think of them as technology companies at all (T. L. Friedman, 2007). All their technology systems are centered on customer fulfillment, on moving and tracking parcels from point to point as efficiently and expediently as possible. A visit to their Web sites reveals a spate of consumer tools, all set up to give customers more power in tracking their parcels, identifying problems, and making new requests quickly and efficiently. Or consider Southwest Airlines' award-winning Web site. This site makes it easy for consumers to identify bargains for travel, make new reservations, and even change reservations as personal priorities change.

Now consider how a new media environment, one that is built on a foundation of interoperable health records, can be marshaled to enhance patient autonomy. Following are just a few of the promising innovations that are currently under development.

- **Self-help tools.** One way of putting control back into the hands of consumers is to provide tools for healthy living. For example, it has been estimated that in the 20th century some 100 million people's lives could have been saved if they had not been exposed to tobacco (President's Cancer Panel, 2007). Yet many who are willing to quit find it difficult and often need the help of a prescribed smoking cessation program combining personal counseling with the use of a graduated nicotine patch. The therapeutic side of these programs can be expensive and can be off-putting to patients who have busy lives and must find time to participate in a smokers' support group or visit with a personal counselor. As part of its Centers of Excellence in Cancer Communication program, the National Cancer Institute has been experimenting with techniques for making the benefits of a personally tailored smoking cessation program available to patients through the Internet

24 hours a day, 7 days a week. Because these programs are computer-based, they can be deployed widely to those who need it for just a fraction of the cost of an expensive counseling program (Saul et al., 2007; Strecher, 2007). Online programs for weight management and exercise are being introduced through the Web, cell phones, personal digital assistants, and other communication devices to help individuals live healthier lives with the behavioral aids that correspond to real-life demands (Pew Research Center, 2005).

- **Personal health records.** One of the reasons why the secretary for the Department of Health and Human Services has identified interoperable health records as a priority in the current decade is so that a foundation for consumer empowerment can be created. Just as interoperable banking records give customers control over their own finances, interoperable health records can give patients control over their own health records. This simple notion that patients should have access to and control over their own health information represents a paradigmatic shift away from the traditional medical model. Behavioral supports that can be put in place with a personal health record include structures that make it easy for patients to set up appointments in a way that is convenient to their schedules; provide age-sensitive reminders for screening, inoculations, and checkups; offer tools for monitoring health status in response to treatment or preventive life changes; improve quality of care by allowing users to track progress of lab results, referrals, and other points of handoff; and offer patients access to state-of-the art health information as needed so that they can make life decisions for themselves and loved ones (Burrington-Brown & Friedman, 2005).

- **Health portals.** It has been argued that information is power, and in the world of health care, accurate medical information means the difference between relying on well-meaning home remedies and using the power of medical science to extend life and live strong. To meet the needs of a surging interest in health information, Web portals have begun to emerge that offer health advice on everything from anthrax to SARS. The trusted sites can be comprehensive one-stop shops for all the information a patient wishes to digest before or after visiting the doctor's office. The availability of current evidence-based health information 24 hours a day, 7 days a week, can make a real-time difference in the "hurry up and wait" world of medical care (Fox & Rainie, 2002). There is, however, one caveat in the availability of real-time health information within the unfettered environs of the Web (Kemper & Mettler, 2002). Undirected searches could lead consumers to sites that are neither usable nor trustworthy (Berland et al., 2001). Consumers and media watchdog groups should remain vigilant as to the authenticity, credibility, and accuracy of the information they uncover on the Web (Eng & Gustafson, 1999; Eng, Maxfield, Patrick, Deering, Ratzan, & Gustafson, 1998).

- **Connective journalism.** One of the perennial problems in health communication lies in the way in which stories are selected by editors for publication (Royal Institution of Great Britain, 2001). Stories that appear to be new or controversial have a greater chance of being published than stories that appear to be old or common knowledge; this situation creates an environment of misrepresentation for health stories (S. M. Friedman, Dunwoody, & Rogers, 1999). This creates difficulties for the public, as news media gravitate to those findings from research laboratories that are preliminary or anomalous in nature and ignore recommendations that are supported by consensus or that represent standards of care (Woloshin & Schwartz, 2006). In one content analysis of news stories, there was an inverse relationship between the number of stories on a particular health topic and the importance of information about that topic for healthy living. The stories about rare conditions and preliminary findings were numerous, while the stories about evidence-supported prevention behaviors (diet, exercise, nutrition, early detection) were infrequent (Frost, Frank, & Maibach, 1997). New media sites can allow newspapers to go beyond the headlines and to link readers to the information and resources they need for healthy living. In fact, some of the online sites are themselves becoming trusted health portals with embedded links from the stories that take the reader back to national public health recommendations. Locally relevant sites can link readers to community resources or offer easy applications to government assistance programs for crucial medical services.

- **Ubiquitous health care.** In the financial industry, customers were given self-directed access to their money any time of the week through automatic teller machines. In the travel industry, consumers can receive travel and weather updates through PDAs or cell phones and they can check in and print their boarding passes from home before going to the airport or at self-standing kiosks in the lobbies of most airports. A new trend enabled by an infrastructure based on connective health information technology will be the ability to offer urgent care services or pharmaceutical products ubiquitously in consumer-friendly environments. As these services get "commoditized," one hope is that the marketplace will force providers to make their services more compatible with consumer needs and lifestyle choices (Crounse, 2007). For example, a well-known retail outlet has recently been credited with finally "reinventing" the pill bottle to make it safer and easier for consumers across all levels of health literacy to use (Bernard, 2005; "A Better Pill Bottle," 2005; Davis et al., 2006; Parker, Baker, Williams, & Nurss, 1995). As with health portals, policy makers and the public should pay close attention to these changes. The quality and accreditation procedures should be in place to assure customers that the care being given adheres to accepted standards.

Need for Competency

Another long-standing area of emphasis in thinking about consumer involvement in health care concerns the need people have to acquire and improve essential life skills. It is one of the reasons why the *For Dummies* book series has been so popular among consumers, and why how-to sites have found a place on the World Wide Web. The problem has been that once most people complete formal schooling, they do not have access to the kinds of training environments that can help them gain control over their own health care. This is especially true for patients, who must move from the comfortable role of a well person into the unfamiliar role of a sick person. In fact, the prevailing culture has encouraged patients to assume a role of passivity and subservience when interacting with the health system. "Good patients" are those who appear passive and compliant; "bad patients" are those who appear assertive and questioning (Taylor et al., 1996).

It is these stereotypes, from a human factors perspective, that need to change. The proactive patient is essential for helping to solve the health care problems that will confront the United States in the next several decades (Atienza et al., 2007; Institute of Medicine, 2001; Wagner, 2004). This is not to say that patients must be up to the task entirely on their own. Rest is essential to the healing process, and when sick, people do not always make the best judgments. It is equally important to consider the skills of family members and caregivers as partners invested in the patient's health. Patients can, in turn, depend on their caregivers to be assertive on their behalf, to ask questions, and to learn what to do with them (Taylor et al., 1996).

There are many ways in which new media can be used to support competency in healthy living and in dealing with the health care systems. The following areas merit special consideration:

- **Functional health literacy.** The Institute of Medicine declared the problem of health illiteracy to be one of the most devastating challenges to public health in existence today (Nielsen-Bohlman & Institute of Medicine Committee on Health Literacy, 2004). One aspect of the health literacy problem is having the knowledge to act appropriately when it comes to preserving health, an aspect referred to as "functional health literacy." Fortunately, problems of functional health literacy can be addressed through better design of the information environment. For example, a recent review by the Cochrane Collaboration identified non-adherence to treatment regimens as a serious medical problem (Haynes et al., 2005). Adherence rates for prescription medicines in the United States typically hover around 50%, and lack of adherence has been identified as the principal cause of death in up to a third of cases in a recent study of geriatric patients (Baker, Wolf, Feinglass, Thompson, Gazmararian, & Huang 2007). Solutions are possible with the aid of information technology (Paasche-Orlow, Schillinger, Greene, & Wagner, 2006). Instructional systems can easily be made available through multimedia (Wofford, Smith, & Miller, 2005), reminder systems can be put in place through monitoring and tracking systems (Thomas et al., 2007), social networks can be mobilized to encourage compliance and provide vigilance as part of their social support (Magai, Consedine, Neugut, & Hershman, 2007), and so on.
- **Information Prescriptions.** Corporations have long recognized the importance of "just in time training" as a tool for building employee competencies. Health educators have argued that it is time to consider ways of applying the same principles to patients. In a book titled *Information Therapy*, Kemper and his colleagues argued that physicians should be remunerated for giving patients

prescriptions to go to a sanctioned Web site and learn about their conditions between visits (Kemper & Mettler, 2002). The information prescription can go a long way in helping patients build their knowledge base relevant to their diagnosis, treatment, and side effects, thus enabling them to make more informed decisions and be more participative in their own care (D'Alessandro, Kreiter, Kinzer, & Peterson, 2004). New media tutorials can offer pedagogical advantages over simple brochures by providing a more in-depth review of processes along with personalized layers of access for novices as well as advanced learners. The sites can also be shared easily with caregivers and loved ones, no matter where they live. Offering professional recommendations for vetted and credible information sources will take the guesswork out of deciding what information on the Web can be trusted. It can also make recommendations equally transparent to patients and providers, as illustrated by the Cancer.gov Web site hosted by the National Cancer Institute (see Figure 6.3).

■ **Skill augmentation.** At their best, information technology solutions can help augment an individual's own knowledge and experience. For example, grammar and spell checking in word-processing programs can offer real-time support for poor spellers, real-time car navigation systems can help travelers cope with unfamiliar street systems, personal financial software can make up for a person's lack of familiarity with complex tax laws, and powerful new graphics programs are giving consumers the power to create professional quality video, photographs, and pictures (Shneiderman, 2002). An exciting area of development in the next generation of consumer health applications will be in thinking through ways of helping patients develop proactive solutions to life challenges. An age-sensitive health record can help remind patients when screening tests are recommended, even if those recommendations seem to have been changing over time. Exercise monitors and meal planners can give dieters real-time advice and support, while smoking cessation aids can help inoculate those in the developing world against the threat of exploitation by international tobacco sales. Personal management programs can be extended beyond simple task management and financial record-keeping functions to include mechanisms for developing a personalized approach to managing risk and building health.

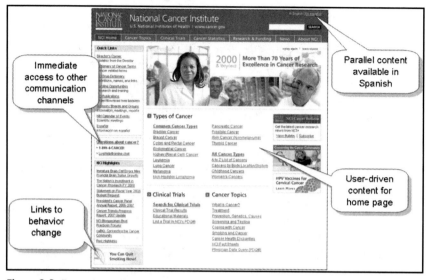

Figure 6.3 Example of Web Content From a National Government Agency, Designed to Support Consumer Needs While Transparently Supporting Health Care Practitioners (Oncologists) and Scientists.

Relatedness

The third ubiquitous need that most people express is a need for relatedness. Humans, as social organisms, have a strong need to cultivate and maintain social relationships with others. This is especially the case when it comes to health. When people fall ill, they look to others for expressions of emotional support as a buffer against the stress they feel in coping with health-threatening situations (Taylor, Falke, Shoptaw, & Lichtman, 1986). They also look to others for clarification for how they should be feeling under atypical circumstances and for what to do to cope (Croyle & Hunt, 1991). They use family members and friends as sounding boards on when to interact with the health care system, and where to go to seek help. These caregivers provide instrumental help as well by taking their loved ones to the hospital or helping them make some of the vital decisions that influence their care (Taylor et al., 1996).

Once connected to the health care system, patients and their loved ones look to their medical teams to help them manage their diagnosis and the course of their treatment. A comprehensive literature review funded by the National Cancer Institute has suggested that there are six fundamental communication needs that must be met by a health care system in order to support a patient's health care needs (Epstein & Street,

2007). These are exchanging information vital to shared management of the health condition, eliciting and validating emotions, managing uncertainty, making decisions, navigating the health care system, and building a sense of trust and continuity in the provider–patient relationship.

One of the most powerful aspects of the Internet as a new medium is not just its ability to link information, but its ability to support connections between people. Not long after the first data packet was sent between machines over early electronic networks, people began using the networks to communicate socially between each other. In the 1980s and 1990s e-mail, discussion groups, chat rooms, instant messaging, and other forms of socially connecting technologies escalated as some of the most important uses of network technology. In the current decade, the so-called Web 2.0 applications have elevated support for social interactions and sharing to new levels. It is easy to envision a new media environment in which these elements are optimized in order to enhance prospects for a healthier, longer, and more fulfilling life. Some examples to watch for are:

- **Health advocacy groups.** In the political arena, the connective capacity of the Internet allows people to organize online and bypass overt attempts to control communication through propaganda or suppression. Some observers credit the transparent qualities of communication on the Internet with fostering a peaceful buffer to the potentially dangerous situation that could have occurred during the political dissolution of the Soviet Union in 1989–1990. In the same way, many observers have suggested that online advocacy groups will play an active role in exerting pressure on traditional power structures of medicine, insurance, and regulation. These groups will demand investment of political and financial capital into attempts to solve some of the major health issues of the new century. They will contribute funding and volunteer their time to encourage political attention to health issues but will be demanding of results from the research and practice communities to improve quality and length of life. Health communication specialists can take advantage of the trend by encouraging biomedical scientists to "opt in" to the conversation, communicating their results in ways that will support understanding and patients' goals for healthy decision making. Health care practitioners and medical systems can take advantage of the trend by refocusing their services to fit within the values expressed by the burgeoning health communities.

■ **Networks of care.** With an electronic health information infrastructure in place, new media applications can be developed to bolster the supportive interpersonal connections needed by patients and the public to prevent, preempt, and control the effects of disease before function is lost. Communication engineers are creating a new generation of telemedicine applications that will upload medical data from portable devices and even home sensors to an electronic repository for monitoring (Wilson, 1999). Distributed communication technologies will allow the patient to access medical records and review medical progress in partnership with a health care team. On the medical system side, these communities of care can be extended to include coordinated input from primary care physicians, specialty physicians, advice nurses, laboratory specialists, case managers, urgent care facilities, and even employer-based health management programs. For patients, giving permission for others to view some of their online medical information will allow family members, caregivers, and significant others to support patients' health while away from the hospital—a godsend for adult children dealing with the challenges of an aging parent wishing to remain active at home while confronting declines in function and health. "Care Pages," an application gaining popularity as a way to keep concerned friends and family apprised of the progress of someone struggling with a serious disease, can help extend the advantages of emotional connectedness in ways that are not intrusive to the patient's own need for rest or recuperation (Garcia-Lizana & Sarria-Santamera, 2007).

■ **Shared communities of knowledge.** Another phenomenon that is gaining momentum is the development of self-organizing communities of knowledge. Electronic publishing pioneer Tim O'Reilly suggested that after the dot-com bubble burst, the Web companies that survived learned from the mistakes of their predecessors. The second generation, or Web 2.0, is characterized by architectures that promote user participation, that harness the power of collective intelligence, and that use data as the next "Intel inside." Physician-entrepreneur Matthew Holt, who convened the first "Health 2.0" conference on user-generated content in 2007, suggested that these new patterns of Web-enabled interaction are catalyzing change in the health care arena. In the new health care market, he explained, patients are coming to understand that they need to work as partners with their health care providers. "You could almost argue that healthcare is being produced by patients to some extent," he speculated (Conn, 2007).

CAVEATS AND RESEARCH OPPORTUNITIES

When Engelbart and his colleagues laid the foundation for a new technological infrastructure back in 1961, what they were really doing was outlining the steps for evolutionary change in human thinking. They referred to the process as "bootstrapping," literally the process by which a whole system can evolve to new levels by "picking itself up by the bootstraps" (Bardini, 2000). Admittedly, the seeds of change planted in those early years took a long time to germinate and grow. They are flourishing now, though, and the implications of change are widespread and global. Some media experts speculate that there will be more change precipitated by advances in the new media environment within the next 5 years than there has been in overall communication environment over the previous 50 (Brown, 2006).

Taking Health Communication Research to the Next Level

The challenge for a new generation of health communications researchers is to understand how to harness this transformation in productive ways that are beneficial to society, to move individual and public health to the next level. It took millennia for the practice of medicine to evolve from folk wisdom to evidence-based treatment and prevention. As sobering as it may sound, the first randomized controlled trial in medicine was not published until 1952 (Daniels & Hill, 1952). Today, the National Library of Medicine adds thousands of empirically based medical studies to its online holdings each week (U.S. National Library of Medicine, 2007) with advances in medical technology leading to real, observable differences in people's lives. From 1900 to 2000, average life expectancy at birth rose from a mere 49 years to almost 80 years due in no small part to the translation of biomedical science into public health outreach and policy (Centers for Disease Control and Prevention, 1999).

Health systems researchers caution that the advances accrued during an era of industrial age medicine may have reached their limit (Cayton, 2006). Along with individual successes in medical treatment has come an epidemic of medical errors that exceeds threats from breast cancer,

AIDS, or automobile accidents (Institute of Medicine, 2001). As one observer put it, "medicine used to be simple, ineffective, and relatively safe; now it is complex, effective, and potentially dangerous" (Chantler, 1999). Moreover, the sheer magnitude of new studies published each year has created a type of "data smog" clouding the understanding of the public, policy makers, and practitioners (Shenk, 1997). Scientists recognize that in the absence of better collaboration, individually based laboratories appear to be reinventing the same wheel simultaneously without moving the knowledge base on complex problems forward. Inefficiencies in industrial age translation mechanisms have created a backlog in getting the benefits of biomedical research out of the laboratory and into practice. By some counts, it currently takes an average of 17 years to move the benefits of medical science from bench to bedside (Westfall, Mold, & Fagnan, 2007).

With the recent mapping of the three billion (plus) base pairs comprising the human genome—an accomplishment made possible by advances in connective information technology—the potential for tackling previously insurmountable problems such as cancer, aging, and the unequal burden of disease is great. Those advances can only come if we bootstrap improvements in the ways in which we conduct biomedical science research, and the ways in which we move the benefits of that science into improved health at individual and population levels.

Collaboration Is the Key

Collaboration lies at the heart of this bootstrapped transformation. What is new about the evolution of new media technologies in the era of Web 2.0 is the development of highly successful "architectures for participation." These architectures rely on data in the way that industrialized medicine relied on intuition and expertise to enable a new era of evidence-based, participative health care. Each member of the participative enterprise will play a crucial role. Patients will bring with them an intuitive understanding of their own physiologies and medical histories and will be motivated by vested self-interest in protecting their own health as well as the welfare of their loved ones. Medical providers will bring a professional understanding of symptoms, processes, and treatments interpreted through the lens of medical science. Payers will continue to maintain their role in diffusing risk across populations, while insisting on systemic changes that reduce overall costs through approaches that are preventive, preemptive, and personalized. Governments and advocacy groups will participate transparently to ensure that benefits from the new transformation reach all parts of society equitably.

The time is right for new media researchers to step into the fray to influence the development of these architectures. This, too, must be a participative enterprise. Computer scientists are essential to the development of the computational architectures necessary to translate data into informed decision making. Biomedical scientists form the backbone of an enterprise that is doubling life expectancy, while communication scientists must focus on ways of enabling a push-pull architecture for participative discussion. Cognitive scientists must take on the role of reducing cognitive burden by developing interfaces that are user friendly and facilitative, while social psychologists are needed to improve group processes in team science and participative medicine. Health economists can evaluate overall trends in the search for returns on investment, while human factors specialists look for systemic changes to reduce error. In all these collaborations, evidence must trump speculation and data must serve as the lingua franca for a new transdisciplinary science (Abrams, 2006).

CONCLUSION

The theme in this chapter is that advances in information technology have enabled an era of massive change in the ways the global community organizes and communicates. For health care, that world changed the day patients began looking to new media as a way of becoming more actively involved in the stewardship of their own care. The course of that change is still undetermined. The technologies themselves are benign; it is what the scientists, practitioners, governments, and the public do with the technology that will be important. Left unattended, the benefits of the new media may easily be squandered in a cacophony of commercial self-interests, and public health may be abandoned to the chicanery of folk wisdom specialists and snake oil salesmen. Riveted on a new, rigorous communication science, the new system can be used to improve the reach, effectiveness, and efficiency of 21st-century medicine. It can be used to take health care to the next level, ensuring progress against the most perplexing public health challenges in ways that benefit the global community.

REFERENCES

Abrams, D. B. (2006). Applying transdisciplinary research strategies to understanding and eliminating health disparities. *Health Education and Behavior, 33*(4), 515–531.

Arora, N. K., Hesse, B. W., Rimer, B. K., Viswanath, K., Clayman, M. L., & Croyle, R. T. (2007). Frustrated and confused: The American public rates its cancer-related information-seeking experiences. *Journal of General Internal Medicine, 23*(3), 223–228.

Atienza, A. A., Hesse, B. W., Baker, T. B., Abrams, D. B., Rimer, B. K., Croyle, R. T., et al. (2007). Critical issues in eHealth research. *American Journal of Preventive Medicine, 32*(5 Suppl.), S71–74.

Baker, D. W., Wolf, M. S., Feinglass, J., Thompson, J. A., Gazmararian, J. A., & Huang, J. (2007). Health literacy and mortality among elderly persons. *Archives of Internal Medicine, 167*(14), 1503–1509.

Bardini, T. (2000). *Bootstrapping: Douglas Engelbart, coevolution, and the origins of personal computing.* Stanford, CA: Stanford University Press.

Beckjord, E. B., Finney Rutten, L. J., Squiers, L., Arora, N. K., Volckmann, L., Moser, R. P., et al. (2007). Use of the Internet to communicate with health care providers in the United States: Estimates from the 2003 and 2005 Health Information National Trends Surveys (HINTS). *Journal of Medical Internet Research, 9*(3), e20.

Berland, G. K., Elliott, M. N., Morales, L. S., Algazy, J. I., Kravitz, R. L., Broder, M. S., et al. (2001). Health information on the Internet: Accessibility, quality, and readability in English and Spanish. *Journal of the American Medical Association, 285*(20), 2612–2621.

Bernard, S. (2005, April 18). The perfect prescription: How the pill bottle was remade—sensibly and beautifully. *New York Magazine.* Retrieved January 19, 2007, from http://nymag.com/nymetro/health/features/11700/

Berners-Lee, T., & Fischetti, M. (1999). *Weaving the Web: The original design and ultimate destiny of the World Wide Web by its inventor.* San Francisco: HarperSanFrancisco.

A better pill bottle from Target. (2005). *Consumer Reports, 70*(8), 7.

Bhattacharya, J., Choudhry, K., & Lakdawalla, D. (2008). Chronic disease and severe disability among working-age populations. *Medical Care, 46*(1), 92–100.

Brailer, D. (2005). Action through collaboration: A conversation with David Brailer. *Health Affairs, 24*(5), 1150–1157.

Brown, J. (Interviewer). (2006, October 19). NBC Universal undergoes restructuring that will cut 700 at the network. *NewsHour with Jim Lehrer* [Television broadcast]. New York and Washington, DC: Public Broadcasting Services.

Burrington-Brown, J., & Friedman, B. (2005). Educating the public about personal health records. *Journal of AHIMA, 76*(9), 94–95.

Cayton, H. (2006). The flat-pack patient? Creating health together. *Patient Education and Counseling, 62*(3), 288–290.

Centers for Disease Control and Prevention. (1999). Decline in deaths from heart disease and stroke—United States, 1900–1999. *Journal of the American Medical Association, 282*(8), 724–726.

Chantler, C. (1999). The role and education of doctors in the delivery of health care. *Lancet, 353*(9159), 1178–1181.

Collins, J. C. (2001). *Good to great: Why some companies make the leap—and others don't.* New York: HarperBusiness.

Conn, J. (2007). Health 2.0: The next generation of Web enterprises. *Modern Health Care Online.* Retrieved December 20, 2007, from http://www.modernhealthcare.com/apps/pbcs.dll/article?AID=/20071211/FREE/312110003/1029/FREE

Creamer, M. (2006). *P&G CEO to ANA: Just let go; A. G. Lafley tells marketers to cede control to consumers to be "in touch."* Retrieved January 13, 2008, from http://adage.com/ana06/article?article_id=112311

Crounse, B. (2007). The newspaper, the wristwatch, and the clinician. *American Journal of Preventive Medicine, 32*(5 Suppl.), S134.

Crowston, K., Sawyer, S., Wigand, R., & Allbritton, M. (2000). How do information and communication technologies reshape work? Evidence from the residential real estate industry. *In Proceedings of the International Conference on Information Systems* (pp. 612–617). Brisbane, Queensland, Australia.

Croyle, R. T., & Hunt, J. R. (1991). Coping with health threat: Social influence processes in reactions to medical test results. *Journal of Personality and Social Psychology, 60*(3), 382–389.

Culliton, B. J. (2006). Extracting knowledge from science: A conversation with Elias Zerhouni. *Health Affairs, 25*(3), w94–w103.

D'Alessandro, D. M., Kreiter, C. D., Kinzer, S. L., & Peterson, M. W. (2004). A randomized controlled trial of an information prescription for pediatric patient education on the Internet. *Archives of Pediatric Adolescent Medicine, 158*(9), 857–862.

Daniels, M., & Hill, A. B. (1952). Chemotherapy of pulmonary tuberculosis in young adults: An analysis of the combined results of three Medical Research Council trials. *British Medical Journal, 1*(4769), 1162–1168.

Davis, T. C., Wolf, M. S., Bass, P. F., III, Thompson, J. A., Tilson, H. H., Neuberger, M., et al. (2006). Literacy and misunderstanding prescription drug labels. *Annals of Internal Medicine, 145*(12), 887–894.

Deci, E. L., & Ryan, R. M. (2000). The "what" and "why" of goal pursuits: Human needs and the self-determination of behavior. *Psychological Inquiry, 11*(4), 227–268.

Deci, E. L., & Ryan, R. M. (2002). *Handbook of self-determination research.* Rochester, NY: University of Rochester Press.

Deci, E. L., & Vansteenkiste, M. (2004). Self-determination theory and basic need satisfaction: Understanding human development in positive psychology. *Ricerche di Psicologia, 27*(1), 23–40.

Dentzer, S. (Writer). (2001). Health on the Web. *NewsHour with Jim Lehrer* [Television broadcast]. New York and Washington, DC: Public Broadcasting Services.

Eng, T. R., & Gustafson, D. H. (1999). *Wired for health and well-being: The emergence of interactive health communication.* Washington, DC: Office of Disease Prevention and Health Promotion, U.S. Department of Health and Human Services.

Eng, T. R., Maxfield, A., Patrick, K., Deering, M. J., Ratzan, S. C., & Gustafson, D. H. (1998). Access to health information and support: A public highway or a private road? *Journal of the American Medical Association, 280*(15), 1371–1375.

Engelbart, D. C. (1962). *Augmenting human intellect: A conceptual framework* [Summary report]. Palo Alto, CA: Stanford Research Institute.

Epstein, R., & Street, R. (2007). *Patient-centered communication in cancer care: Promoting healing and reducing suffering* (NIH Publication No. 07–6225). Bethesda, MD: National Cancer Institute.

Fox, S. (2007). *E-patients with a disability or chronic disease.* Washington, DC: Pew Internet & American Life Project.

Fox, S., & Rainie, L. (2002). *Vital decisions: How Internet users decide what information to trust when they or their loved ones are sick.* Unpublished manuscript, Washington DC.

Friedman, S. M., Dunwoody, S., & Rogers, C. L. (Eds.). (1999). *Communicating uncertainty: Media coverage of new and controversial science.* Mahwah, NJ: Erlbaum.

Friedman, T. L. (2007). *The world is flat: A brief history of the twenty-first century* (Rev. ed.). New York: Picador.

Frost, K., Frank, E., & Maibach, E. (1997). Relative risk in the news media: A quantification of misrepresentation. *American Journal of Public Health, 87*(5), 842–845.

Garcia-Lizana, F., & Sarria-Santamera, A. (2007). New technologies for chronic disease management and control: A systematic review. *Journal of Telemed Telecare, 13*(2), 62–68.

Grantham, C. E., & Carr, J. A. (2002). *Consumer evolution: Nine effective strategies for driving business growth.* New York: Wiley.

Grantham, C. E., & Nichols, L. D. (1993). *The digital workplace: Designing groupware platforms.* New York: Van Nostrand Reinhold.

Haynes, R., Yao, X., Degani, A., Kripalani, S., Garg, A., & McDonald, H. (2005). Interventions for enhancing medication adherence (review). *Cochrane Collaboration, 4.*

Hesse, B. W. (2005). Harnessing the power of an intelligent health environment in cancer control. *Studies in Health Technology and Informatics, 118,* 159–176.

Hesse, B. W., & Grantham, C. E. (1991). The emergence of electronically distributed work communities: Implications for research on Telework. *Electronic Networks: Research Applications and Policy, 1*(1), 4–17.

Hesse, B. W., Nelson, D. E., Kreps, G. L., Croyle, R. T., Arora, N. K., Rimer, B. K., et al. (2005). Trust and sources of health information: The impact of the Internet and its implications for health care providers: Findings from the first Health Information National Trends Survey. *Archives of Internal Medicine, 165*(22), 2618–2624.

Hesse, B. W., & Shneiderman, B. (2007). eHealth research from the user's perspective. *American Journal of Preventive Medicine, 32*(5 Suppl.), S97–103.

Hesse, B. W., Werner, C. W., & Altman, I. (1988). Temporal aspects of computer-mediated communication. *Computers in Human Behavior, 4*(2), 147–165.

Institute of Medicine. (2001). *Crossing the quality chasm: A new health system for the 21st century.* Washington, DC: National Academy Press.

Johnson, J. D. (1997). *Cancer-related information seeking.* Cresskill, NJ: Hampton Press.

Kemper, D. W., & Mettler, M. (2002). *Information therapy: Prescribed information as a reimbursable medical service.* Boise, ID: Healthwise.

Kiesler, S. (1997). *Culture of the Internet.* Mahwah, NJ: Erlbaum.

Kiesler, S., & Sproull, L. (1987). *Computing and change on campus.* New York: Cambridge University Press.

Kreps, G. L., & Thornton, B. C. (1992). *Health communication: Theory & practice* (2nd ed.). Prospect Heights, IL: Waveland Press.

Magai, C., Consedine, N., Neugut, A. I., & Hershman, D. L. (2007). Common psychosocial factors underlying breast cancer screening and breast cancer treatment adherence: A conceptual review and synthesis. *Journal of Women's Health, 16*(1), 11–23.

Markoff, J. (2005). *What the dormouse said—: How the sixties counterculture shaped the personal computer industry.* New York: Viking.

Mazur, D. J. (2003). *The new medical conversation: Media, patients, doctors, and the ethics of scientific communication.* Lanham, MD: Rowman & Littlefield.

Napolli, P. M. (2001). Consumer use of medical information from electronic and paper media: A literature review. In R. E. Rice & J. E. Katz (Eds.), *The Internet and health communication: Experiences and expectations* (pp. 79–98). Thousand Oaks, CA: Sage.

National Science Foundation. (2007). *Cyberinfrastructure vision for 21st century discovery* (No. NSF 07–28). Arlington, VA: Author.

Nelson, D. E., Kreps, G. L., Hesse, B. W., Croyle, R. T., Willis, G., Arora, N. K., et al. (2004). The Health Information National Trends Survey (HINTS): Development, design, and dissemination. *Journal of Health Communication, 9*(5), 443–460.

Niederdeppe, J., & Levy, A. G. (2007). Fatalistic beliefs about cancer prevention and three prevention behaviors. *Cancer Epidemiology Biomarkers and Prevention, 16*(5), 998–1003.

Nielsen-Bohlman, L., & Institute of Medicine Committee on Health Literacy. (2004). *Health literacy: A prescription to end confusion.* Washington, DC: National Academies Press.

O'Reilly, T. (2005). *What is Web 2.0? Design patterns and business models for the next generation of software.* Retrieved January 19, 2008, from http://www.oreillynet. com/pub/a/oreilly/tim/news/2005/09/30/what-is-web-20.html

Paasche-Orlow, M. K., Schillinger, D., Greene, S. M., & Wagner, E. H. (2006). How health care systems can begin to address the challenge of limited literacy. *Journal of General Internal Medicine, 21*(8), 884–887.

Parker, R. M., Baker, D. W., Williams, M. V., & Nurss, J. R. (1995). The test of functional health literacy in adults: A new instrument for measuring patients' literacy skills. *Journal General Internal Medicine, 10*(10), 537–541.

Pew Charitable Trust. (2007). *Percentage of U.S. adults online.* Retrieved August 5, 2008, from http://www.pewinternet.org/trends/Internet_Adoption_3.18.08.pdf

Pew Research Center. (2005). *Trends 2005: Information for the public interest.* Washington, DC: Author.

President's Cancer Panel. (2007). *Promoting healthy lifestyles: Policy, program, and personal recommendations for reducing cancer risk.* Washington, DC: U.S. Department of Health and Human Services.

Prochaska, J. J., Teherani, A., & Hauer, K. E. (2007). Medical students' use of the stages of change model in tobacco cessation counseling. *Journal of General Internal Medicine, 22*(2), 223–227.

Quam, L., Smith, R., & Yach, D. (2006). Rising to the global challenge of the chronic disease epidemic. *Lancet, 368*(9543), 1221–1223.

Royal Institution of Great Britain. (2001). *Guidelines on science and health communication.* London: Author.

Rutten, L. J., Moser, R. P., Beckjord, E. B., Hesse, B. W., & Croyle, R. T. (2007). *Cancer communication: Health information national trends survey* (NIH Pub. No. 07–6214). Bethesda, MD: National Cancer Institute.

Saul, J. E., Schillo, B. A., Evered, S., Luxenberg, M. G., Kavanaugh, A., Cobb, N., et al. (2007). Impact of a statewide Internet-based tobacco cessation intervention. *Journal of Medical Internet Research, 9*(3), e28.

Seligman, M. E. P., Rashid, T., & Parks, A. C. (2006). Positive psychotherapy. *American Psychologist, 61*(8), 774–788.

Shenk, D. (1997). *Data smog: Surviving the information glut.* San Francisco: Harper Edge.

Shneiderman, B. (2002). *Leonardo's laptop: Human needs and the new computing technologies.* Cambridge, MA: MIT Press.

Sproull, L., & Kiesler, S. (1991). *Connections: New ways of working in the networked organization.* Cambridge, MA: MIT Press.

Stokols, D., Montero, M., Bechtel, R. B., & Churchman, A. (2002). Toward an environmental psychology of the Internet. In R. Bechtel & A. Churchman (Eds.), *Handbook of environmental psychology* (pp. 661–675). Hoboken, NJ: John Wiley & Sons.

Strecher, V. (2007). Internet methods for delivering behavioral and health-related interventions (eHealth). *Annual Review of Clinical Psychology, 3,* 53–76.

Strong, K., Mathers, C., Epping-Jordan, J., & Beaglehole, R. (2006). Preventing chronic disease: A priority for global health. *International Journal of Epidemiology, 35*(2), 492–494.

Taylor, S. E., Aspinwall, L. G., Costa, P. T., Jr., & VandenBos, G. R. (1996). Psychosocial aspects of chronic illness. In P. T. Costa Jr. & G. R. VandenBos (Eds.), *Psychological aspects of serious illness: Chronic conditions, fatal diseases, and clinical care* (pp. 3–60). Washington, DC: American Psychological Association.

Taylor, S. E., Falke, R. L., Shoptaw, S. J., & Lichtman, R. R. (1986). Social support, support groups, and the cancer patient. *Journal of Consult Clinical Psychology, 54*(5), 608–615.

Thomas, K. G., Thomas, M. R., Stroebel, R. J., McDonald, F. S., Hanson, G. J., Naessens, J. M., et al. (2007). Use of a registry-generated audit, feedback, and patient reminder intervention in an internal medicine resident clinic—a randomized trial. *Journal of General Internal Medicine, 22*(12), 1740–1744.

Toffler, A. (1990). *Powershift: Knowledge, wealth, and violence at the edge of the 21st century.* New York: Bantam Books.

Toffler, A., & Toffler, H. (1993). *War and anti-war: Survival at the dawn of the 21st century.* Boston: Little, Brown.

U.S. National Library of Medicine. (2007). *Fact sheet: Medline.* Retrieved January 5, 2008, from http://www.nlm.nih.gov/pubs/factsheets/medline.html

Viswanath, K. (2005). Science and society: The communications revolution and cancer control. *Nature Reviews Cancer, 5*(10), 828–835.

Wagner, E. H. (2004). Chronic disease care. *British Medical Journal, 328*(7433), 177–178.

Weinstein, N. D., Lyon, J. E., Sandman, P. M., & Cuite, C. L. (1998). Experimental evidence for stages of health behavior change: The precaution adoption process model applied to home radon testing. *Health Psychology, 17*(5), 445–453.

Westfall, J. M., Mold, J., & Fagnan, L. (2007). Practice-based research—"blue highways" on the NIH roadmap. *Journal of the American Medical Association, 297*(4), 403–406.

Whorf, B. L. (1956). *Language, thought, and reality: Selected writings.* Cambridge, MA: Technology Press of Massachusetts Institute of Technology.

Wilson, C. B. (1999). Sensors 2010. *British Medical Journal, 319*(7220), 1288.

Wofford, J. L., Smith, E. D., & Miller, D. P. (2005). The multimedia computer for office-based patient education: A systematic review. *Patient Education and Counseling, 59*(2), 148–157.

Woloshin, S., & Schwartz, L. M. (2006). Media reporting on research presented at scientific meetings: More caution needed. *Medical Journal of Australia, 184*(11), 576–580.

World Health Organization. (2006). *Preventing chronic diseases: A vital investment.* Geneva, Switzerland: Author.

Zuboff, S. (1988). *In the age of the smart machine: The future of work and power.* New York: Basic Books.

Zuboff, S., & Maxmin, J. (2002). *The support economy: Why corporations are failing individuals and the next episode of capitalism.* New York: Viking.

7

E-Health Self-Care Interventions for Persons With Chronic Illnesses: Review and Future Directions

ROBERT L. GLUECKAUF AND MIA LIZA A. LUSTRIA

The growing complexity of today's health care environment has made it increasingly important for consumers to take a more active role in making health decisions and in self-care management. This is particularly urgent for the 1 in 10 Americans who have debilitating chronic conditions, such as diabetes, heart disease, and mental illness. Chronic illnesses cost the United States approximately $1.3 trillion annually—of this amount, $1.1 trillion per year is associated with lost productivity and $277 billion is spent on treatment (DeVol et al., 2007). Since the prevalence of chronic conditions tends to increase with age, these figures are estimated to increase exponentially as the baby boomer generation ages (Garrett & Martini, 2007; Thorpe, 2006).

Active engagement in self-management strategies is critical for the treatment and effective long-term care of chronic diseases (Bodenheimer, Lorig, Holman, & Grumbach, 2002; Woolf et al., 2005). Effective self-management hinges not only on promoting informed decision making, but also on engaging individuals with chronic illnesses collaboratively in their own care through the development of problem-solving skills and coping strategies (Bodenheimer et al., 2002). There is a growing body of research supporting the importance of the role of patient-centered care for long-term illness on a number of health outcomes, such as reduced hospital visits, improved coping, improved quality of life, disease control, and reduced risk for complications (Del Sindaco et al., 2007; Gately, Rogers, & Sanders, 2007; Hurley et al., 2007; Kennedy et al., 2007; Lorig, Ritter, Laurent, & Fries, 2004; McManus et al., 2005; Monninkhof et al., 2004; Richardson et al., 2006; Smeulders, van Haastregt, van Hoef, van Eijk, & Kempen, 2006; Strong, Von Korff, Saunders, & Moore, 2006; Williams et al., 2004; Wilson & Mayor, 2006). Key components of effective self-management include the development of behavioral skills in performing recommended strategies for optimal health (e.g., blood pressure monitoring, glucose monitoring, exercise, and problem-solving skills), as well as adherence to treatment regimens (Bodenheimer et al., 2002; Del Sindaco et al., 2007; C. Griffiths et al., 2005; Hurley et al., 2007; Kennedy et al., 2003; Lamers, Jonkers, Bosma, Diederiks, & van Eijk, 2006; Lorig et al., 2004; McCarthy et al., 2004; McManus et al., 2005; Richardson et al., 2006; Strong et al., 2006).

Telecommunication technologies, especially Internet- and telephone-based systems, have the ability to extend the reach of self-management education programs to individuals with chronic illnesses in a number of ways. Both the Internet and telephone are viable and low-cost media that can be used to access health information and health care services and are capable of overcoming geographic and time barriers. Despite ongoing concerns about the quality of health information and accessibility of tele-communication-mediated resources, a growing number of individuals with chronic illnesses are going online to seek information about specific diseases and their treatment, as well as to do research on prescription and over-the-counter drugs (Fox, 2007). The Pew Internet & American Life Project reported in 2007 that 86% of Internet users with a disability or chronic illness went online to research at least 1 of 17 health topics (Fox, 2007). This information influenced their medical decision making, led them to ask more questions of their providers, enhanced their ability to cope with chronic illness, and changed the way they thought about and managed their diet, nutrition, and physical activities (Fox, 2007; T. H. Wagner, Baker, Bundorf, & Singer, 2004). Persons with stigmatized diseases (e.g., HIV/AIDS, epilepsy, mental illness) find the Internet and telephone particularly appealing due to the increased privacy they offer for discussing sensitive, often taboo topics in a "safe, non-judgmental" environment (Berger, Wagner, & Baker, 2005). Caregivers of individuals with chronic illnesses also use the Internet and telephone to seek support with others going through similar experiences (Lasker, Sogolow, & Sharim, 2005; Patsos, 2001; Rossi et al., 2006; Stakisaitis, Spokiene, Juskevicius, Valuckas, & Baiardi, 2007).

The primary objectives of this chapter are to conduct a review of e-health outcome research on persons with chronic illnesses and to highlight issues that require further attention and development. First, specific procedures and inclusionary criteria used in performing the current review are described. Second, the findings of randomized controlled trials on the effects of e-health interventions on health status, and in influencing health-promoting activities, and psychosocial functioning are analyzed. Third, key conceptual and methodological problems that limit the validity, generalizability, and utility of e-health outcome research are delineated. Finally, the practice implications of e-health intervention studies are addressed.

METHODOLOGY

An extensive search of e-health outcome interventions published from 2002 to 2007 in peer-reviewed journals across three databases, Medline, PsycINFO, and CINAHL, was performed. The descriptors used in our search queries were as follows: "World Wide Web," "Internet," "telephone," "health," "intervention," "randomized controlled trial," cancer," "depression," "diabetes," "cardiovascular disease," "obesity," and "chronic disease." Titles and abstracts of studies retrieved in the initial search then were examined for relevance. This process facilitated a reduction of the list to a total of 150 Internet and 393 telephone studies. These articles were obtained and subsequently subjected to a more thorough qualitative review. We formulated strict exclusion and inclusion criteria to guide selection of relevant articles in order to minimize selection bias. These criteria are summarized in Table 7.1.

The authors coded the articles independently, and the results were compared for accuracy. Any disparities in judgment that emerged during the coding process were resolved through discussion and consensual agreement. Of the 543 potentially relevant studies, only 27 Internet- and 44 telephone-based articles satisfied all four inclusion criteria.

RESULTS

Telecommunication and Technology-Based Health Interventions

What makes e-health interventions appealing to people with chronic illnesses and health educators? Cassel et al. (1998) aptly described the

Table 7.1

INCLUSION CRITERIA FOR SYSTEMATIC REVIEW

INCLUSION CRITERIA	OPERATIONAL DEFINITION
1. Contained a substantial e-health intervention component	The intervention must have had a substantial e-health component in that the major delivery mode must have been either via telephone, videoconferencing, or via the Web (e.g., Web site, e-mail, online discussion group).
2. Focused on patients with a chronic illness	The intervention had to be focused on individuals diagnosed with a chronic, recurrent condition or illness (e.g., diabetes, cancer, cardiovascular disease, PTSD) for an average of 1 year. Studies that focused primarily on caregivers of individuals with chronic illnesses were excluded. Studies that largely focused on prevention and targeted a general sample population were also excluded (e.g., anti-smoking, alcoholism, eating disorders, physical activity).
3. Focused on self-management	The intervention must have been focused on self-management. This included studies that actively involved patients in decision making and treatment planning and that focused on developing strategies to improve health outcomes (e.g., cognitive-behavioral therapy that has a problem-solving component or focuses on adherence), personalized planning and treatment, and patient feedback or tracking of target outcomes (e.g., through journaling, discussion groups/forums, communication with experts and peers).
4. Randomized controlled trial	Only studies that used true experimental designs (i.e., random assignment to conditions and at least one control group) were included in the review.

Internet as a "hybrid channel" that combines the broad reach of mass communication channels with the persuasive capabilities of interpersonal channels. Synchronous Web technologies such as chat and computer conferencing allow real-time interactions that approach the reflexivity of face-to-face encounters (Street, 2003). Games, simulations, and other interactive online activities can be used to model healthy behaviors and teach proper management and prevention skills in engaging environments (Walther, Pingree, Hawkins, & Buller, 2005). Web delivery also allows for the presentation of information in a variety of formats (e.g., graphics, audio, video) to suit different learning styles and literacy levels.

The power of Web technologies for supporting self-help behavioral interventions, however, largely rests in the ability to automate delivery of self-regulatory tools tailored to meet particular patients' needs. Computerized implementation of theory-based approaches for changing individual health behaviors has become more sophisticated over the years as we continue to learn about what Web features contribute the most to efficacy.

Although Web-based technologies have the distinct advantage of simulating real-time, face-to-face transactions, interventions using these applications have been restricted to community organizations and to individuals who have the financial resources to afford computers and Internet access. Populations that are economically disadvantaged and those who live in rural communities typically have not been included in Web-based health care intervention studies. Furthermore, persons with chronic illnesses, especially those over 60 with low technology comfort and skill, may be reluctant to use the Internet to participate in e-health clinical trials. Thus, the telephone provides a low-cost, easy-to-use, and universally available option for delivering health care information and services.

The overall findings of this review indicate that technology-based delivery of self-care programs for managing chronic illnesses is a viable alternative to traditional methods of delivery (see Table 7.2 at the end of the chapter for a summary). The majority of studies reported that e-health intervention was significantly more effective than routine medical care. Lack of success was largely due to problems of engagement, with high attrition rates. The majority of the studies showed positive results on target health outcomes or were partially successful (e.g., reported positive or improved outcomes only on some targeted outcomes). The following section reviews e-health outcome studies in four major categories: mental health conditions, diabetes, cardiac-related disorders, and other chronic illnesses. Within each category, we focus separately on the findings of Web-based and telephone-based interventions.

Telecommunications-Based Self-Care Intervention for Mental Health Conditions

Eleven of 71 telecommunication-based outcome studies focused on mental health: 6 in the area of depression, 3 on panic disorder, and 1 each in the areas of posttraumatic stress disorder and complicated grief. Technology-based delivery is especially promising for this health context for several reasons. The privacy of Web- and telephone-based delivery encourages open communication about topics participants may feel uneasy discussing freely face-to-face. Telecommunication-based delivery also has the potential of increasing people's access to a limited pool of skilled mental health professionals trained in evidence-based therapies (e.g., cognitive-behavioral therapy or interpersonal therapy). These modalities have the distinct advantage of bringing together peers with similar stigmatizing conditions across different geographic locations and walks of life, thus increasing their exposure to positive role models and creative problem-solving efforts (C. M. Andersson, Bjaras, Tillgren, & Ostenson, 2005; K. M. Griffiths & Christensen, 2006; T. H. Wagner et al., 2004). Computing technology, particularly Web-based applications, can also facilitate automation of routine aspects of therapy, such as patient assessment and monitoring and gathering of patient feedback, all of which can be conducted either synchronously or asynchronously.

Results of Web-Based Mental Health Interventions

Similar to the findings of Griffiths and Christensen (2006), our review revealed an overall positive pattern of results for Web-based mental health interventions. Six of the seven Web-based psycho-educational interventions for persons with mental health conditions reported success on all or most of the targeted outcomes. One trial found no significant effects of the Web-based program on participants' depressive symptoms; the authors of the article attributed their null findings to lack of participant engagement and limited contact with therapists (see Clarke et al., 2002).

Web-based mental health outcome studies relied heavily on multimodal methods of delivery using a combination of educational Web sites, online discussion forums, and minimal mediated contact with experts either via phone or e-mail. Only Wagner et al. (2006) used a single intervention modality (i.e., e-mail communication). Improvements in targeted symptoms (e.g., depressive symptoms and panic attacks) were ascribed to participant self-management through the use of a combination of cognitive-behavioral training, coping and stress management exercises, journaling, and feedback. Feedback was provided through moderated discussion forums and mediated contact with an expert either via phone or e-mail. Lack of engagement and high dropout rates were observed in studies that lacked substantial feedback mechanisms or contact with experts (e.g., Clark, 2002). This concern was highlighted in two randomized controlled trials of ODIN (Overcoming Depression on the Internet), a Web-based self-help program designed to reduce depression among individuals suffering from mild to moderate depression. In the first trial of ODIN, Clarke (2002) found that only patients with low baseline levels of depression showed modest improvements in depressive symptoms following treatment in the Web intervention. Clarke attributed this finding to limited participant engagement with the purely self-help Web-based program. This problem was mitigated in a subsequent randomized controlled trial of ODIN (Clarke et al., 2005). In this trial, participation in the online cognitive-behavior self-help therapy program was boosted through the use of reminders delivered via e-mail and postcards. As a result, participants in the treatment group showed significantly greater improvements in depressive symptoms than those in the control group. There were no significant between-subject differences based on the type of reminder provided.

Although the ODIN trials provided evidence for the efficacy of purely self-help online programs, the provision of even minimal therapist feedback via e-mail was shown to boost the effects of treatment on target outcomes. For example, Andersson (2005) found that participants exposed to a self-help Web site and moderated online discussion group with minimal therapist feedback showed significantly greater improvements in mental health outcomes than a comparison group with no therapist contact. The incremental effect of minimal therapist contact in an online cognitive-behavioral self-help program was likewise tested by Klein et al. (2005), who compared three groups: an information-only control group, Web-based cognitive behavioral treatment for agoraphobia with e-mail expert support, and Web-based cognitive-behavioral treatment without e-mail support. They found both cognitive-behavioral approaches were effective in improving physical health ratings and reducing physician visits compared to the control condition. Furthermore, attrition rates were lowest among participants who had access to minimal therapist contact via e-mail.

Results of Telephone-Based Mental Health Interventions

Similar to the findings of Web-based mental health interventions, telephone-based cognitive-behavioral approaches showed significantly greater improvements on target outcomes from baseline to follow-up than those of routine medical care. All four telephone-based outcome studies showed significant positive effects across several mental health outcomes.

It should be noted, however, that participants in telephone interventions typically had fewer options for seeking out mental health information and interactions with peers than their Web-based counterparts. Telephone protocols included an educational workbook focusing on self-care skills (e.g., exercise and socialization) and ongoing medication management, as well as one-on-one telephone-based cognitive-behavioral intervention with an experienced clinician emphasizing the development of problem-solving skills, relapse prevention, effective thinking, and the need to increase pleasant daily activities. The modal number of individual sessions was 12, each lasting approximately 15 to 30 minutes. In contrast, Web-based interventions included educational Web sites, online discussion forums, and e-mail contact with experts. However, direct contact with therapists over the telephone was generally more time intensive than that offered by Web-based interventions.

The outcomes of the four telephone-based mental health interventions were uniformly positive. Across the three depression treatment studies (Dietrich et al., 2004; Hunkeler et al., 2006; Simon, Ludman, Tutty, Operskalski, & Korff, 2004), participants who received telephone-based training showed significantly greater decreases in depressive symptoms from baseline to follow-up than routine care controls (i.e., pharmacotherapy and routine office visits). In the one study on anxiety disorders (i.e., generalized anxiety and panic disorder), significantly greater reductions in anxiety and depression were obtained in the telephone-based cognitive-behavioral intervention than in the routine care group (Rollman et al., 2005).

Although the findings of telephone-based mental health intervention outcome studies were promising, three of four studies used a single routine care control condition, thus limiting the strength of causal conclusions about the benefits of telephone-based cognitive-behavioral therapy. It is entirely plausible that increased contact with treatment staff in itself may have resulted in differential improvements in the telephone interventions. However, in the one study that used a contact control group, Simon et al. (2004) found that the telephone care management had significantly smaller effects on improvement in depressive symptoms and patient satisfaction than the telephone-based cognitive-behavioral intervention program. Thus, preliminary evidence was obtained supporting the incremental advantages of telephone-based mental health intervention in reducing depression in patients with diagnosable mental health problems over standard treatment and follow-up. Future outcome research in this domain needs to incorporate control conditions that permit the testing of alternative rival hypotheses for the benefits of e-health treatment.

Diabetes Management via Telecommunication-Based Self-Help Programs

In recent years, Web and telephone delivery of self-management programs have emerged as popular approaches to the management of diabetes. Self-management is particularly important for individuals with diabetes, given the complexity of the disease and the numerous comorbid conditions associated with it. In order to successfully manage their disease, diabetes patients must not only take medications and maintain a healthy lifestyle but also monitor a number of variables (i.e., blood glucose values, blood pressure, cholesterol levels, weight, food intake, and physical activity) in order to reduce risk factors. As a result, Web- and telephone-based interventions focused on diabetes self-management are more complex than others, and most have, in addition to an educational component, built-in self-regulatory activities such as tools for uploading and monitoring blood glucose levels or means for calculating food intake or body mass index, strategies for enhancing adherence to the diabetes regimen, and message framing to tailor treatment to the specific needs of the individual with diabetes.

Fourteen of the 71 articles reviewed here focused on diabetes self-management. Seven were primarily Web-based, and 7 were telephone-based interventions. In contrast to the self-care interventions for mental health, the proportion of diabetes studies reporting positive outcomes was substantially lower, particularly among those that were telephone-based interventions. Of the 14 studies, 8 showed incremental benefits for the telecommunication-based approaches, whereas the remainder reported null findings. There was also a substantial discrepancy between the outcomes of Web- and telephone-based interventions. Six of 7 Web-based studies showed positive effects, whereas only 2 of 7 telephone interventions led to substantial changes on key outcomes, such as HbA_{1c} levels. In addition, problems with participant engagement and retention were noted across both intervention modalities.

Results of Web-Based Diabetes Self-Care Management Studies

Web-based diabetes intervention programs typically included (1) instructional support for patients via letters advocating lifestyle modification; (2) physician and/or patient education on the importance of taking medication, how to read medical instructions, and how to organize medication regimens, as well as structural supports such as regular reminders from providers either during routine visits or via phone or mail; (3) information on how to collect blood glucose levels at different times in the day to help identify peaks in glycemic levels as well as to help monitor triggers; and (4) tailoring of health messages to suit the unique needs, information-processing styles, and stages of disease, culture, values, and risk factors of individual patients. Tailored materials have been shown to be more effective in motivating patients to make general dietary changes (e.g., increase intake of fruit and vegetables and to reduce intake of dietary fat) than non-tailored materials (Brug, Oenema, & Campbell, 2003; Brug, Oenema, Kroeze, & Raat, 2005; De Bourdeaudhuij & Brug, 2000; Kroeze, Werkman, & Brug, 2006; Oenema, Brug, & Lechner, 2001; Oenema, Tan, & Brug, 2005).

In their conceptually driven investigation, McKay et al. (2002) and Glasgow et al. (2003) tested the efficacy of D-Net, a Web-based diabetes self-management intervention, on a group of older Type 2 diabetes patients. The first trial involved testing the efficacy of four interventions on a subset of patients ($n = 160$). The first group was an information-only control. The second group received individualized feedback through computer-mediated access to a coach trained to provide personalized dietary advice. In addition, participants were able to input their daily intake of fruits, vegetables, and saturated fats and graph this information. This allowed them to receive real-time feedback and track their progress. The third group had access to a peer-directed (but professionally moderated) online support group that allowed them to exchange diabetes-related information, coping strategies, and emotional support. Participants also had access to a more structured conference area that featured targeted forums on particular topic areas. The final group received combined interventions 3 months after the trial. The second trial tested the same conditions on a larger group ($N = 320$) 10 months after the original trial. All conditions demonstrated moderate success at 3 months as well as at 10 months on targeted behavioral, psycho-social, and some biological outcomes. There were no significant differences between the groups, although the group receiving tailored self-management had the lowest overall cholesterol levels. The addition of tailoring and peer support did not seem to significantly improve Web use or engagement over time. Logons to the D-Net Web site gradually decreased beginning in the third month of the trial, and the lowest usage was observed during months 7 to 10 (Glasgow et al., 2003).

The remaining four Web-based diabetes management interventions reported more positive results and better engagement overall than the D-Net studies (see Cho et al., 2006; C. Kim et al., 2007; Kwon et al., 2004; Tatti & Lehmann, 2003). The major focus of these studies was support for blood glucose monitoring with substantive feedback from experts to help interpret results of glucose-level values. Tatti and Lehmann's study largely focused on patient education by providing a small group of Type 1 diabetes patients ($n = 24$) with access to AIDA, a free online diabetes simulator. The simulator was used to demonstrate realistic scenarios that might result from different plasma insulin and blood glucose levels. At 6-week follow-up, HbA_{1c} and hypoglycemic episodes (e.g., dizziness, nausea, vomiting) decreased more for the treatment group than for the control.

To address the issue of engagement, Kwon (2004; $n = 110$) and Cho (2006; $n = 80$) tested the effects of a Web-based blood glucose monitoring system after 12 weeks and 30 months, respectively. Participants in each trial had access to an online blood glucose monitoring system as well as trained clinical instructors who, upon reviewing uploaded glucose values, provided stage-based recommendations on a biweekly basis. Significant reductions in HbA_{1c} levels were observed in the treatment group and sustained over time (after 30 months). More notable decreases were observed among participants with HbA_{1c} levels below 7% at baseline than among those with HbA_{1c} levels above 7%. A similar trend was demonstrated by C. Kim et al. (2007; $n = 40$) in a trial testing the efficacy of a Web-based blood glucose monitoring system with tailored medical advice and brief reminders sent through a messaging system. Noteworthy is the fact that all three glucose monitoring systems were tested on a Korean population, which may suggest that the differential compliance rates may be based more on cultural differences than on the intervention itself.

Results of Telephone-Based Diabetes Interventions

Telephone intervention typically provided one-on-one training with a diabetes educator focusing on (1) meal planning, information about diabetes complications, exercise programs, and the risks of smoking and alcohol for people with diabetes; (2) collaborative problem solving to enhance diabetes management; and (3) monitoring insulin, carbohydrate intake, and blood glucose values. Consistent with the findings of the telephone-based mental health outcome studies (see results of Telephone-Based Mental Health Interventions section, p. 158), participants in telephone-based diabetes interventions had access to fewer educational and peer support options than those offered by Web-based diabetes training. Note, also, that the average duration of a diabetes-focused telephone session was substantially shorter than its mental health counterpart.

As mentioned above, 7 of 14 articles used the telephone as the major format for delivering diabetes self-care management to adults and children with diabetes. In contrast to the positive pattern of findings of the Web-based studies, only 2 of 7 telephone-based interventions led to significantly greater improvements on key outcomes than the control groups. Two possible reasons may explain the discrepant pattern of the findings between the two treatment modalities and the limited impact of the telephonic self-care interventions. First, economically disadvantaged and disruptive living conditions were noted more frequently among participants of telephone-based diabetes interventions than among samples of Web-based diabetes interventions. Investigators reported that such living circumstances made it difficult to schedule telephone sessions on a regular basis, leading to high rates of no-shows and cancellations (see, e.g., Krein et al., 2004). This factor may have led to disproportionately lower success rates in telephone-based diabetes outcome studies. A second limiting factor may be the duration of diabetes telephone counseling sessions. Telephone-based diabetes interventions were 7.5 minutes in average length, approximately 50% the duration of a typical telephone-based mental health counseling session. This may have contributed to the substantially weaker effects of this mode of intervention on physiological markers, such as HbA_{1c} and lipid ratios. The third factor was the higher illness severity and comorbidity rates reported in telephone-based diabetes studies. Patients with poor glycemic control and/or comorbidities (e.g., severe hypertension and renal disease) may have presented difficult challenges to telephone interventionists, requiring coordination efforts beyond the scope of their brief 7.5-minute interactions with diabetes participants. Thus, diabetes investigators should take into account potential barriers associated with participants' lifestyles, the logistics of treatment implementation, and illness severity in designing future diabetes telephone-based interventions.

Telecommunications-Based Self-Care Intervention for Cardiac Conditions

Twelve of 71 articles in this review focused on telecommunications-based self-help interventions for adults with cardiac conditions. Eleven studies used the telephone as the primary mode of treatment delivery. Only 1 study evaluated the effects of Web-based cardiac self-care on participants' health functioning (Southard et al., 2003).

Web-Based Self-Care Intervention for Cardiac Conditions

Cardiac rehabilitation and secondary prevention programs have evolved as an accepted therapy for patients of cardiovascular diseases. These programs are endorsed as effective and useful by the American Heart Association and the American College of Cardiology in the treatment of patients with coronary artery disease and chronic heart failure (Balady et al., 2007).

A meta-analysis found that secondary prevention programs positively affect processes of care (reducing risk and improving use of proven efficacious therapies) and quality of life and reduce incidence of myocardial infarctions by 17% over a median follow-up of 12 months (Clark, Hartling, Vandermeer, & McAlister, 2005). Traditional cardiac rehabilitation and secondary prevention programs have evolved from largely exercise-based training programs to more comprehensive and multifaceted interventions with the following core components: baseline patient assessment, nutritional counseling, risk factor management (lipids, blood pressure, weight, diabetes mellitus, and smoking), psychosocial interventions, and physical activity counseling (Balady et al., 2007; Thomas et al., 2007). Delivery of cardiac rehabilitation programs also has evolved from clinic-based outpatient programs to include home-, telephone-, and Web-based delivery approaches.

There was, however, a dearth of Web-based self-care interventions for cardiac rehabilitation found in this review. There are several potential reasons for this. During the initial screening, we discovered that most interventions dealing with cardiovascular disease were preventive in nature. Cardiovascular disease prevention and secondary risk management were often folded into efficacy studies of self-care management interventions for comorbid conditions such as diabetes and cancer. Cardiac rehabilitation services also usually involve more substantial supervision from trained health care professionals, given the vulnerability of patients who are typically referred for such services, for example, following nonfatal heart attack. These interventions were excluded from the current review because of their-less-than substantial self-care components. Even the single Web-based cardiac rehabilitation self-management outcome study included in this study by Southard et al. (2003), while qualifying as self-care, still had significant involvement from a nurse-therapist.

Southard et al. (2003) compared usual care patients to those involved in a 6-month Web-based case management program involving e-mail and telephone contact with a nurse–case manager and dietitian. Self-care components included an online community that enabled patients to communicate through discussion groups and e-mail as well as online assessments, interactive education modules, and dynamic self-monitoring tools. Participants in the intervention group experienced significantly fewer cardiovascular events and greater weight loss than the usual care group. No significant differences in depressive symptoms, blood pressure levels, and dietary habits were found between groups. Significant cost savings ($413 per patient) and a return on investment of 213% were also estimated for the patients assigned to the Web-based intervention. While this study provides preliminary evidence for the efficacy and cost-effectiveness of Web-based cardiac rehabilitation programs, the small sample and limited diversity in the patient sample (e.g., 97% White, 52% with college degree or higher level of education, 64.2% with annual incomes of more than $40,000) limit generalizability of the results.

Telephone-Based Self-Care Intervention for Cardiac Conditions

The diversity of target problems and populations was substantially greater in the cardiac outcome studies than in the diabetes and mental health outcome studies. Of the 11 cardiac studies, 5 evaluated the impact of health failure management, and one each tested the impact of smoking cessation treatment, depression/anxiety reduction training, and self-care management after cardiac rehabilitation, cardiac surgery, implantation of a cardioverter defibrillator, and heart transplantation. Seven studies showed significant differential positive effects for telephone-based intervention, whereas 4 reported no significant post-treatment differences on target outcomes between groups. The remainder of this section will focus on the pattern of results for heart failure management ($n = 5$), the only cardiac intervention category for which a comparison between a minimum of two outcome studies could be performed. The treatment approach typically consisted of health care educator–facilitated training on weight management, diet, and exercise. Participants also were encouraged to discuss over the telephone recent exacerbations of heart failure symptoms, and any concerns they encountered in adhering to their medication regimen and other facets of treatment. The results of the heart failure management studies were mixed. On the positive side, three of five studies (DeWalt et al., 2006; Dunagan et al., 2005; Sisk et al., 2006) reported that telephone-based interventions led to significantly lower rates of hospitalization for older adults with heart failure than did routine care control groups. In contrast, only one study (Sisk et al., 2006) found significant improvements in participants' daily functioning or health-related quality of life from baseline to the 12-month follow-up. This pattern of results has been described in previous reviews (McAlister, Lawson, Teo, & Armstrong, 2001). Traditional face-to-face disease management programs have significantly reduced hospitalization rates for adults with heart failure but have had a less clear impact on quality of life. Various factors such as variations in illness severity and treatment intensity (i.e., amount of direct patient contact) have been proposed in previous studies to account for limited improvement in quality of life in heart failure self-care interventions, but the evidence supporting this hypothesis has been inconsistent (cf., Dunagan et al., 2005).

OTHER ONLINE SELF-HELP PROGRAMS FOR VARIOUS CHRONIC DISEASES

This section discusses the use and efficacy of Web- and telephone-based self-management programs for other chronic diseases. A total of 28 articles focused on a wide range of other health conditions. Eight focused on pulmonary disorders ($n = 8$), 8 on cancer ($n = 8$), and 5 on chronic pain; the remaining 7 articles covered a variety of health conditions (e.g., HIV/AIDS, stroke, multiple sclerosis, and head injury). Although a review of the findings of this wide range of studies is beyond the scope of this chapter, we highlight notable trends and major issues in the use of Internet and telephone modalities in self-care management across these conditions.

Telecommunication-Based Self-Care Intervention for Pulmonary Conditions

Studies of three Web-based interventions and one telephone-based intervention focused on self-management of asthma, all of which had a significant patient education component focusing on understanding asthma and environmental triggers, as well as strategies to control attacks and manage asthma via medication adherence and self-monitoring. Three Web-based studies yielded positive outcomes. In contrast, one telephone-based intervention yielded mixed results. Krishna et al. (2003) evaluated a multimedia interactive educational program on asthma patients and their caregivers through the use of animated vignettes depicting real-life scenarios requiring decisions about alternative behaviors that would likely affect asthma. This educational program resulted in increased asthma knowledge, and concomitant declines in asthma symptom days, emergency visits to physicians, and use of rescue medications. Similarly successful, Jan et al. (2007) tested a telemonitoring approach via the Blue Angel monitoring program. Patients were encouraged to monitor their peak expiratory flows and asthma symptoms daily on the Internet. These values were assessed by their physicians, who then communicated a tailored self-management program to their patients via e-mail and telephone. Joseph et al. (2007) tested the efficacy of Puff-City, a culturally tailored program based on theory-based models that addresses negative asthma management behaviors among African American asthma patients in an urban area. Messages were framed based on users' beliefs, attitudes, and personal barriers to change.

In the one telephone-based self-care intervention, Khan and associates (2004) compared the effects of a comprehensive asthma education program to those of routine asthma care on the development and use of action plans and the frequency of asthma symptoms. The program trained parents to recognize and avoid triggers, to use written asthma action plans, and to seek help as appropriate. On the positive side, the intervention group children were significantly more likely than controls to possess a written asthma action plan. However, no significant differences in post-treatment improvement were found between the intervention and control groups in the frequency of asthma symptoms. Khan and associates attributed this null finding to the unanticipated strength of the usual care condition. Seventy percent of parents in the usual care group had a written asthma action plan at follow-up, and follow-up symptoms in this group were half of baseline values.

Telecommunication-Based Self-Care Intervention for Chronic Pain

Five articles—four on Web-based interventions and one on a telephone-based intervention—focused on self-management of chronic pain. One was on rheumatoid arthritis (van den Berg et al., 2006), one on osteoarthritis (Blixen, Bramstedt, Hammel, & Tilley, 2004); one on chronic back pain (Buhrman, Fältenhag, Ström, & Andersson, 2004), and two on chronic headache (G. Andersson, Lundstrom, & Ström, 2003; Devineni & Blanchard, 2005). The overall findings of the Web-based interventions were promising, with most studies showing significant post-treatment improvement. In contrast, Blixen and associates (2004) found no incremental benefit for telephone intervention on pain complaints.

Web-based interventions involved symptom monitoring and some form of tailored supervision via communication with experts. In addition to these main components, van den Berg and associates (2006) held group meetings every 3 months during the 48-week intervention. During these meetings, patients were able to meet with other group members and got demonstrations of new exercises from physical therapists. Despite this more substantive contact with patients, van den Berg and associates (2006) only reported success on self-reported outcomes (patients' perceptions of their ability to meet physical activity recommendations), but not on actual physical activity as measured by an activity monitor. The other three interventions reported greater success, which might be attributed to a more significant cognitive-behavior therapy component. For example, Devineni and Blanchard (2005) found greater decreases in headache and other symptoms with the treatment group (who received training in significant progressive relaxation, limited biofeedback with autogenic training, and stress management training) than with the wait-list control. While one might argue that minimal therapist contact might be a major contributor to success, Andersson and associates (2003) found no significant incremental effects from the addition of telephone support to a Web-based cognitive-behavior therapy intervention for headache sufferers.

In Blixen and associates' (2004) telephone study, the intervention group received six weekly mailings of osteoarthritis health education modules, a relaxation audiotape, and six weekly 45-minute follow-up telephone self-management sessions. The control group received usual care from their rheumatologists. No significant post-treatment differences were found in pain severity, quality of life, health status, or depression. Only differences in self-efficacy in managing pain were found between the intervention and usual care groups at the 3-month assessment phase. However, this between-group effect was not maintained at the 6-month follow-up.

Telecommunication-Based Self-Care Intervention for Cancer

Eight articles on telecommunication-based cancer care intervention met criteria for inclusion in the review. The two Web-based and three telephone-based interventions focused on self-care management for women with breast cancer. The remaining three telephone-based interventions targeted men with prostate cancer, survivors of childhood cancer, and adult cancer survivors. The remainder of this section will focus on the pattern of findings from five breast cancer intervention studies, the only cancer intervention category for which a comparison between a minimum of two outcome studies could be performed. These breast cancer studies provided coping skills training using two different approaches. Owen and associates (2005) examined the effects of a self-guided online support group for early-stage breast cancer patients over a 12-week period ($n = 62$). Winzeberg and associates (2003) assessed the psychosocial impact of Bosom Buddies, a 12-week Web-based professionally moderated, social support group for breast cancer survivors ($n = 72$). Of the two approaches, Winzelberg and associates' moderated social support group was more efficacious in terms of reducing depression, perceived stress, and cancer-related trauma among breast cancer survivors. Compared to the self-guided online social support group, patients involved with Bosom Buddies viewed the intervention more positively and were more engaged, logging onto the Web site about three times a week and posting an average of three messages per week. Participants in Bosom Buddies used the discussion forum more actively than they did an online journaling tool provided on the same site.

All three telephone-based interventions showed significant incremental benefits for telephone-based intervention over the control conditions. Pinto and associates (2005) studied the effects of a telephone-based moderate-intensity physical activity program on fitness, mood, physical symptoms, and body image in women with breast cancer. The telephone-based intervention group reported significantly more total minutes of physical activities, more minutes of moderate-intensity physical activity, and higher energy expenditure per week than did controls. The intervention group also outperformed controls on a field test of fitness. Mishel and associates (2005) tested the effects of a telephone-based cognitive-behavioral intervention to increase effective coping with the uncertainties of breast cancer in a combined African American and non-Hispanic White sample. The treatment group reported a significant increase in positive cognitive reframing, whereas the routine care control group showed no change from baseline to the 10-month follow-up. There was also a significant treatment-by-ethnicity effect on the women's tendencies to catastrophize about the outcomes of breast cancer. African American women showed a significant decline in catastrophic thinking about breast cancer from baseline to 10 months compared to the control group, which experienced no change over time. In contrast, no substantial differences in the levels of catastrophizing were noted for non-Hispanic White women in both the cognitive-behavioral and routine care condition over time. Finally, Allen and associates (2002) compared the effects of a telephone-based problem-solving training intervention versus usual care on improvement in coping skills for women with breast cancer. The intervention consisted of two in-person and four telephone sessions with an oncology nurse, who provided problem-solving skills training and informational materials to the women over a 12-week period. Women in the problem-solving group reported significantly lower unmet needs and better mental health than usual care participants at the 4-month assessment, but this effect was not maintained at the 8-month assessment. Thus, considerable support was obtained for the efficacy of both Web- and telephone-based intervention for women with breast cancer. Further research is needed to evaluate the effectiveness of telephone-based cognitive-behavioral interventions in routine oncological practice and the cost savings of this approach.

Summary

This review of interventions for self-management of chronic diseases clearly demonstrates the usefulness and efficacy of the use of telecommunication-based modalities for educating patients and helping them manage their diseases. A key issue in the medical management of chronic conditions is the problem of maintaining patient engagement in their own care, which has been addressed in several ways. Tailoring and individualized problem-solving techniques have been used to facilitate the creation of personally relevant health messages and individualized approaches to self-management. When persons with chronic illnesses perceive messages to be personally relevant, they are more likely to process this information thoughtfully and be more open to persuasive efforts. Minimal expert feedback through computer- and telephone-mediated communication (e.g., e-mail, discussion forums, short messaging services, telephone counseling) has also been helpful in maintaining patient engagement in the long term. Information and communication technologies widen access to and reach of trained and skilled health professionals, which may be particularly relevant for vulnerable populations in hard-to-reach areas or who are experiencing rare debilitating diseases. Key to the success of any online intervention is thoughtful use of health behavior theory to guide design. This review reveals that knowledge alone does not change behaviors, and that it is important to provide self-regulating tools deemed important to building efficacy to engage in the behaviors being targeted or changed. Web and telephone delivery approaches provide an opportunity to provide self-regulating tools in a number of interactive formats (e.g., animation, simulations, graphics) that can suit many different learning styles. Self-monitoring tools also allow for real-time demonstrations of how specific behaviors can affect outcomes. In addition, Web uploads can help health care professionals provide individualized feedback that patients can use to track their progress on certain goals.

CONCEPTUAL AND METHODOLOGICAL ISSUES

Several key conceptual and methodological issues were noted in our review of e-health intervention research for individuals with chronic illnesses. First, we address the conceptual limitations of current e-health studies; this is followed by a discussion of methodological pitfalls. One of the key conceptual shortcomings of current e-health outcome studies is the failure to incorporate meaningful control or comparison groups into the overall research design. Most investigators have employed routine medical care as the control condition against which the effects of telehealth interventions have been compared. Although this design is appropriate for initial clinical trials of the efficacy of telehealth interventions, it severely restricts the range of research questions that can be addressed. Similar to other forms of program evaluation (Glueckauf, 1990; Glueckauf & Ketterson, 2004), advances in e-health outcome research are predicated upon the ability to test conceptually and pragmatically meaningful rival hypotheses. For example, McKay et and associates (2002) compared the effects of Internet-based peer support, professional coaching, and the provision of information alone on the psychosocial and physiological functioning of adults with Type 2 diabetes. This design permitted a rigorous test of the differential impact of two empirically validated theory-driven interventions (i.e., professional coaching and peer support) against a third alternative (i.e., provision of information only) that had shown only limited effects in previous intervention research (e.g., Clement, 1995). In addition to hypothesis testing, e-health investigators should strive to include comparison groups that allow them to assess the differential effects of a variety of potentially efficacious technologies. For example, in a family therapy intervention for rural teens with epilepsy, Glueckauf and associates (2002) tested the effects of desktop family videoconferencing against a less expensive, more widely available plain old telephone system (POTS)-based speakerphone alternative, rather than exclusively comparing the target delivery mode to traditional face-to-face family therapy.

A second conceptual shortcoming of e-health outcome research was found in the limited understanding of the relationship between consumer perceptions of the desirability, ease of use, and utility of e-health interventions and treatment outcome. We continue to lack basic information about the social-psychological mechanisms that link intervention processes to telehealth outcomes. To our knowledge, there are only a few studies to date that have examined the factors that enhance and reduce the quality (e.g., clarity, ease of use, distractibility, and comfort) of telehealth communications across modalities, age groups, minorities, and ethnic groups, and in turn, their relationship with treatment outcome (Glueckauf & Ketterson, 2004; Glueckauf, Pickett, Ketterson, & Nickelson, 2006). Furthermore, the relationship between potential mediators/moderators of treatment (e.g., adherence to treatment, therapeutic alliance, and session attendance) and treatment outcome remains poorly understood.

Third, despite its important theoretical and practical implications, one of the most neglected conceptual issues in e-health research is that of "optimal fit." This crucial issue was raised many years ago by behavior-ist Gordon Paul (1967), who asked, which interventions are most effec-tive for what types of problems and for which consumer populations. Although matching telehealth technology to the person and his or her specific health concerns has long been the fundamental philosophical stance of assistive technology and telehealth advocates, this tenet cannot be accepted as inherently veridical and should be subjected to empirical investigation (Scherer, 2002). It is entirely plausible that certain types of health concerns may be treated more efficaciously with Web-based solu-tions than by telephone among certain populations (e.g., urban-dwelling adults with anxiety disorders). However, the opposite may be the case in the provision of health information and support services to rural con-stituencies (e.g., rural older adults with heart failure), who may report greater health care benefits from telephone or POTS-based videocon-ferencing interactions than from services rendered over the Internet. It is also possible that persons with chronic illnesses may show equivalent outcomes across several different health care delivery approaches.

The issue of optimal fit is especially significant in the development and evaluation of the impact of e-health interventions across different ethnic minority populations. As noted previously, we currently have only limited knowledge about the influence of ethnic and cultural factors on the efficacy and perceived utility of telecommunication-mediated outreach programs. Furthermore, we continue to lack basic informa-tion regarding the influence of attitudinal factors, such as discomfort with technology and preferences for same-race providers on acceptance of alternative health care delivery approaches (Glueckauf et al., 2004). Thus, a key future direction for e-health research is to compare the effects of different telehealth technologies for specific types of health care problems across different consumer populations, particularly those of ethnic minority origin.

In terms of methodological issues, a major shortcoming was found in the limited number and poor quality of cost-effectiveness analyses per-formed in current telehealth evaluations. Although a few studies (e.g., Emmons et al., 2005; Rotheram-Borus et al., 2004; Southard et al., 2003) provided preliminary evidence of cost savings, the cost-effectiveness anal-yses performed in these investigations were poorly delineated and overly simplistic. Formal cost-effectiveness, cost-benefit, cost-offset and oppor-tunity cost, or disease-adjusted life years analyses (Whitten et al., 2002) should be included routinely in all e-health outcome studies, particularly those that focus on improving health status and psychosocial adjustment.

A second methodological shortcoming lies in the limited recruitment of ethnic minorities in e-health intervention research. Only a few of the studies reviewed here compared the effects of self-care management across different ethnic groups (e.g., Mishel et al., 2005). Two possible explanations for this limitation may be located in well-known barriers to recruitment of minorities and in culturally-based preferences in the delivery of health care services. E-health researchers typically have not incorporated minority recruitment coordinators into their subject accrual plans. It is critical to employ same-culture role models to reduce fear and distrust about technology as well as perceived negative intentions of investigators (e.g., Glueckauf & Ketterson, 2004; Sue & Sue, 1999). Involvement of key community leaders (e.g., church leaders and local politicians) also may be required to engender enthusiasm and participation in telehealth program initiatives. E-health researchers may benefit from exposure to previous studies conducted by health services researchers who have tested several different models of engagement and retention (e.g., Gorelick, Harris, Burnett, & Bonecutter, 1998; Hautman & 1995; Stoy et al., 1995).

IMPLICATIONS FOR PRACTICE

Although further data are needed to justify their widespread use, the current review suggests that Web- and telephone-based resources that provide options for engagement with experts and peer interaction may serve as helpful adjuncts to traditional therapies. A key issue in health care management of chronic conditions is the problem of maintaining patient engagement in treatment, which has been addressed in several ways. As noted across several studies, one-on-one interaction with health educators, Web site bulletin boards, and monitored chat groups are among the preferred uses of e-health among adults with chronic illnesses. These modalities have the potential to provide consumers with increased social support and useful information enabling them to better understand their conditions.

Regarding the routine use of e-health technologies, we want to emphasize that, similar to other clinical proficiencies, e-health requires specific competencies and skills, such as knowledge about telecommunication systems, telehealth equipment, and data security protocols, as well as practical skills in the use of telehealth technologies. Health care professionals also need to be cognizant of the ethical dilemmas and licensure and regulatory requirements related to the practice of tele-health. Glueckauf and associates (2003) and others (e.g., Maheu, Whit-ten, & Allen, 2001) have discussed the need for practitioner training in the delivery of e-health and have provided self-assessment questions that highlight important technical and practice issues in e-health and help professionals identify areas where their knowledge and skills may require further development. Note that these self-study guidelines are only a beginning point in preparing professionals to deploy telehealth technologies in their daily practice. Research on practitioner education in telehealth is needed both to identify the key elements (i.e., critical content areas) of educational training packages and to assess the impact of such educational initiatives on provider and client outcomes.

FINAL NOTE

In conclusion, one of the greatest challenges to the viability of e-health is the need for scientific rigor and creativity in the design and evaluation of the impact of self-care training and support for people with chronic illnesses. If the field is to advance, investigators must strive to recruit adequate samples of ethnic minority populations, employ meaningful comparison conditions, and evaluate the goodness of fit between tech-nology and specific health care problems. There is also a dire need for research that assesses the cost-effectiveness, cost utility, and cost offsets of e-health interventions.

Table 7.2

SUMMARY OF E-HEALTH INTERVENTIONS FOR SELF-MANAGEMENT OF CHRONIC DISEASES

AUTHORS	DESIGN	MEDICAL CONDITION	MODALITIES	RESEARCH OBJECTIVES	RESULTS
Ahles et al. (2006)	1,337 patients from 14 rural primary care practices who reported diverse pain problems with ($n = 644$) or without ($n = 693$) psychosocial problems were randomized to usual care ($n = 516$) or intervention groups ($n = 821$). All patients in the intervention groups received information tailored to their problems and concerns. Their physicians also received computerized feedback about their specific pain problems. A nurse educator telephoned patients with pain and psychosocial problems to teach problem-solving strategies and basic pain management skills. Outcomes were assessed with the Medical Outcomes Study 36-Item Short Form and the Functional Interference Estimate at baseline, 6 months, and 12 months.	Chronic pain	Telephone, computerized feedback to physicians	The objective of this study was to compare the effects of a telephone-based, pain-management intervention versus usual primary care practice.	Patients with pain and psychosocial problems randomized to the telephone-based, pain-management intervention significantly improved on ratings of bodily pain, role functioning, vitality, and functional interference compared with usual-care patients who showed little change at the 6-month post-testing. These gains were maintained at the 12-month follow-up.

(continued)

Table 7.2

SUMMARY OF E-HEALTH INTERVENTIONS FOR SELF-MANAGEMENT OF CHRONIC DISEASES

AUTHORS	DESIGN	MEDICAL CONDITION	MODALITIES	RESEARCH OBJECTIVES	RESULTS
Allen et al. (2002)	164 women with breast cancer were randomly assigned to either a 12-week problem-solving intervention ($n = 87$) or usual care ($n = 77$). The intervention consisted of two in-person and four telephone sessions with an oncology nurse who provided problem-solving skills training and informational materials to the women over a 12-week period. Usual care included routine medical intervention from the participant's physician. Participants were assessed for physical and psychosocial adjustment through telephone and mailed surveys at baseline, at 4 months, and at 8 months.	Cancer	Telephone	To compare the effects of a problem-solving training intervention versus usual care on improvement in coping skills for women with breast cancer.	Problem-solving group participants had significantly lower unmet needs and better mental health than usual-care participants at the 4-month assessment, but this effect was not maintained at the 8-month assessment. The intervention also significantly decreased the number and severity of difficulties experienced by women with average or good problem-solving skills at 8 months as compared to the control group. In contrast, no differences were obtained between intervention and control groups in alleviating problems in women with poor baseline problem-solving skills at the 8-month assessment.

Andersson et al. (2005)	Two-group randomized trial with individuals suffering with mild-to-moderate depression; treatment group ($n = 57$) had access to a self-help Web site and participated in a monitored online discussion group while control group ($n = 60$) only had access to the online discussion group.	Mental health	Web site, online discussion group	Assess efficacy of a 10-week Web-based cognitive behavioral self-help intervention with therapist-monitored discussion group compared to wait-list condition involving participation in an online moderated discussion group only.	Improvement in depressive symptoms including anxiety symptoms and quality of life in intervention group persisted through 6-month follow-up. Attrition was high in treatment group. Participation in the Web-based discussion group only had no effect on depressive symptoms.
Andersson et al. (2003)	This 6-week study compared self-recruited headache sufferers randomized to either a Web-based self-help program with e-mail support ($n = 20$), or to a group receiving, in addition, weekly individual telephone calls ($n = 24$).	Chronic pain (headache)	Web site, e-mail, telephone	Investigate supplemental effects of adding minimal therapist contact via telephone to a stand-alone Web-based self-help program for headache sufferers.	Results showed significant reductions in headache-related disability, depression, maladaptive coping strategies, and perceived stress but little to indicate any superior performance and little improvement in the headache index in the Internet-only group with or without expert contact via phone.

(continued)

Table 7.2

SUMMARY OF E-HEALTH INTERVENTIONS FOR SELF-MANAGEMENT OF CHRONIC DISEASES (*continued*)

AUTHORS	DESIGN	MEDICAL CONDITION	MODALITIES	RESEARCH OBJECTIVES	RESULTS
Andersson et al. (2002)	Tinnitus patients were randomized to a 6-week cognitive behavioral therapy intervention through an online self-help manual and mediated contact with expert (*n* = 53) or to a waiting-list control group (*n* = 64).	Other chronic conditions (tinnitus)	Web site, e-mail, mediated contact with expert	Investigate efficacy of a Web-based cognitive behavior therapy (CBT) in decreasing distress in individuals with tinnitus.	Tinnitus-related distress, depression, and diary ratings of annoyance decreased significantly in the treatment group compared to the control. These improvements persisted even at 1-year follow-up.
Bailey et al. (2004)	Watchful waiting intervention (WWI) participants received 5 weekly intervention calls from a nurse. WWI designed to help men integrate uncertainty into their lives by teaching them to cognitively reframe the way in which they viewed their illness and the uncertainty it produced. Control subjects received usual care. Outcomes were: new view of life, mood state, quality of life, and cognitive reframing.	Cancer	Telephone	To compare the effects of a telephone-based WWI versus usual care on men with prostate cancer's capacity to cognitively reframe and manage the uncertainty of their condition.	WWI participants were significantly more likely than controls to view their lives in a new light and experience a decrease in confusion following the intervention. Additionally, intervention subjects reported greater improvement in their quality of life than did controls and believed their quality of life in the future would be better than did controls.

| Bambauer et al. (2005) | Hospitalized acute coronary syndrome survivors with mild to severe depression and/or anxiety at 1-month post-discharge were randomized to either telephone-based counseling intervention or a routine care control group. Intervention patients ($n = 53$) received up to 6 30-minute telephone-counseling sessions focused on cardiac-related fears, including loss of control, loss of self-image, dependency, stigma, abandonment, anger, isolation, and fear of death. Counseling was goal-oriented, time-limited, and issue-focused. Control patients ($n = 47$) received usual care. | Cardiovascular disease | Telephone | To compare the effects of a telephone-based counseling intervention versus usual care on improvement in self-rated health among distressed patients with heart disease. | Patients in the intervention group reported significantly greater improvements in self-rated health (SRH) between baseline and month 3 than the control group. Although gains in the intervention group were maintained at the 6-month follow-up, no significant differences in SRH improvements were observed between the control and intervention groups from baseline to the 6-month assessment phase. |

(continued)

Table 7.2

SUMMARY OF E-HEALTH INTERVENTIONS FOR SELF-MANAGEMENT OF CHRONIC DISEASES (*continued*)

AUTHORS	DESIGN	MEDICAL CONDITION	MODALITIES	RESEARCH OBJECTIVES	RESULTS
Bell et al. (2005)	Participants with traumatic brain injury (TBI) were randomly assigned to receive telephone calls at 2 and 4 weeks and 2, 3, 5, 7, and 9 months after discharge ($n = 85$) or standard follow-up ($n = 86$). The calls consisted of brief motivational interviewing, counseling, and education, plus facilitating usual care or usual care alone through follow-up appointments and therapy prescriptions. A composite outcome was used as the primary endpoint on an intent-to-treat basis. The primary outcome was an overall composite based on the scores on the FIM, DRS, CIQ, FSE, GOS-E, EuroQol, NFI, PQOL, SF-36, and BSI.	Other chronic conditions (TBI)	Telephone	To compare the effects of a scheduled telephone intervention offering counseling and education to people with TBI on behavioral outcomes compared with standard follow-up at 1-year post-injury.	The primary outcome was significantly better for patients assigned to the scheduled telephone intervention. Further analyses of the specific composite variables showed that the group receiving telephone counseling scored significantly better on the functional status and perceived quality of well-being composites than did the group assigned to standard follow-up care.

| Bennett et al. (2007) | 56 physically inactive adult cancer survivors (mean = 42 months since completion of treatment) were assigned randomly to intervention (*n* = 28) and control groups (*n* = 28). The motivational interviewing (MI) intervention consisted of one in-person counseling session followed by two MI telephone calls over 6 months. Control group participants received two telephone calls without MI content. Outcomes measures included the Community Healthy Activities Model Program for Seniors questionnaire, 6-minute walk evaluation, Medical Outcomes Study Short-Form 36, and the Schwartz Cancer Fatigue Scale and were administered at baseline, 3 months, and 6 months. | Cancer | Telephone | To evaluate the effect of an MI intervention on increasing physical activity and on improving aerobic fitness, health, and fatigue in cancer survivors. | Controlling for time since completion of cancer treatment, MI intervention participants reported a significantly high level of regular physical activity than that of control participants. In contrast, no significant mean differences were reported on aerobic fitness, physical and mental health, and fatigue between the two groups. In the intervention group, individuals with high self-efficacy for exercise at baseline increased their physical activity more than those with low self-efficacy. This relationship, however, was not obtained in the control group. |

(*continued*)

Table 7.2

SUMMARY OF E-HEALTH INTERVENTIONS FOR SELF-MANAGEMENT OF CHRONIC DISEASES (*continued*)

AUTHORS	DESIGN	MEDICAL CONDITION	MODALITIES	RESEARCH OBJECTIVES	RESULTS
Blixen et al. (2004)	32 participants with osteoarthritis (OA) were randomized to a control or intervention group. The intervention group received 6 weekly mailings of OA health education modules, a relaxation audiotape and 6 weekly 45 minute follow-up telephone self-management sessions. Participants in the control group received usual care for their OA with their rheumatologists. Outcome measures were administered at baseline, and at 3 and 6 months following entry in the study.	Other chronic conditions (osteoarthritis)	Telephone	To compare the effects of a nurse-run telephone self-management program versus usual care on self-efficacy, functional status and depression for older adults with OA.	No significant post-treatment differences were found on the primary outcome measures. Only self-efficacy in managing pain differentiated between the intervention and usual care groups at the 3-month assessment phase. However, this between-group effect was not maintained at the 6-month follow-up.

| **Blumenthal et al. (2006)** | 389 patients with end-stage lung disease awaiting lung transplantation were randomly assigned to either 12 weeks of telephone-based coping skills training ($n = 200$) or to usual medical care ($n = 189$). Patients completed a battery of quality-of-life instruments and were followed for up to 3.4 years to assess all-cause mortality. | Other chronic conditions (lung disease) | Telephone | To compare the effects of a telephone-based psychosocial intervention versus routine medical on quality of life and survival in patients awaiting lung transplantation. | The telephone-based psychosocial intervention group reported significantly greater improvements in emotional distress, anxiety, depression, feelings of vitality, and perceived social support than the routine care control group. There were 29 deaths (9%) over a mean follow-up period of 1.1 years. Survival analyses revealed that there was no difference in survival between the two groups. |

(continued)

Table 7.2

SUMMARY OF E-HEALTH INTERVENTIONS FOR SELF-MANAGEMENT OF CHRONIC DISEASES (*continued*)

AUTHORS	DESIGN	MEDICAL CONDITION	MODALITIES	RESEARCH OBJECTIVES	RESULTS
Boter (2004)	536 stroke patients were randomized at discharge to standard care (*n* = 273) or standard care plus outreach care (*n* = 263). The outreach program included a problem-solving component and education about stroke consequences. The outreach care consisted of three telephone calls and one home visit within 5 months after discharge by stroke nurses. Six months after discharge, they assessed the two primary outcomes: quality of life (SF-36) and dissatisfaction with care.	Other chronic conditions (lung disease)	Telephone	To compare the effects of a telephone-based outreach nursing care program plus usual care versus usual care post-stroke on quality of life and dissatisfaction with treatment.	Outreach care patients had significantly better scores on the SF-36 domain "Role Emotional" than controls. No statistically significant differences were found on the other primary outcome measures. For secondary outcomes, no statistically significant differences were found, except that intervention patients used fewer rehabilitation services and had lower anxiety scores.

Source	Design	Domain	Media	Objective	Results
Buhrman et al. (2004)	Chronic back pain sufferers were randomly assigned to a Web-based cognitive behavioral self-help program (n = 22) or to a waiting-list control condition (n = 29).	Chronic pain (back pain)	Web site, e-mail, interactive CD-ROM, telephone	Investigate effects of an Internet-based cognitive-behavioral intervention with telephone support for chronic back pain.	Results showed statistically significant improvements in catastrophizing, control over pain, and ability to decrease pain in treatment versus control groups. On the other hand, there was no significant interaction between group and time on the secondary outcome measures: multidimensional pain inventory; pain and impairment relationship scale; and hospital anxiety scale.
Carlbring et al. (2005)	Two-group randomized controlled trial for patients suffering from panic disorder (PD). Patients were randomized to a Web-based self-help group (n = 25) or to a live-help therapy session group (n = 24).	Mental health	Web site, e-mail, face-to-face contact with expert	Compare 10 individual weekly sessions of cognitive-behavior therapy for PD with or without agoraphobia with a 10-module self-help program on the Internet.	Results suggest that Internet-administered self-help plus minimal therapist contact via e-mail can be equally effective as traditional individual cognitive-behavior therapy. This outcome was confirmed after 1 year.

(continued)

Table 7.2

SUMMARY OF E-HEALTH INTERVENTIONS FOR SELF-MANAGEMENT OF CHRONIC DISEASES (*continued*)

AUTHORS	DESIGN	MEDICAL CONDITION	MODALITIES	RESEARCH OBJECTIVES	RESULTS
Cho et al. (2006)	Two-arm randomized controlled trial comparing diabetes patients treated with the Web-based monitoring system ($n = 40$) and a usual care control group ($n = 40$).	Diabetes	Web site, blood glucose monitoring system, charts, telephone, face-to-face, note system	Investigate the long-term effectiveness of the Internet-based glucose monitoring system (IBGMS) on glucose control in patients with type 2 diabetes.	The mean A1C and HFI were significantly lower in the intervention group than in the control group, showing a significant decrease during first 3 months of the RCT and remaining stable throughout the study. Close monitoring via a Web-based glucose monitoring system is effective in controlling blood glucose and achieving glucose stability over time.

| Chouinard & Robichaud-Ekstrand (2005) | Participants ($N = 168$) were randomly assigned by cohorts to inpatient counseling with telephone follow-up, inpatient counseling, and usual care. The inpatient intervention consisted of a 1-hour counseling session, and the telephone follow-up included six calls during the first 2 months after discharge. The nursing intervention was tailored to the individual's stage of change. End points at 2 and 6 months included actual and continuous smoking cessation rates (measured by biochemical markers) and increased motivation (progress through stages of change). | Cardiovascular disease | Telephone | To test whether smokers with cardiovascular disease (CVD) receiving a nurse-delivered inpatient smoking cessation counseling intervention with telephone follow-up (Group 1) or without (Group 2) will present higher point-prevalent smoking abstinence, higher rates of continuous abstinence, and a better progression to ulterior stages of change at 2 and 6 months after hospital discharge than the usual care group (Group 3). | Assuming that surviving patients lost to follow-up were smokers, the 6-month smoking abstinence rate was significantly higher (41.5%) in the inpatient counseling with telephone follow-up group (Group 1), compared with both the inpatient counseling without follow-up (30.2%) (Group 2) and usual care groups (20%) (Group 3). Progress through more advanced stages of change was also significantly greater for Group 1 (43.3%) than both Group 2 (32.1%) and Group 3 (18.2%) at the 2- and 6-month follow-ups. Stage of change at baseline and intervention predicted smoking status at 6 months. |

(continued)

Table 7.2

SUMMARY OF E-HEALTH INTERVENTIONS FOR SELF-MANAGEMENT OF CHRONIC DISEASES (*continued*)

AUTHORS	DESIGN	MEDICAL CONDITION	MODALITIES	RESEARCH OBJECTIVES	RESULTS
Clarke et al. (2002)	Participants in this 28-week trial were randomized to an Internet-based, cognitive therapy, self-help program for depression ($n = 144$) or a no-access control group ($n = 155$). Participants in both groups were free to obtain nonexperimental, usual care services for their depression.	Mental health	Web site, e-mail, snail mail	Evaluate effects of an Internet-based cognitive therapy self-help program for depression on levels of depression of self-reported depressed and nondepressed individuals.	Results showed no significant effects of the Internet program on depression members across the entire sample. However, post-hoc, exploratory analyses revealed a modest effect among persons reporting low levels of depression at intake. Authors explained that the negative results might have resulted from infrequent patient use of the Internet site, or a more seriously depressed sample than the intervention was intended to help.

| Clarke et al. (2005) | Three-arm randomized trial for adults with self-reported depression. Participants were randomized to one of three groups: (1) treatment as usual control group without access to the ODIN website ($n = 100$), (2) ODIN program group with postcard reminders ($n = 75$), and (3) ODIN program group with telephone reminders ($n = 80$). | Mental health | Web site, e-mail, telephone | Examine the supplemental effects of reminders on a Web-based cognitive therapy self-help program for depression (ODIN) among adults with self-reported depression. | Results showed overall significant relationship between improved mental state (reduced depression rates) of patients sent reminders compared to the control group. There was no significant difference between methods by which reminders were sent. |
| DeBusk et al. (2004) | 462 adults with heart failure were randomly assigned (228 to intervention and 234 to usual care). The nurse care management intervention included coordination of care across disciplines, patient and caregiver education, enhancement of self-management skills, effective follow-up, and guidelines-based medications for heart failure. Time to first rehospitalization for heart failure or for any cause and time to a combined end point of first rehospitalization, emergency department visit, or death were the primary outcome measures. | Cardiovascular disease | Telephone | To compare the effects of a telephone-mediated nurse care management program for heart failure versus routine care on rate of rehospitalization for heart failure and for all causes over a 1-year period. | No significant differences were found on rate of first rehospitalization for heart failure between the intervention and routine care conditions. Furthermore, rate of all-cause rehospitalization did not significantly differentiate between the groups. |

(continued)

Table 7.2

SUMMARY OF E-HEALTH INTERVENTIONS FOR SELF-MANAGEMENT OF CHRONIC DISEASES (*continued*)

AUTHORS	DESIGN	MEDICAL CONDITION	MODALITIES	RESEARCH OBJECTIVES	RESULTS
Devineni & Blanchard (2005)	Chronic headache sufferers were randomized to a Web-based intervention involving minimal therapist e-mail contact (*n* = 39) and to a symptom monitoring waitlist control group (*n* = 47).	Chronic pain (tension/headache)	Web site, e-mail, print	Evaluate an Internet-delivered behavioral regimen composed of progressive relaxation, limited biofeedback with autogenic training, and stress management versus a symptom monitoring waitlist control.	Treatment led to a significantly greater decrease in headache activity and headache-related disability than symptom monitoring alone. Attrition rates were typical of behavioral self-help programs (38.1% and 64.8% during treatment and at 2 months post treatment).
DeWalt et al. (2006)	127 heart failure patients taking furosemide were randomly assigned to either telephone-based self-management training (*n* = 62) or routine care (*n* = 65). Self-care training consisted of daily weight measurement, diuretic dose self-adjustment, and symptom recognition and response. Picture-based educational materials, and telephone follow-up were provided to reinforce adherence. Control patients received a generic heart failure brochure and usual care.	Cardiovascular disease	Telephone	To perform a randomized controlled trial comparing a telephone-based self-management training program versus usual care on hospitalization rates and health quality of life of heart failure patients with low literacy skills.	Patients in the telephone-based self-management group had a lower rate of hospitalization or death than patients in the control group. At 12 months, a significantly larger number of patients in the intervention group monitored their weight daily than in the routine care group. In contrast, no significant difference in heart failure–related quality of life was found between the two groups at the 12-month follow-up.

Dietrich et al. (2004)

405 outpatients were randomly assigned to either telephone-based intervention ($n = 224$) or routine depression care ($n = 181$). Intervention included telephone-based for increasing adherence to depression treatment, and teaching of self-management practices such as exercise or engaging in social activities. In addition, treating mental health clinicians at participating primary care practices received ongoing progress reports over the telephone. Usual care participants received routine outpatient treatment from outpatient clinicians. The latter were administered a 45–60 minute program on depression diagnosis and assessment of suicidal thoughts prior to the initiation of the study.

Mental health

Telephone

To compare the effects of a telephone-mediated self-management intervention versus usual care on targeted processes for management of depression and outcomes at 6 months.

Although mean depression scores declined among patients in both groups, the decline was significantly greater in intervention patients at both the 3- and 6-month follow-ups. At 6 months, 37% of intervention patients showed remission compared with 27% for usual care patients. In regard to targeted treatment processes, the intervention clinicians significantly more often asked patients about suicidal thoughts, offered educational materials, and assisted in setting self-management goals, than usual care patients. Of intervention patients, 90% rated their depression care as good or excellent at 6 months compared with 75% of usual care patients.

(continued)

Table 7.2

SUMMARY OF E-HEALTH INTERVENTIONS FOR SELF-MANAGEMENT OF CHRONIC DISEASES (*continued*)

AUTHORS	DESIGN	MEDICAL CONDITION	MODALITIES	RESEARCH OBJECTIVES	RESULTS
Dougherty et al. (2005)	168 individuals who received ICD implantation for either a first sudden cardiac arrest or life-threatening arrhythmia were randomly assigned to either telephone-based psychoeducation intervention ($n = 85$) or usual care ($n = 83$). Measures were obtained at baseline, 6 and 12 months post hospitalization.	Cardiovascular disease	Telephone	To compare the benefits of a structured, 8-week educational telephone intervention versus usual care on physical functioning, psychological adjustment, self-efficacy, and health care utilization 12 months after ICD implantation.	The telephone-based, psychoeducation intervention group showed significantly greater improvement on physical concerns, anxiety, fear of dying, self-confidence, and knowledge in managing ICD recovery than the usual care control group at both 6 and 12 months after ICD implantation. In contrast, no statistically significant differences between the groups were found on total outpatient visits, hospitalizations, or ER visits for both assessment intervals.

| Dunagan et al. (2005) | 151 patients hospitalized with heart failure (HF) were randomized to scheduled telephone calls by specially trained nurses promoting self-management and guideline-based therapy plus a written education packet (*n* = 76) or to usual care (*n* = 75). Nurses also screened patients HF exacerbations, which they managed with supplemental diuretics or by contacting the primary physician for instructions. Usual care participants received a written educational packet describing the causes of HF, the basic principles of treatment, their role in routine care and monitoring of their condition, and strategies for managing a HF exacerbation. | Cardiovascular disease | Telephone | To compare the impact of a nurse-administered, telephone-based disease management program versus usual care for adults with health failure on need for hospital-based care, mortality, functional status, and satisfaction with care. | The intervention group had significantly fewer hospital admissions and total hospital days, and lower hospital costs during the first 6 months of the program than usual care patients. None of the differences remained statistically significant at the 1-year follow-up. There were modest but statistically significant changes in physical functioning scores on both the SF-12 and the Minnesota Living with Heart Failure Questionnaire (MLHFQ) at 6 months, but not at 12 months. Changes in scores for the SF-12 mental functioning scale, MLHFQ emotional health subscale, and BDI were not significantly different at 6 or 12 months. |

(*continued*)

Table 7.2

SUMMARY OF E-HEALTH INTERVENTIONS FOR SELF-MANAGEMENT OF CHRONIC DISEASES (*continued*)

AUTHORS	DESIGN	MEDICAL CONDITION	MODALITIES	RESEARCH OBJECTIVES	RESULTS
Emmons et al. (2005)	796 participants were randomly assigned to either a peer-delivered telephone counseling intervention (PC; $n = 398$) or a self-help intervention (SH; $n = 398$). PC participants were assigned a peer counselor who was trained in motivational interviewing principles; a maximum of six calls were provided within a 7-month period. SH participants received a letter from the study physicians highlighting the importance of smoking cessation to reduce the risk of secondary cancers, and a cessation manual, "Clearing the Air: How to Quit Smoking and Quit for Keeps."	Cancer	Telephone and postal service mail	To compare the effects of a peer-based telephone counseling versus self-help on smoking among childhood cancer survivors.	The quit rate was significantly higher in the telephone-based PC group compared with the SH group at both the 8- and 12-month follow-ups. Controlling for baseline self-efficacy and readiness to change, the PC group was twice as likely to quit smoking than the SH group. The total intervention delivery cost per person was $298.17 for the PC group, and $1.25 for the SH group. The incremental cost-effectiveness of the PC group compared with the SH control group [(CostPC – CostSH)/(Quit ratePC – Quit rateSH)] was $5,371 per additional quit at 12 months.

| Farmer et al. (2005) | 93 young adults with Type 1 diabetes were randomly assigned to either: (a) real-time graphical phone-based feedback plus nurse-initiated support and problem solving ($n = 47$) or (b) minimal patient feedback consisting of a graphical time series of blood glucose readings for the previous 24 hours ($n = 46$). The length of both intervention and control conditions was 9 months. | Diabetes | General packet radio system, mobile phone (Motorola T720i), blood glucose monitor (One Touch Ultra) | To compare the effects of a mobile phone–based telemedicine system, including real-time feedback, phone diary recordings, and nurse-initiated support and problem solving versus a minimal feed-back control condition on glycemic control. | There was a reduction in HbA1c in the intervention group after 9 months from 9.2% to 8.6% and a reduction in HbA1c in the control group from 9.3 to 8.9. This difference in change in HbA1c between groups was not statistically significant. |

(continued)

Table 7.2

SUMMARY OF E-HEALTH INTERVENTIONS FOR SELF-MANAGEMENT OF CHRONIC DISEASES (*continued*)

AUTHORS	DESIGN	MEDICAL CONDITION	MODALITIES	RESEARCH OBJECTIVES	RESULTS
Glasgow et al. (2002)	320 adults with Type 2 diabetes were randomly assigned to 1 of 4 conditions (Note: telephone follow-up = TF; community resources utilization component = CR): (1) TF ($n = 80$), (2) TF + CR ($n = 80$), (3) CR ($n = 80$) or (4) no CR + no TF ($n = 80$). The TF condition received telephone-based, tailored support for behavior changes and problem-solving training to facilitate dietary self-care. The CR group received information on community resources (e.g., eating at local restaurants and grocery shopping). The TF + CR group received a combination of TF and CR treatments. The no CR + no TF group received a general pamphlet about low-fat eating and usual care from their physicians. Outcome measures were assessed at baseline and 12-months later.	Diabetes	Telephone, office-based multimedia touchscreen computer	To evaluate the incremental effects of adding TF versus a CR utilization component to a computer-assisted dietary goal-setting intervention for Type 2 diabetes patients.	All conditions showed significant improvement from baseline to the 12-month follow-up across behavioral (e.g., Kristal fat and fiber behavioral scale), biological (e.g., lipid ratio, HbA1C), and psychosocial (e.g., quality of life, self-efficacy) measures. However, participants who received TF (i.e., TF and TF + CR) showed significantly greater improvement on lipid ratio than the CR and no TF + no CR participants. In contrast, the TF conditions made significantly lower improvement on use of community resources than the CR and no TF + no CR groups.

Glasgow et al. (2003)	Randomized trial with Type 2 diabetes patients; All participants ($n = 320$) had access to a basic nutrition information Web site, with one group receiving additional tailored self-management training via mediated contact with experts and the other receiving additional online social support. Study assessed multiple measures within each of three different domains: behavioral, biological, and psychosocial outcomes after 10 months exposure to the intervention. (a) Information only condition (basic Web site) $n = 80$, (b) Web site with telephone support $n = 80$, (c) Web site with community support $n = 80$, (d), Combined condition $n = 80$.	Diabetes	Web site, e-mail, chat, discussion group, print	Evaluate incremental effects of adding (1) tailored self-management training or (2) peer support components to a basic Internet-based, information-focused comparison intervention.	All conditions significantly improved from baseline on behavioral, psychosocial, and some biological outcomes; but there were few differences between conditions. Total cholesterol was lowest in the tailored self-management condition. There were difficulties in maintaining usage over time and additions of tailored self-management and peer-support components generally did not significantly improve results.

(continued)

197

Table 7.2

SUMMARY OF E-HEALTH INTERVENTIONS FOR SELF-MANAGEMENT OF CHRONIC DISEASES (*continued*)

AUTHORS	DESIGN	MEDICAL CONDITION	MODALITIES	RESEARCH OBJECTIVES	RESULTS
Howells et al. (2002)	91 young people with Type 1 diabetes were randomly assigned to continued routine managed plus negotiated telephone support (NTS) (*n* = 31), annual clinic with NTS (*n* = 29), or continued routine management (*n* = 31).	Diabetes	Telephone	To compare the effects of an NTS plus routine care versus annual clinic plus NTS versus routine care on HbA1c levels, self-efficacy, barriers to adherence, problem solving, and diabetes knowledge in young people with Type 1 diabetes.	Self-efficacy for diabetes self-management was found to increase significantly in the combined intervention group compared with the routine management control from baseline to the 1-year assessment. Over the year, the mean HbA1c increased significantly (8.6%–9.0%). The deterioration in HbA1c was observed across the groups. NTS with or without CR did not improve overall glycaemic control. Note that no attempt was made to intensify insulin therapy. Normalization of glycaemia, while the goal, was approached by using twice-daily regimens. The NTS sessions were designed to be driven by the young person.

Study	Condition	Technology	Objective	Findings
Hunkeler et al. (2006)	Mental health	Telephone	To determine the long-term effectiveness of collaborative care management for depression in late life.	Across the 12-, 18-, and 24-month follow-up evaluations, IMPACT patients showed significantly higher levels of improvement on depression (SCL-20), quality of life (SF-12), physical functioning (PCS-12), and satisfaction with care than their control group counterparts. Only overall functional impairment failed to differentiate between the two groups at the 24-month follow-up. IMPACT patients also reported significantly greater confidence in managing their depression (self-efficacy) at 24 months than control participants.
				1,801 patients were randomly assigned to either a 12-month collaborative care intervention (IMPACT; $n = 906$) or usual care for depression ($n = 895$). Participants in the IMPACT arm received an initial face-to-face visit with a depression care manager, followed by 12 monthly telephone sessions focusing on problem solving and relapse prevention. The usual care group included antidepressant medication, counseling by the doctor, and referral to specialty mental health care.
Jan et al. (2007)	Asthma	Web-based asthma monitoring system, e-journal, telephone, e-mail, print diaries	Determine whether the addition of a Web-based multimedia asthma educational and monitoring program to a traditional clinic-based patient educational program would improve children's and caregivers' management of asthma symptoms.	Intervention group decreased nighttime and daytime symptoms; improved morning and night PEF; increased adherence rates ($p < 0.05$); improved well-controlled rates; improved knowledge regarding self-management; and improved quality of life when compared with conventional management.
				Two-group randomized controlled trial. Asthma patients were randomized to a physician-managed online interactive asthma monitoring tool treatment group ($n = 99$) or a usual care control group receiving a traditional asthma care plan consisting of a written asthma diary supplemented with instructions for self-management ($n = 97$).

(continued)

Table 7.2

SUMMARY OF E-HEALTH INTERVENTIONS FOR SELF-MANAGEMENT OF CHRONIC DISEASES (*continued*)

AUTHORS	DESIGN	MEDICAL CONDITION	MODALITIES	RESEARCH OBJECTIVES	RESULTS
Joseph et al. (2007)	Two-arm randomized controlled trial. High school students with asthma were randomized to a tailored Web site (treatment; $n = 162$) or to a generic asthma Web site (control; $n = 152$).	Asthma	Web site, expert coordinator	Evaluate a multimedia, Web-based asthma management program to specifically target urban high school students.	At 12 months, intervention students demonstrated more positive behaviors, reported fewer symptom days, symptom nights, school days missed, restricted-activity days, and hospitalizations for asthma compared to the control students.

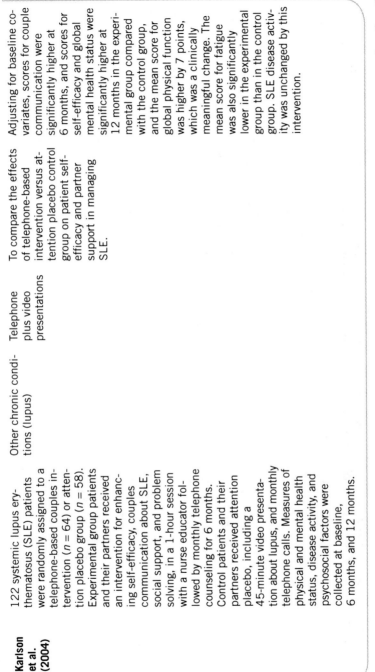

| Karlson et al. (2004) | Other chronic conditions (lupus) | Telephone plus video presentations | To compare the effects of telephone-based intervention versus attention placebo control group on patient self-efficacy and partner support in managing SLE. | 122 systemic lupus erythematosus (SLE) patients were randomly assigned to a telephone-based couples intervention (n = 64) or attention placebo group (n = 58). Experimental group patients and their partners received an intervention for enhancing self-efficacy, couples communication about SLE, social support, and problem solving, in a 1-hour session with a nurse educator followed by monthly telephone counseling for 6 months. Control patients and their partners received attention placebo, including a 45-minute video presentation about lupus, and monthly telephone calls. Measures of physical and mental health status, disease activity, and psychosocial factors were collected at baseline, 6 months, and 12 months. | Adjusting for baseline covariates, scores for couple communication were significantly higher at 6 months, and scores for self-efficacy and global mental health status were significantly higher at 12 months in the experimental group compared with the control group, and the mean score for global physical function was higher by 7 points, which was a clinically meaningful change. The mean score for fatigue was also significantly lower in the experimental group than in the control group. SLE disease activity was unchanged by this intervention. |

(continued)

Table 7.2

SUMMARY OF E-HEALTH INTERVENTIONS FOR SELF-MANAGEMENT OF CHRONIC DISEASES (*continued*)

AUTHORS	DESIGN	MEDICAL CONDITION	MODALITIES	RESEARCH OBJECTIVES	RESULTS
Khan et al. (2004)	The parents were randomized to receive either standard care (155 children) or standard care plus education by telephone (155 children) from a trained asthma educator. The conceptual framework was theory of empowerment with reinforcement by telephone reminder to improve the skills of parents to recognize and avoid triggers, to use written asthma action plans, and to seek help appropriately. Symptoms, parental asthma knowledge, parental quality of life, and use of asthma action plans and preventer therapy were collected at baseline and 6 months later. The primary measure was days of wheeze in last 3 months.	Asthma	Telephone	To compare the effects of asthma education by telephone versus routine care on asthma symptoms, use of written asthma action plans, increase regular use of preventer therapy, increase parental asthma knowledge and improve parental quality of life.	At follow-up, the intervention group children were significantly more likely than controls to possess a written asthma action plan. Possession of action plans increased from baseline in the intervention group but tended to decrease in the control group. Use of action plans was greater in the intervention group but decreased from baseline in both groups. Both intervention and control groups showed significant decreases in asthma symptoms.

| Kim & Oh (2003) | 20 patients were randomly assigned to an intervention group and 16 to a control group. The 12-week telephone intervention consisted of education and reinforcement of diet, exercise, medication adjustment, as well as frequent self-monitoring of blood glucose levels. Telephone intervention was performed twice per week for the first month and then weekly for the second and third month. Participants were requested to write self-management logs including blood glucose levels, diet, and an exercise diary. The control group received routine care consisting of one office visit to a physician. The HbA1c and diabetes adherence were measured before and after the intervention. | Diabetes | Telephone | To compare the effects of nurse telephone-based intervention on glycosylated haemoglobin (HbA1c) levels and adherence to diabetes control recommendations for Type 2 diabetic adults. | Patients in the intervention group showed significantly greater improvement in mean HbA1c levels than control group participants. The intervention group exhibited greater diet and blood glucose testing adherence than the control group. |

(continued)

Table 7.2

SUMMARY OF E-HEALTH INTERVENTIONS FOR SELF-MANAGEMENT OF CHRONIC DISEASES (*continued*)

AUTHORS	DESIGN	MEDICAL CONDITION	MODALITIES	RESEARCH OBJECTIVES	RESULTS
Kim et al. (2007)	Two-arm randomized controlled trial. Diabetes patients in the intervention group used the diabetes monitoring system for 12 weeks without any outpatient visits ($n = 35$). Patients in the control group were given glucometers and received their usual outpatient management from their physicians ($n = 36$).	Diabetes	Web site, cellphone, SMS, glucometer, pedometer	Evaluate effectiveness of Web-based diabetes management system with short messaging system on diabetes self-management.	At 12 weeks, the intervention group demonstrated significant decreases in body weight, A1C levels, fasting, and postprandial glucose levels compared to the control group. Total cholesterol, triglyceride, and LDL and HDL cholesterol levels in the intervention group were not significantly different compared with those in the control group.
Klein, Richards, & Austin (2005)	Subjects with panic disorder were randomized to one of three groups: using a block design to: Internet-based treatment ($n = 19$), treatment with a self-help manual with limited therapist assistance ($n = 18$), or an Internet-based information control (IC) ($n = 18$) condition for 6 weeks. Internet subjects were able to access therapist daily.	Mental health	Web site, e-mail, print, telephone, video, snail mail	Evaluate effects of Internet-based cognitive behavioral panic treatment (CBT) (with e-mail contact), therapist-assisted CBT manual or information-only control (both with telephone contact) on panic disorder patients.	Internet treatment was more successful than the CBT manual in reducing clinician-rated agoraphobia and number of physician visits. Attrition was lower than other Internet studies.

| Krein et al. (2004) | 246 poorly controlled Type 2 diabetes patients were randomly assigned to either telephone-based collaborative case management (n = 123) or usual care plus education materials (n = 123). In the telephone-based, case management intervention nurse practitioners monitored and coordinated care, and engaged in collaborative goal setting (e.g., changing diet and exercise routines). Control patients received educational materials and usual care from their primary care providers. Outcome measures were collected at baseline and 18 months after entry into the study. | Mental health | Telephone, semiautomatic blood pressure monitor device | To compare the effects of a telephone-based, collaborative case management intervention versus usual care plus education materials on glycemic control, intermediate cardiovascular outcomes (e.g., blood pressure and lipid control), satisfaction with care, and resource utilization for adults with poorly controlled Type 2 diabetes. | At the 18-month follow-up, both case management and control patients showed poor glycemic control. No significant group differences were found in mean exit HbA(1C) level. There was also no evidence that the intervention resulted in improvements in low-density lipoprotein cholesterol level or blood pressure control. Furthermore, no difference in resource utilization was obtained between the groups on resource utilization between study groups. Intervention and control patients averaged 0.5 hospitalizations and six primary care outpatient visits during the study period. However, intervention patients were substantially more satisfied with their diabetes care, with 82% rating their providers as better than average compared with 64% of patients in the control group. |

(continued)

SUMMARY OF E-HEALTH INTERVENTIONS FOR SELF-MANAGEMENT OF CHRONIC DISEASES (*continued*)

Table 7.2

AUTHORS	DESIGN	MEDICAL CONDITION	MODALITIES	RESEARCH OBJECTIVES	RESULTS
Krishna et al. (2003)	Two-arm randomized controlled study. Both groups were exposed to a National Asthma Education and Prevention Program. The intervention group received self-management education via an Internet-enabled multimedia program ($n = 119$) while the control group received printed and verbal asthma education only ($n = 127$). Data were collected at baseline, 3 months, and 12 months.	Asthma	Web site, online games, print, telephone	Evaluate effects of supplementing conventional asthma care with interactive multimedia education on asthma knowledge and self-management of children and their caregivers.	Children and caregivers in the intervention group increased their knowledge and demonstrated decreased asthma symptom days from 81 to 51 days/year and emergency room visits from 1.93 to 0.62 per year. Asthma knowledge in 7–17 year old children correlated ($r = 0.37$) with fewer urgent physician visits and decreased use of rescue medications ($r = 0.30$).
Kwon et al. (2004)	Two-group randomized controlled trial with diabetes patients randomized to a Web-based blood glucose monitoring system (IBGMS; $n = 51$) group or usual care control group ($n = 50$). Pre- and postprandial blood glucose readings were uploaded to the Web site. Physicians reviewed data and responded via Web postings.	Diabetes	Web site, e-mail, print	Investigate effectiveness of an Internet-based blood glucose monitoring system (IBGMS) on controlling the changes in HbA1c levels of Type 2 diabetes patients.	There was a significant decrease in Hemoglobin A1c at $p < 0.001$ in the treatment group at 3-month follow-up. There was also a differential response between subjects with initial A1c < 7.0% versus those > 7.0%.

Lange et al. (2003)	Randomized controlled trial of standardized treatment of posttraumatic stress delivered through the Internet compared to a wait-list control.	Mental health	Web site, online risk assessment tool, mediated contact with expert	Compared symptoms of posttraumatic stress sufferers randomized to a standardized treatment of posttraumatic stress delivered through the Internet versus a wait-list control.	Participants in treatment group improved significantly more than wait-list controls. Decreases in symptoms of posttraumatic stress were statistically significant. There was no relapse at 6-week follow-up. Treatment was a success on all or most major points.
Logue et al. (2005)	665 overweight or obese men and women from 15 primary care sites were randomly assigned to either augmented usual care (AUC) (n = 336) consisting of dietary and exercise advice, prescriptions, and three 24-hour dietary recalls every 6 months, or transtheoretical model-chronic disease (TM-CD) care (n = 329) composed of AUC elements plus stage-of-change (SOC) assessments for five target behaviors every other month, mailed SOC and target behavior-matched workbooks, and monthly telephone calls from a weight-loss advisor. Weight change was the primary outcome for the 2-year study.	Other chronic conditions (obesity)	Telephone	To compare the effects of a TM-CD telephone and mailed assignments intervention for obesity versus AUC on weight change in adults with obesity.	Repeated measures analyses showed nonsignificant adjusted differences between the AUC and TM-CD groups for weight change, waist circumference, energy intake or expenditure, blood pressure, and blood lipids. The pattern of change over time suggested that TM-CD participants were trying harder to impact target behaviors during the first 6 to 12 months of the trial but relapsed afterward. 60% of trial participants maintained their baseline weights for 18 to 24 months.

(continued)

Table 7.2

SUMMARY OF E-HEALTH INTERVENTIONS FOR SELF-MANAGEMENT OF CHRONIC DISEASES (*continued*)

AUTHORS	DESIGN	MEDICAL CONDITION	MODALITIES	RESEARCH OBJECTIVES	RESULTS
Lorig et al. (2006)	Two-group randomized trial with chronic disease patients (heart, lung, or Type 2 diabetes). Patients participated in a small-group Chronic Disease Self-Management Program (CDSMP) with or without an interactive Web-based component including references and discussion groups on chronic diseases, medication, and also illustrations of suggested exercises. The efficacy of the Internet-based CDSMP was compared with usual-care controls at 1 year. Treatment group $n = 457$ Usual care $n = 501$	Chronic disease	Web site, e-mail, discussion group, print	Determine efficacy of an Internet-based CDSMP in changing health-related behaviors and improving health statuses.	At 48 weeks, the intervention group had significant improvements in health status compared with usual care control patients. The intervention group had similar results to the small-group CDSMP participants. Change in self-efficacy at 6 months was found to be associated with better health status outcomes at 1 year.

| Maljanian et al. (2005) | Two-arm RCT with diabetes comprehensive care versus diabetes comprehensive care plus telephone-based follow-up The intervention consisted of 12 weekly phone calls to reinforce education and self-management skills. The calls included adherence with self-management activities, and attendance at MD office visits. Education focused on glycemic control and prevention of complications. The initial clinic-based diabetes management program included three 4-hour classes on the basics of diabetes, nutrition and exercise, the importance of adherence to the American Diabetes Association (ADA) care standards, and collaborative care management. Outcomes were evaluated at 3- and 12-month follow-ups. | Diabetes | Telephone | To assess the incremental effects of an intensive telephone follow-up in a diabetes disease management program on improving glycemic control, adherence with ADA standards of care, and health-related quality of life (HRQOL). | Adherence to ADA standards of care, specifically annual eye exams, physician foot exams, foot self-exams, and pneumonia vaccination, were significantly better with the added telephone intervention, but there were no differences between the groups on glycemic control, HRQOL, or patient satisfaction. The additional telephone intervention further improved adherence to ADA guidelines for self-care and medical care but did not affect glycemic control or HRQOL. |

(continued)

Table 7.2

SUMMARY OF E-HEALTH INTERVENTIONS FOR SELF-MANAGEMENT OF CHRONIC DISEASES (*continued*)

AUTHORS	DESIGN	MEDICAL CONDITION	MODALITIES	RESEARCH OBJECTIVES	RESULTS
McKay et al. (2002)	Randomized trial comparing four conditions: Information-Only Condition (IOC; $n = 33$), Personalized Self-Management Coach Condition (PMSCC; $n = 30$), Peer Support Condition (PSC; $n = 37$) and the Combined Condition (CC; $n = 33$). Measures included demographics, Web site uses, glycated hemoglobin, eating behaviors, and mental health status.	Diabetes	Web site, e-mail, discussion group, online support group, chat, mediated contact with expert	Evaluate 12-week individual and combined effects of diabetes self-management instruction and peer-support in the Internet-based Diabetes Network (D-Net) on the following outcomes: physiologic, behavioral, mental health, and Web site usage.	Article is a 3-month follow-up report on the D-Net project on first 160 patients recruited for the study. Improvement was observed on all measures but there were no significant differences between conditions.

| Middleton et al. (2005) | Patients undergoing carotid endarterectomy (CEA) ($N = 133$) were randomized to either the intervention ($n = 66$) or control group ($n = 67$). The intervention consisted of telephone liaison between the participant and a RN at 2, 6, and 12 weeks following CEA, combined with education about stroke risk-factor management and structured liaison with the patient's surgeon and referring general practitioner. The control group did not receive any RN postoperative telephone contact, but their general practitioners were informed that their patient had undergone a CEA and given details of their immediate postoperative recovery 2 weeks following the procedure. | Cardiovascular disease | Telephone | To compare the short-term impact of nursing-led, telephone-mediated care for patients after CEA versus routine treatment following CEA. | The telephone-based postdischarge intervention showed significantly greater improvements on patient knowledge of stroke warning signs, patient self-reported changes to improve lifestyle, and diet modification than the routine care control group from baseline to the 3-month follow-up. In addition, statistically significant improvements were found from baseline to follow-up for the intervention group ratings of their general health status and sufficient time and sessions per week spent in physical activity, as compared to control participants who showed no change over time. |

(continued)

Table 7.2

SUMMARY OF E-HEALTH INTERVENTIONS FOR SELF-MANAGEMENT OF CHRONIC DISEASES (*continued*)

AUTHORS	DESIGN	MEDICAL CONDITION	MODALITIES	RESEARCH OBJECTIVES	RESULTS
Mishel et al. (2005)	Breast cancer survivors were randomly assigned to either the intervention or usual care control condition. The intervention was delivered during four weekly telephone sessions, focusing on cognitive-behavioral strategies to manage uncertainty about recurrence, and a self-help manual designed to help women understand and manage long-term treatment side effects and other symptoms. Treatment outcome data on uncertainty management were gathered at preintervention and a 10-month follow-up.	Cancer	Telephone	To test the efficacy of a theoretically based uncertainty management intervention delivered to older long-term breast cancer survivors versus usual care on knowledge of long-term treatment effects, problem solving, social support, cognitive coping strategies, and emotional distress.	The treatment group had an increase in cognitive reframing while the control group did not change from baseline to 10 months. This difference was most pronounced for African American women where the treatment group increased and the control group decreased between baseline and 10 months. There was no difference between groups for problem solving. While all the groups increased in cancer knowledge, the treatment group had the greatest increase from baseline to 10 months. There was no difference between groups for problem solving. Follow-up analyses revealed that there was a significant treatment by ethnicity increase in use of coping self-statements. There was

| Napolitano et al. (2002) | 81 adults awaiting lung transplantation were randomly assigned to either telephone-based cognitive-behavioral (CB) intervention ($n = 41$) or usual care ($n = 40$). CB treatment included education about stress and health, specific coping techniques (e.g., relaxation training, problem solving, and calming self-statements), and relapse prevention. Usual care included clinic visits with transplant team pulmonologists and nurse coordinators. Health-related quality of life (both general and disease-specific), general psychological well-being, and social support were assessed at baseline and 8 weeks following entry in the study. | Other chronic conditions (lung) | Telephone | To compare the efficacy of an 8-week, tailored, telephone-based CB intervention versus usual care on measures of quality of life and general well-being for individuals awaiting lung transplantation. | a significant treatment by ethnicity effect for the catastrophizing subscale with a decrease from baseline to 10 months post baseline for African American women in the treatment group and no change in their control group over time.

Adjusting for pretreatment baseline scores, age, gender, and time waiting on the transplant list, the telephone-based CB group reported greater general well-being, better general quality of life, better disease-specific quality of life, and higher levels of social support than participants in the usual care group. |

(continued)

Table 7.2

SUMMARY OF E-HEALTH INTERVENTIONS FOR SELF-MANAGEMENT OF CHRONIC DISEASES (*continued*)

AUTHORS	DESIGN	MEDICAL CONDITION	MODALITIES	RESEARCH OBJECTIVES	RESULTS
Nunn et al. (2006)	123 children with Type 1 diabetes, ages 3–16 years, were randomly assigned to either an intervention group receiving normal care and bimonthly telephone support ($n = 63$) or to a control group receiving normal care only ($n = 60$). The intervention group received bimonthly 15–30 minute, telephone-based education and support sessions for 7 months. The primary outcome was change in the HbA1c levels. Admission rates and changes in diabetes knowledge, psychological parameters, compliance, and patient perception also were measured.	Diabetes	Telephone	To compare the effects of telephone intervention from a diabetes educator plus routine care versus routine care only on improvements in childrens' hemoglobin A1c (HbA1c) level, hospital admissions, diabetes knowledge, compliance, and psychological well-being.	There were no significant differences between the intervention and the control groups on improvement for HbA1c levels from baseline to posttreatment. Both groups showed equivalent gains on this measure over time. Furthermore, there were no significant improvements in diabetes knowledge, compliance, or psychological function between and within the two groups.

| Owen et al. (2005) | Two-group randomized trial with early-stage breast cancer patients. Participants were randomized into either a small online coping group ($n = 32$) or a waiting-list control condition ($n = 30$). | Cancer | Web site, discussion group, on-line support group, e-mail | This 12-week study examined the effects and potential mechanisms of action of a self-guided, Internet-based coping-skills training group on quality of life outcomes in women with early-stage breast cancer. | Results were mixed: no significant main effects were observed for the treatment on primary dependent variables. However, there was greater improvement in emotional well-being for treatment relative to control participants, and effect sizes for overall quality of life, emotional well-being, and breast-specific concerns were modest. In addition, participants with low health status at the beginning of the study who were provided with access to the treatment showed significantly greater improvement. |

(*continued*)

Table 7.2

SUMMARY OF E-HEALTH INTERVENTIONS FOR SELF-MANAGEMENT OF CHRONIC DISEASES (*continued*)

AUTHORS	DESIGN	MEDICAL CONDITION	MODALITIES	RESEARCH OBJECTIVES	RESULTS
Park et al. (2003)	Adult heart transplant candidates were randomly assigned to a bibliotherapy plus telephone-based, cognitive-behavioral weight-loss program ($n = 21$) or bibliotherapy only ($n = 22$). In the telephone-based condition, a bachelor's-level clinician delivered intervention in 12 15–20 minute sessions focusing on stimulus and impulse control, problem solving, assertiveness, positive thinking, and reinforcement. In the bibliotherapy condition, participants received a 20-lesson manual focusing on the same skills as the telephone-based cognitive-behavioral intervention group. Primary outcome measures were assessed at baseline and 3 months following the onset of treatment.	Cardiovascular disease	Telephone	To assess the relative effectiveness of a bibliotherapy weight-loss program or a bibliotherapy plus telephone contact weight-loss program on weight loss for heart transplant candidates.	An intent-to-treat analysis showed a significant weight loss at post-treatment for the entire sample. Within-group analyses indicated that a significant weight change in the telephone group, but not the bibliotherapy-only group. Participants in the telephone group returned more 3-day food diaries and self-monitoring postcards, with pounds lost significantly correlated with the number of completed self-monitoring postcards.

| Pinto et al. (2005) | Cancer | Telephone | To compare the effects of a home-based moderate-intensity telephone-based PA versus contact control on PA, fitness, mood, physical symptoms (e.g., fatigue and weight gain), and body esteem in breast cancer patients. | The telephone-based PA group reported significantly more total minutes of PA, more minutes of moderate-intensity PA, and higher energy expenditure per week than controls. The PA group also outperformed controls on a field test of fitness. Changes in PA were not reflected in objective activity monitoring. The PA group was more likely than controls to progress in motivational readiness for PA and to meet PA guidelines. No significant group differences were found in body mass index and percent body fat. Posttreatment group comparisons revealed significant improvements in vigor and a reduction in fatigue in the PA group. |

86 sedentary women who had completed treatment for stage 0 to II breast cancer were randomly assigned to a physical activity program (PA) ($n = 43$) or contact control group ($n = 43$). Participants in the PA group received 12 weeks of PA counseling (based on the Transtheoretical Model) delivered via telephone, as well as weekly exercise tip sheets. Assessments were conducted at baseline, after treatment (12 weeks), and 6 and 9 month after baseline follow-ups. The control participants were asked not to change their current level of activity during the 12 weeks. They received a weekly phone call from research staff for 12 weeks. These women received the same cancer survivorship tip sheets as the PA group.

(continued)

Table 7.2

SUMMARY OF E-HEALTH INTERVENTIONS FOR SELF-MANAGEMENT OF CHRONIC DISEASES (*continued*)

AUTHORS	DESIGN	MEDICAL CONDITION	MODALITIES	RESEARCH OBJECTIVES	RESULTS
Riegel et al. (2006)	Hospitalized Hispanic participants with chronic heart failure ($N = 134$) were randomized to a telephone case management emphasizing patient self-care ($n = 69$) or usual care ($n = 65$). Bilingual/bicultural Mexican-American registered nurses provided 6 months of telephone case management. Data on hospitalizations were collected from automated systems at 1, 3, and 6 months after the index hospital discharge. Health-related quality of life and depression were measured by self-report at baseline, 3, and 6 months.	Cardiovascular disease	Telephone	Compared the impact of telephone case management ($n = 69$) versus usual care ($n = 65$) in decreasing hospitalizations and improving health-related quality of life and depression in Hispanics of Mexican origin with chronic heart failure.	Intention to treat analysis was used. No significant between-group differences were found in heart failure (HF) hospitalizations. In addition, no significant group differences were found in HF readmission rates, HF days in the hospital, HF cost of care, all-cause hospitalizations or cost, mortality, health-related quality of life, and depression.

| Ries et al. (2003) | Other chronic conditions (lung) | Telephone | To compare the effects of a combined telephone and face-to-face pulmonary rehabilitation maintenance program versus routine care on physiologic and psychosocial outcomes in adults with chronic lung disease. | 172 patients with chronic lung disease were randomly assigned to a 12-month maintenance intervention with weekly telephone contacts and monthly supervised reinforcement sessions ($n = 87$) or standard care ($n = 85$). Weekly telephone sessions elicited data on compliance with home treatment, information about recent health problems, as well as advice and assistance. Supervised reinforcement included respiratory care instruction, exercise, and support. Standard care included care by the primary provider, a written home treatment plan, and monthly group meetings. Measures were obtained before and after pulmonary rehabilitation and 6, 12, and 24 months later. | During the 12-month intervention, exercise tolerance and overall health status were significantly better maintained in the intervention group than in the usual care condition. Intervention group participants also had significantly fewer hospital days than usual care patients following pulmonary rehabilitation. In contrast, no group differences for other measures of pulmonary function, dyspnea, self-efficacy, generic and disease-specific quality of life, and health care use at the 12-month assessment phase. By 24 months, there were no significant group differences. Patients returned to levels that approached, but remained above pre-rehabilitation measures. |

(continued)

Table 7.2

SUMMARY OF E-HEALTH INTERVENTIONS FOR SELF-MANAGEMENT OF CHRONIC DISEASES (*continued*)

AUTHORS	DESIGN	MEDICAL CONDITION	MODALITIES	RESEARCH OBJECTIVES	RESULTS
Ritterband et al. (2003)	Two-group randomized control trial. Children were randomized to Internet intervention group (Web; $n = 12$) or no Internet intervention group (no-Web; $n = 12$).	Other chronic conditions (encopresis)	Web site, face-to-face contact with expert	Evaluate the benefits of enhanced toilet training delivered through the Internet for children with encopresis.	Web subjects demonstrated greater improvements in reduced fecal soiling, increased defecation in toilet, and increased unprompted trips to the toilet $p < 0.02$. Treatment was a success on all or most major points.
Rodrigue et al. (2005)	35 adults were randomized to telephone-based Quality-of-Life Therapy (QOLT; $n = 17$) or telephone-based supportive therapy (ST; $n = 18$). QOL, mood and social intimacy assessments were conducted at baseline and at 1 and 3 months after treatment. QOLT focused on problem-solving training with information and specific suggestions tailored to the identified concerns of the patient. ST provided patients with information about the transplant experience, listening actively to their concerns and worries, and promoting the use of other support systems.	Other chronic conditions (lung)	Telephone	To compare the effects of telephone-based QOLT versus telephone-based social support on QOL, mood disturbance, and social intimacy in adults awaiting lung transplantation.	When compared to ST patients, QOLT patients had significantly higher QOL scores at the 1- and 3-month assessments, lower mood disturbance scores at the 3-month assessment, and higher social intimacy scores at the 1-month assessment.

| Rollman et al. (2005) | 191 individuals with panic and/or generalized anxiety disorder were randomly assigned to a telephone-based care management intervention ($n = 116$) or to usual care ($n = 75$). For the telephone intervention group, two trained care managers provided psychoeducation, monitored treatment responses, and informed physicians of their progress via an electronic medical record system. The usual care group received a disorder-specific brochure on their anxiety diagnosis plus routine care from their physicians. | Mental health | Telephone | To examine whether telephone-based collaborative care for panic and generalized anxiety disorders improves clinical and functional outcomes more than the usual care provided by primary care physicians. | At the 12-month follow-up, the telephone intervention group reported significantly greater improvements on anxiety, depressive symptoms, and mental health-related quality of life than usual care patients. In addition, intervention participants made larger improvements relative to baseline in hours worked per week and fewer work days absent in the past month than usual care participants. |

(continued)

Table 7.2

SUMMARY OF E-HEALTH INTERVENTIONS FOR SELF-MANAGEMENT OF CHRONIC DISEASES (*continued*)

AUTHORS	DESIGN	MEDICAL CONDITION	MODALITIES	RESEARCH OBJECTIVES	RESULTS
Rotheram-Borus et al. (2004)	Young people living with HIV (YPLH) participants were randomly assigned to a 3-module intervention totaling 18 sessions delivered by telephone ($n = 59$), in person ($n = 61$), or a delayed-intervention condition ($n = 55$). Similar across intervention delivery format (in-person or telephone sessions), 3 modules of 6 sessions each focused on a different target behavior: improving physical health, reducing sexual and substance use acts, and improving mental health.	Other chronic conditions (HIV)	Telephone	To compare the cost-effectiveness of individual in-person versus individual telephone delivery self-management intervention versus a delayed control group for YPLH.	The total cost of the in-person intervention for the 3 modules was $3,500 per participant, which was higher than the cost of $2,692 per participant for the telephone intervention. The excess cost of traveling time and expenses for in-person sessions accounted for this difference. In addition, intention-to-treat analyses found that the in-person intervention resulted in a significantly higher proportion of sexual acts protected by condoms overall and with HIV-seronegative partners. The in-person group significantly increased their proportion of protected sexual acts compared with the delayed group over time. The proportion

					of protected sexual acts in the telephone group was not significantly different from that in the delayed or in the in-person intervention over time.
Simon et al. (2004)	600 primary care patients beginning antidepressant treatment for depression were randomly assigned to either usual primary care (*n* = 195); usual care plus a telephone care management program including at least three outreach calls, feedback to the treating physician, and care coordination (*n* = 207); usual care plus care management integrated with a structured 8-session cognitive-behavioral therapy program delivered by telephone (*n* = 198).	Mental health	Telephone	To compare telephone care management versus telephone care management plus telephone psychotherapy versus routine depression care on changes in depression severity and patient-rated improvement on depressive symptoms.	Compared with usual care, the telephone psychotherapy intervention led to lower mean Hopkins Symptom Checklist Depression Scale depression scores, a higher proportion of patients reporting that depression was "much improved," and a higher proportion of patients "very satisfied" with depression treatment. The telephone care management program had smaller effects on patient-rated improvement and satisfaction than the telephone psychotherapy intervention, but these were nonetheless statistically significant. Note, however, effects on mean depression scores did not differentiate significantly between the telephone care management and routine depression care groups.

(continued)

Table 7.2

SUMMARY OF E-HEALTH INTERVENTIONS FOR SELF-MANAGEMENT OF CHRONIC DISEASES (*continued*)

AUTHORS	DESIGN	MEDICAL CONDITION	MODALITIES	RESEARCH OBJECTIVES	RESULTS
Sisk et al. (2006)	406 adults who met diagnostic criteria for systolic dysfunction were randomly assigned to either a telephone-based education and self-management intervention ($n = 203$) or usual care ($n = 203$). During the 12-month intervention, bilingual nurses counseled patients on diet, medication adherence, and self-management of symptoms through an initial visit and regularly scheduled follow-up telephone calls. Usual care patients received federal consumer guidelines for managing systolic dysfunction but no other intervention apart from routine medical care.	Cardiovascular disease	Telephone	To compare the effects of a nurse-led intervention focused on specific management problems versus usual care among ethnically diverse heart failure patients with systolic dysfunction in ambulatory care practices.	The intervention group had significantly fewer hospitalizations than the usual care group over the 12-month period of the nurse-facilitated, self-management program. Furthermore, at the 18-month follow-up, intervention patients had 55 fewer cumulative hospitalizations than their usual care counterparts. The intervention group also rated their overall daily functioning significantly higher than the control group.

| Southard et al. (2003) | Two-group randomized controlled trial. CVD patients were randomized to the Web-based intervention (n = 53); and usual care (n = 51) for 6 months. | Cardiovascular disease | Web site, e-mail, discussion group, online support group, online risk assessment tool, mediated contact with expert, snail mail, telephone | Evaluate efficacy of an Internet-based 24-week clinical trial that provided risk-factor management training, risk-factor education, and monitoring to CVD patients as compared to usual care. | Fewer cardiovascular events occurred in intervention group $p = 0.053$ as compared to usual care. Cost $453 per patient with return on investment estimated at 213%. Weight loss was statistically significant in intervention group. No statistically significant differences between intervention and control groups were found for depression scores, blood pressure, and dietary habits. |

(continued)

SUMMARY OF E-HEALTH INTERVENTIONS FOR SELF-MANAGEMENT OF CHRONIC DISEASES (*continued*)

Table 7.2

AUTHORS	DESIGN	MEDICAL CONDITION	MODALITIES	RESEARCH OBJECTIVES	RESULTS
Stuifbergen et al. (2003)	142 women with multiple sclerosis (MS) were randomly assigned to either a combined face-to-face and telephone-based cognitive-behavioral (CB) intervention (*n* = 76) or to waiting-list control group (*n* = 66). The two-phase intervention included face-to-face CB classes for 8 weeks, then 3 months of telephone follow-up reinforcing patient self-efficacy and goal attainment. Participants were followed over an 8-month	Other chronic conditions (multiple sclerosis)	Telephone	To compare the effects of a wellness intervention program versus a waiting list control condition for women with MS on self-efficacy, use of health-promoting behaviors, and QOL.	A statistically significant group by time effect for self-efficacy for health behaviors, health-promoting behaviors, and the mental health and pain scales of the SF-36. Telephone-based CB intervention led to significant increases in self-efficacy, use of health-promoting behaviors, and perceptions of mental health and pain from baseline to the 8-month follow-up, whereas little or no change was found for the waiting-list control group.

| **Tatti & Lehmann (2003)** | period. Control group participants had contact only with the project manager during the 8-month duration of the study. Principal outcomes measures were health-promoting behaviors and quality of life (QOL). Two-group randomized study involving Type 1 diabetes patients. Treatment group was exposed to the online interactive diabetes simulator (AIDA) ($n = 12$), while the control group ($n = 12$) received conventional lessons with slides and transparencies for a total of six lessons over a 6-week period. | Diabetes | Web site, face-to-face contact with expert | Investigate effects of a 6-week educational intervention with or without supplemental use of AIDA. AIDA is a free Web-based program that provides interactive simulation of plasma insulin and blood glucose profiles for demonstration, teaching, and self-learning purposes. | HbA1c and number of symptomatic hypoglycemic episodes dropped significantly in the treatment group exposed to the Web-based diabetes simulator compared to the control. Treatment was a success on all or on most major points. |

(continued)

Table 7.2

SUMMARY OF E-HEALTH INTERVENTIONS FOR SELF-MANAGEMENT OF CHRONIC DISEASES (*continued*)

AUTHORS	DESIGN	MEDICAL CONDITION	MODALITIES	RESEARCH OBJECTIVES	RESULTS
Tranmer & Parry (2004)	Cardiac surgery patients ($N = 200$) were randomly allocated to two groups: (a) an intervention group ($n = 102$) who received telephone calls from an advanced practice nurse (APN) twice during the first week following discharge then weekly thereafter for 4 weeks, and (b) a usual care group ($n = 98$). The intervention approach included ongoing information and assessment, self-management of common symptoms, and referrals to appropriate health care resources. The usual care group received standard outpatient preparation, an education booklet, and home care follow-up, as necessary. Measures of health-related quality of life (HRQL), symptom distress, and unexpected health care contacts were obtained at 5 weeks following discharge.	Cardiovascular disease	Telephone	To compare the effects of APN telephone-delivered support and self-management training versus usual care on HRQL, symptom distress, and unplanned contacts with the hospital following discharge from cardiac surgery.	There were no significant group differences in HRQL, unexpected contacts with the health care system, or symptom distress.

van den Berg et al. (2006)	Physically inactive patients with rheumatoid arthritis were randomly assigned to an Internet-based physical activity program with individual guidance, a bicycle ergometer, and group contacts (individualized training [IIT] group; $n = 82$) or to an Internet-based program providing only general information on exercises (general training [GT] group; $n = 78$).	Chronic pain (rheumatoid arthritis)	Web site, e-mail, face-to-face contact with expert	Compare effectiveness of a general Internet-based physical activity intervention and a Web-based intervention with tailored supervision and training for patients with rheumatoid arthritis (RA).	The study found a greater proportion of patients in the IT group reported meeting physical activity recommendations than the general group. No differences were found with respect to the total amount of physical activity as measured with an activity monitor. There were also no sustained differences between the two programs regarding functional ability and quality of life.
Verheijden et al. (2004)	Randomized controlled trial comparing usual care ($n = 73$) to usual care plus Web-based nutrition counselling and social support ($n = 73$). Both groups had access to usual care for 8 months after which the treatment group had access to a nutrition counselling and social support Web site (Heartweb).	Diabetes	Web site, online discussion forum, face-to-face contact with expert	Evaluate impact of Web-based nutrition counseling and social support on social support measures, anthropometry, blood pressure, and serum cholesterol in patients at increased cardiovascular risk.	No statistically significant differences were found between intervention and control groups in terms of social support, anthropometry, blood pressure, and serum cholesterol levels. Use of the Web site was very low.

(continued)

Table 7.2

SUMMARY OF E-HEALTH INTERVENTIONS FOR SELF-MANAGEMENT OF CHRONIC DISEASES (*continued*)

AUTHORS	DESIGN	MEDICAL CONDITION	MODALITIES	RESEARCH OBJECTIVES	RESULTS
Vidrine et al. (2006)	Current smokers from a large, inner-city HIV/AIDS care center were randomly assigned to either a cellular telephone smoking-cessation intervention ($n = 48$) or usual care ($n = 47$). The intervention group received eight counseling sessions delivered via cellular telephone in addition to the usual care components. The usual care group received brief physician advice to quit smoking, targeted self-help written materials, and nicotine replacement therapy. Smoking-related outcomes were assessed at a 3-month follow-up.	Other chronic conditions (HIV)	Cellular telephone	To compare the efficacy of a telephone-based, smoking-cessation intervention versus usual care on quit rates in a multiethnic, economically disadvantaged HIV-positive population.	Biochemically verified point prevalence smoking abstinence rates were 10.3% for the usual care group and 36.8% for the cellular telephone group; participants who received the cellular-telephone intervention were 3.6 times more likely to quit smoking compared with participants who received usual care.

Wagner et al. (2006)	Two-arm randomized controlled trial. Individuals suffering complicated grief were randomized to a wait-list control group (*n* = 29) and e-mail–based cognitive-behavioral therapy group.	Mental health	E-mail	Investigate efficacy of an Internet-based cognitive-behavioral therapy program for bereaved people suffering complicated grief.	Compared to the wait-list control group, patients in the Web-based cognitive-behavior therapy group improved significantly on symptoms of intrusion, avoidance, maladaptive behavior, and general psychopathology with results maintained at 3-month follow-up. Study also and showed a large treatment effect.
Winzelberg et al. (2003)	Two-group randomized control trial with breast cancer survivors randomized to an Internet-based coping skills training group (*n* = 36) versus a wait-listed control (*n* = 36). The group was semistructured, moderated by a health care professional, and delivered in an asynchronous newsgroup format.	Cancer	Web site, discussion group, on-line support group, e-mail	Examine effects of a 12-week Web-based coping skills training program, Bosom Buddies, on reducing breast cancer survivors' scores on depression, perceived stress, and cancer-related trauma measures.	Depression, perceived stress, and cancer-related trauma scores improved in intervention group. Measures of anxiety and specific ways of responding to cancer did not improve. The results were independent of the amount of time spent online.

(continued)

Table 7.2

SUMMARY OF E-HEALTH INTERVENTIONS FOR SELF-MANAGEMENT OF CHRONIC DISEASES (*continued*)

AUTHORS	DESIGN	MEDICAL CONDITION	MODALITIES	RESEARCH OBJECTIVES	RESULTS
Woollard et al. (2003)	212 patients at cardio-vascular (CV) risk were randomized to either: (1) "Low" intervention (*n* = 69), monthly 10–15 minute tele-phone contacts for 1 year followed one face-to-face individual counseling ses-sion; (2) "High" intervention (*n* = 74) individual face-to-face counseling continued over 1 year, taking place monthly for up to 1 hour, or (3) Controls (*n* = 69), usual care only. Both intervention groups received cognitive-behavioral intervention to control weight, increase physical activity, reduce fat and sodium intake, moder-ate alcohol intake, and en-courage smoking cessation. Participants were assessed at baseline with follow-up 12 and 18 months later.	Cardiovascular disease	Telephone	To compare the ef-fects among individual face-to-face counsel-ing, telephone-based counseling, and usual care on dietary intake, body mass index and blood lipids in patients at CV risk.	Significant improvements in diet and lipid profiles were found across all con-ditions from baseline to the 18-month follow-up. Total serum cholesterol fell by 3%, 3%, and 2% in the High, Low, and Control groups, respec-tively, at 12 months and by 7%, 5%, and 8% at 18 months. Contrary to expectation, no group x time interactions were found for the primary outcomes. Fat intake and serum cholesterol did not differ significantly among the groups for either the 12- or 18-month assess-ment phases. Body mass index also increased in all groups with no significant changes among the three groups.

| **Yates et al. (2005)** | A repeated measures experimental design was used to examine outcomes at baseline (completion of cardiac rehabilitation [CRI]) and at 3 and 6 months. During booster sessions, the subject's individualized goals, negotiated in CR, were used as a basis for intervening. Subjects who reported progress toward goal achievement were encouraged to attribute accomplishments to their own abilities. Factors inhibiting achievement of target goals were also discussed to deal with areas of relapse. Usual care for people completing the CR program consisted of one telephone call at 4–6 weeks to assess program satisfaction and current cardiovascular risk reduction behaviors. | Cardiovascular disease | Telephone | To examine the effects of a booster intervention on health, behavioral, and clinical physical status outcomes among CR graduates randomly assigned to one of three groups: structured educational/counseling sessions by telephone ($n = 24$), clinic ($n = 20$), or usual care ($n = 20$). | For subjects who had low physical functioning scores at baseline, the clinic intervention was more effective than either phone or usual care in increasing their physical functioning at 3 months. By 6 months, the differential effect of treatment was no longer evident. No effects of the booster sessions were found for behavioral outcomes, including adherence to the exercise program, frequency of exercise, heart rate, and blood pressure. |

REFERENCES

Ahles, T. A., Wasson, J. H., Seville, J. L., Johnson, D. J., Cole, B. F., Hanscom, B., et al. (2006). A controlled trial of methods for managing pain in primary care patients with or without co-occurring psychosocial problems. *Annals of Family Medicine, 4*(4), 341–350.

Allen, S. M., Shah, A. C., Nezu, A.M., Nezu, C. M., Ciambrone, D., Hogan, J., et al. (2002). A problem-solving approach to stress reduction among younger women with breast carcinoma. *Cancer, 94*(12), 3089–3100.

Andersson, C. M., Bjaras, G., Tillgren, P., & Ostenson, C. G. (2005). A longitudinal assessment of inter-sectoral participation in a community-based diabetes prevention programme. *Social Science and Medicine, 61*(11), 2407–2422.

Andersson, G., Bergstrom, J., Hollandare, F., Carlbring, P., Kaldo, V., & Ekselius, L. (2005). Internet-based self-help for depression: Randomised controlled trial. *British Journal of Psychiatry, 187*, 456–461.

Andersson, G., Lundstrom, P., & Ström, L. (2003). Internet-based treatment of headache: Does telephone contact add anything? *Headache, 43*(4), 353–361.

Andersson, G., Strömgren, T., Ström, L., & Lyttkens, L. (2002). Randomized controlled trial of Internet-based cognitive behavior therapy for distress associated with tinnitus. *Psychosomatic Medicine, 64*(5), 810–816.

Bailey, D. E., Mishel, M. H., Belyea, M., Stewart, J. L., & Mohler, J. (2004). Uncertainty intervention for watchful waiting in prostate cancer. *Cancer Nursing, 27*(5), 339–346.

Balady, G. J., Williams, M. A., Ades, P. A., Bittner, V., Comoss, P., Foody, J. A. M., et al. (2007). Core components of cardiac rehabilitation/secondary prevention programs: 2007 update. *Journal of Cardiopulmonary Rehabilitation & Prevention, 27*(3), 121–129.

Bambauer, K. Z., Aupont, O., Stone, P. H., Locke, S. E., Mullan, M. G., Colagiovanni, J., et al. (2005). The effect of a telephone counseling intervention on self-rated health of cardiac patients. *Psychosomatic Medicine, 67*(4), 539–545.

Bell, K. R., Temkin, N. R., Esselman, P. C., Doctor, J. N., Bombardier, C. H., Fraser, R. T., et al. (2005). The effect of a scheduled telephone intervention on outcome after moderate to severe traumatic brain injury: A randomized trial. *Archives of Physical Medicine and Rehabilitation, 86*(5), 851–856.

Bennett, J. A., Lyons, K. S., Winters-Stone, K., Nail, L. M., & Scherer, J. (2007). Motivational interviewing to increase physical activity in long-term cancer survivors: A randomized controlled trial. *Nursing Research, 56*(1), 18–27.

Berger, M., Wagner, T. H., & Baker, L. C. (2005). Internet use and stigmatized illness. *Social Science & Medicine, 61*(8), 1821–1827.

Blixen, C. E., Bramstedt, K. A., Hammel, J. P., & Tilley, B. C. (2004). A pilot study of health education via a nurse-run telephone self-management programme for elderly people with osteoarthritis. *Journal of Telemedicine and Telecare, 10*, 44–49.

Blumenthal, J. A., Babyak, M. A., Keefe, F. J., Davis, R. D., Lacaille, R. A., Carney, R. M., et al. (2006). Telephone-based coping skills training for patients awaiting lung transplantation. *Journal of Consulting and Clinical Psychology, 74*(3), 535–544.

Bodenheimer, T., Lorig, K., Holman, H., & Grumbach, K. (2002). Patient self-management of chronic disease in primary care. *Journal of the American Medical Association, 288*(19), 2469–2475.

Boter, H. (2004). Multicenter randomized controlled trial of an outreach nursing support program for recently discharged stroke patients. *Stroke, 35*(12), 2867–2872.

Brug, J., Oenema, A., & Campbell, M. (2003). Past, present, and future of computer-tailored nutrition education. *American Journal of Clinical Nutrition, 77*(4 Suppl.), 1028S–1034S.

Brug, J., Oenema, A., Kroeze, W., & Raat, H. (2005). The Internet and nutrition education: Challenges and opportunities. *European Journal of Clinical Nutrition, 59*(Suppl. 1), S130–137; discussion S138–139.

Buhrman, M., Fältenhag, S., Ström, L., & Andersson, G. (2004). Controlled trial of Internet-based treatment with telephone support for chronic back pain. *Pain, 111*(3), 368–377.

Carlbring, P., Nilsson-Ihrfelt, E., Waara, J., Kollenstam, C., Buhrman, M., Kaldo, V., et al. (2005). Treatment of panic disorder: Live therapy vs. self-help via the Internet. *Behaviour Research and Therapy, 43*(10), 1321–1333.

Cassell, M. M., Jackson, C., & Cheuvront, B. (1998). Health communication on the Internet: An effective channel for health behavior change? *Journal of Health Communication, 3*(1), 71–79.

Cho, J.-H., Chang, S.-A., Kwon, H.-S., Choi, Y.-H., Ko, S.-H., Moon, S.-D., et al. (2006). Long-term effect of the Internet-based glucose monitoring system on HbA1c reduction and glucose stability: A 30-month follow-up study for diabetes management with a ubiquitous medical care system. *Diabetes Care, 29*(12), 2625–2631.

Chouinard, M. C., & Robichaud-Ekstrand, S. (2005). The effectiveness of a nursing inpatient smoking cessation program in individuals with cardiovascular disease. *Nursing Research, 54*(4), 243–254.

Clark, A. M., Hartling, L., Vandermeer, B., & McAlister, F. A. (2005). Meta-analysis: Secondary prevention programs for patients with coronary artery disease. *Annals of Internal Medicine, 143*(9), 659–672.

Clarke, G., Eubanks, D., Reid, E., Kelleher, C., O'Connor, E., DeBar, L. L., et al. (2005). Overcoming depression on the Internet (ODIN) (2): A randomized trial of a self-help depression skills program with reminders. *Journal of Medical Internet Research, 7*(2), e16.

Clarke, G., Reid, E., Eubanks, D., O'Connor, E., DeBar, L. L., Kelleher, C., et al. (2002). Overcoming depression on the Internet (ODIN): A randomized controlled trial of an Internet depression skills intervention program. *Journal of Medical Internet Research, 4*(3), e14.

De Bourdeaudhuij, I., & Brug, J. (2000). Tailoring dietary feedback to reduce fat intake: An intervention at the family level. *Health Education Research, 15*(4), 449–462.

DeBusk, R. F., Miller, N. H., Parker, K. M., Bandura, A., Kraemer, H. C., Cher, D. J., et al. (2004). Care management for low-risk patients with heart failure: A randomized, controlled trial. *Annals of Internal Medicine, 141*(8), 606–613.

Del Sindaco, D., Pulignano, G., Minardi, G., Apostoli, A., Guerrieri, L., Rotoloni, M., et al. (2007). Two-year outcome of a prospective, controlled study of a disease management programme for elderly patients with heart failure. *Journal of Cardiovascular Medicine, 8*(5), 324–329.

Devineni, T., & Blanchard, E. B. (2005). A randomized controlled trial of an Internet-based treatment for chronic headache. *Behaviour Research and Therapy, 43*(3), 277–292.

DeVol, R., Bedroussian, A., Charuworn, A., Chatterjee, A., Kim, I. K., Kim, S., et al. (2007). *An unhealthy America: The economic burden of chronic disease—charting a new course to save lives and increase productivity and economic growth.* Retrieved

February 2008, from http://www.milkeninstitute.org/pdf/chronic_disease_report.pdf

DeWalt, D. A., Malone, R. M., Bryant, M. E., Kosnar, M. C., Corr, K. E., Rothman, R. L., et al. (2006). A heart failure self-management program for patients of all literacy levels: A randomized, controlled trial. *BMC Health Services Research, 6*, 30.

Dietrich, A. J., Oxman, T. E., Williams, J. W., Jr., Schulberg, H. C., Bruce, M. L., Lee, P. W., et al. (2004). Re-engineering systems for the treatment of depression in primary care: Cluster randomised controlled trial. *British Medical Journal, 329*(7466), 602–609.

Dougherty, C. M., Thompson, E. A., & Lewis, F. M. (2005). Long-term outcomes of a telephone intervention after an ICD. *Pacing and Clinical Electrophysiology, 28*(11), 1157–1167.

Dunagan, W. C., Littenberg, B., Ewald, G. A., Jones, C. A., Emery, V. B., Waterman, B. M., et al. (2005). Randomized trial of a nurse-administered, telephone-based disease management program for patients with heart failure. *Journal of Cardiac Failure, 11*(5), 358–365.

Emmons, K. M., Puleo, E., Park, E., Gritz, E. R., Butterfield, R. M., Weeks, J. C., et al. (2005). Peer-delivered smoking counseling for childhood cancer survivors increases rate of cessation: The partnership for health study. *Journal of Clinical Oncology, 23*(27), 6516–6523.

Farmer, A. J., Gibson, O. J., Dudley, C., Bryden, K., Hayton, P. M., Tarassenko, L., et al. (2005). A randomized controlled trial of the effect of real-time telemedicine support on glycemic control in young adults with type 1 diabetes. *Diabetes Care, 28*(11), 2697–2702.

Fox, S. (2007, October 8). *E-patients with a disability or chronic disease.* Retrieved February 2008 from http://www.pewinternet.org/pdfs/EPatients_Chronic_Conditions_2007.pdf

Garrett, N., & Martini, E. M. (2007). The boomers are coming: A total cost of care model of the impact of population aging on the cost of chronic conditions in the United States. *Disease Management, 10*(2), 51–60.

Gately, C., Rogers, A., & Sanders, C. (2007). Re-thinking the relationship between long-term condition self-management education and the utilisation of health services. *Social Science and Medicine, 65*(5), 934–945.

Glasgow, R. E., Boles, S. M., McKay, H. G., Feil, E. G., & Barrera, J. M. (2003). The D-Net diabetes self-management program: Long-term implementation, outcomes, and generalization results. *Preventive Medicine, 36*(4), 410–419.

Glasgow, R. E., Toobert, D. J., Hampson, S. E., & Strycker, L. A. (2002). Implementation, generalization and long-term results of the "Choosing well" diabetes self-management intervention. *Patient Education and Counseling, 48*(2), 115–122.

Glueckauf, R. L. (1990). Program evaluation guidelines for the rehabilitation professional. *Advances in Clinical Rehabilitation, 3*, 250–266.

Glueckauf, R. L., Fritz, S. P., Ecklund-Johnson, E. P., Liss, H. J., Dages, P., & Carney, P. (2002). Videoconferencing-based family counseling for rural teenagers with epilepsy: Phase 1 findings. *Rehabilitation Psychology, 47*(1), 49–72.

Glueckauf, R. L., & Ketterson, T. U. (2004). Telehealth interventions for individuals with chronic illness: Research review and implications for practice. *Professional Psychology: Research and Practice, 35*(6), 615–627.

Glueckauf, R. L., Pickett, T. C., Ketterson, T. U., Loomis, J. S., & Rozensky, R. H. (2003). Preparation for the delivery of telehealth services: A self-study framework for expansion of practice. *Professional Psychology: Research and Practice, 34*(2), 159–163.

Glueckauf, R. L., Pickett, T. C., Ketterson, T. U., & Nickelson, D. W. (2006). Telehealth research and practice: Key issues and developments in research. In P. Kennedy & S. Llewelyn (Eds.), *The essentials of clinical health psychology* (pp. 305–331). London: Wiley.

Gorelick, P. B., Harris, Y., Burnett, B., & Bonecutter, F. J. (1998). The recruitment triangle: Reasons why African Americans enroll, refuse to enroll, or voluntarily withdraw from a clinical trial. An interim report from the African-American Antiplatelet Stroke Prevention Study (AAASPS). *Journal of the National Medical Association, 90*(3), 141–145.

Griffiths, C., Motlib, J., Azad, A., Ramsay, J., Eldridge, S., Feder, G., et al. (2005). Randomised controlled trial of a lay-led self-management programme for Bangladeshi patients with chronic disease. *British Journal of General Practice, 55*(520), 831–837.

Griffiths, K. M., & Christensen, H. (2006). Review of randomised controlled trials of Internet interventions for mental disorders and related conditions. *Clinical Psychologist, 10*(1), 16–29.

Hautman, M., & P., Bomer. (1995). Interactional model for recruiting ethnically diverse research participants. *Journal of Multicultural Nursing and Health, 1*, 8–15.

Howells, L., Wilson, A. C., Skinner, T. C., Newton, R., Morris, A. D., & Greene, S. A. (2002). A randomized control trial of the effect of negotiated telephone support on glycaemic control in young people with type 1 diabetes. *Diabetic Medicine, 19*(8), 643–648.

Hunkeler, E. M., Katon, W., Tang, L., Williams, J. W., Jr., Kroenke, K., Lin, E. H. B., et al. (2006). Long term outcomes from the impact randomised trial for depressed elderly patients in primary care. *British Medical Journal, 332*(7536), 259–263.

Hurley, M. V., Walsh, N. E., Mitchell, H. L., Pimm, T. J., Williamson, E., Jones, R. H., et al. (2007). Economic evaluation of a rehabilitation program integrating exercise, self-management, and active coping strategies for chronic knee pain. *Arthritis and Rheumatism, 57*(7), 1220–1229.

Jan, R. L., Wang, J. Y., Huang, M. C., Tseng, S. M., Su, H. J., & Liu, L. F. (2007). An Internet-based interactive telemonitoring system for improving childhood asthma outcomes in Taiwan. *Telemedicine Journal and e-Health, 13*(3), 257–268.

Joseph, C. L., Peterson, E., Havstad, S., Johnson, C. C., Hoerauf, S., Stringer, S., et al. (2007). A Web-based, tailored asthma management program for urban African-American high school students. *American Journal of Respiratory and Critical Care Medicine, 175*(9), 888–895.

Karlson, E. W., Liang, M. H., Eaton, H., Huang, J., Fitzgerald, L., Rogers, M. P., et al. (2004). A randomized clinical trial of a psychoeducational intervention to improve outcomes in systemic lupus erythematosus. *Arthritis and Rheumatism, 50*(6), 1832–1841.

Kennedy, A., Nelson, E., Reeves, D., Richardson, G., Roberts, C., Robinson, A., et al. (2003). A randomised controlled trial to assess the impact of a package comprising a patient-orientated, evidence-based self-help guidebook and patient-centred consultations on disease management and satisfaction in inflammatory bowel disease. *Health Technology Assessment, 7*(28), iii, 1–113.

Kennedy, A., Reeves, D., Bower, P., Lee, V., Middleton, E., Richardson, G., et al. (2007). The effectiveness and cost effectiveness of a national lay-led self care support programme for patients with long-term conditions: A pragmatic randomised controlled trial. *Journal of Epidemiology and Community Health, 61*(3), 254–261.

Khan, M. S. R., O'Meara, M., Stevermuer, T. L., & Henry, R. L. (2004). Randomized controlled trial of asthma education after discharge from an emergency department. *Journal of Paediatrics and Child Health, 40*(12), 674–677.

Kim, C., Kim, H., Nam, J., Cho, M., Park, J., Kang, E., et al. (2007). Internet diabetic patient management using a short messaging service automatically produced by a knowledge matrix system. *Diabetes Care, 30*(11), 2857–2858.

Kim, H. S., & Oh, J. A. (2003). Adherence to diabetes control recommendations: Impact of nurse telephone calls. *Journal of Advanced Nursing, 44*(3), 256–261.

Klein, B., Richards, J. C., & Austin, D. W. (2005). Efficacy of Internet therapy for panic disorder. *Journal of Behavior Therapy and Experimental Psychiatry, 37,* 213–238.

Krein, S. L., Klamerus, M. L., Vijan, S., Lee, J. L., Fitzgerald, J. T., Pawlow, A., et al. (2004). Case management for patients with poorly controlled diabetes: A randomized trial. *American Journal of Medicine, 116*(11), 732–739.

Krishna, S., Francisco, B. D., Balas, E. A., Konig, P., Graff, G. R., & Madsen, R. W. (2003). Internet-enabled interactive multimedia asthma education program: A randomized trial. *Pediatrics, 111*(3), 503(508).

Kroeze, W., Werkman, A., & Brug, J. (2006). A systematic review of randomized trials on the effectiveness of computer-tailored education on physical activity and dietary behaviors. *Annals of Behavioral Medicine, 31*(3), 205–223.

Kwon, H.-S., Cho, J.-H., Kim, H.-S., Song, B.-R., Ko, S.-H., Lee, J.-M., et al. (2004). Establishment of blood glucose monitoring system using the Internet. *Diabetes Care, 27*(2), 478–483.

Lamers, F., Jonkers, C. C., Bosma, H., Diederiks, J. P., & van Eijk, J. T. (2006). Effectiveness and cost-effectiveness of a minimal psychological intervention to reduce non-severe depression in chronically ill elderly patients: The design of a randomised controlled trial. *BMC Public Health, 6,* 161.

Lange, A., Rietdijk, D., Hudcovicova, M., van de Ven, J. P., Schrieken, B., & Emmelkamp, P. M. (2003). Interapy: A controlled randomized trial of the standardized treatment of posttraumatic stress through the Internet. *Journal of Consulting and Clinical Psychology, 71*(5), 901–909.

Logue, E., Sutton, K., Jarjoura, D., Smucker, W., Baughman, K., & Capers, C. (2005). Transtheoretical model-chronic disease care for obesity in primary care: A randomized trial. *Obesity: A Research Journal, 13*(5), 917–927.

Lorig, K. R., Ritter, P. L., Laurent, D. D., & Fries, J. F. (2004). Long-term randomized controlled trials of tailored-print and small-group arthritis self-management interventions. *Medical Care, 42*(4), 346–354.

Lorig, K. R., Ritter, P. L., Laurent, D. D., & Plant, K. (2006). Internet-based chronic disease self-management: A randomized trial. *Medical Care, 44*(11), 964–971.

Maheu, M. M., Whitten, P., & Allen, A. (2001). *E-health, telehealth, and telemedicine: A guide to start-up and success.* San Francisco: Jossey-Bass.

Maljanian, R., Grey, N., Staff, I., & Conroy, L. (2005). Intensive telephone follow-up to a hospital-based disease management model for patients with diabetes mellitus. *Disease Management, 8*(1), 15–25.

McAlister, F. A., Lawson, F. M. E., Teo, K. K., & Armstrong, P. W. (2001). A systematic review of randomized trials of disease management programs in heart failure. *American Journal of Medicine, 110*(5), 378–384.

McCarthy, C. J., Mills, P.M., Pullen, R., Richardson, G., Hawkins, N., Roberts, C. R., et al. (2004). Supplementation of a home-based exercise programme with a class-based programme for people with osteoarthritis of the knees: A randomised controlled trial and health economic analysis. *Health Technology Assessment, 8*(46), iii–iv, 1–61.

McKay, H. G., Glasgow, R. E., Feil, E. G., Boles, S. M., & Barrera, J. M. (2002). Internet-based diabetes self-management and support: Initial outcomes from the diabetes network project. *Rehabilitation Psychology, 47*(1), 31–48.

McManus, R. J., Mant, J., Roalfe, A., Oakes, R. A., Bryan, S., Pattison, H. M., et al. (2005). Targets and self monitoring in hypertension: Randomised controlled trial and cost effectiveness analysis. *British Medical Journal, 331*(7515), 493.

Middleton, S., Donnelly, N., Harris, J., & Ward, J. (2005). Nursing intervention after carotid endarterectomy: A randomized trial of coordinated care post-discharge (CCPD). *Journal of Advanced Nursing, 52*(3), 250–261.

Mishel, M. H., Germino, B. B., Gil, K. M., Belyea, M., LaNey, I. C., Stewart, J., et al. (2005). Benefits from an uncertainty management intervention for African-American and Caucasian older long-term breast cancer survivors. *Psycho-Oncology, 14*(11), 962–978.

Monninkhof, E., van der Valk, P., Schermer, T., van der Palen, J., van Herwaarden, C., & Zielhuis, G. (2004). Economic evaluation of a comprehensive self-management programme in patients with moderate to severe chronic obstructive pulmonary disease. *Chronic Respiratory Disease, 1*(1), 7–16.

Napolitano, M. A., Babyak, M. A., Palmer, S., Tapson, V., Davis, R. D., & Blumenthal, J. A. (2002). Effects of a telephone-based psychosocial intervention for patients awaiting lung transplantation. *Chest, 122*(4), 1176–1184.

Nunn, E., King, B., Smart, C., & Anderson, D. (2006). A randomized controlled trial of telephone calls to young patients with poorly controlled type 1 diabetes. *Pediatric Diabetes, 7*(5), 254–259.

Oenema, A., Brug, J., & Lechner, L. (2001). Web-based tailored nutrition education: Results of a randomized controlled trial. *Health Education Research, 16*(6), 647–660.

Oenema, A., Tan, F., & Brug, J. (2005). Short-term efficacy of a Web-based computer-tailored nutrition intervention: Main effects and mediators. *Annals of Behavioral Medicine, 29*(1), 54–63.

Owen, J. E., Klapow, J. C., Roth, D. L., Shuster, J. L., Jr., Bellis, J., Meredith, R., et al. (2005). Randomized pilot of a self-guided Internet coping group for women with early-stage breast cancer. *Annals of Behavioral Medicine, 30*(1), 54–64.

Park, T. L., Perri, M. G., & Rodrigue, J. R. (2003). Minimal intervention programs for weight loss in heart transplant candidates: A preliminary examination. *Progress in Transplantation, 13*(4), 284–288.

Paul, G. L. (1967). Strategy of outcome research in psychotherapy. *Journal of Consulting Psychology, 31* (2), 109–118.

Pinto, B. M., Frierson, G. M., Rabin, C., Trunzo, J. J., & Marcus, B. H. (2005). Home-based physical activity intervention for breast cancer patients. *Journal of Clinical Oncology, 23*(15), 3577–3587.

Richardson, G., Sculpher, M., Kennedy, A., Nelson, E., Reeves, D., Roberts, C., et al. (2006). Is self-care a cost-effective use of resources? Evidence from a randomized trial in inflammatory bowel disease. *Journal of Health Services Research Policy, 11*(4), 225–230.

Riegel, B., Carlson, B., Glaser, D., & Romero, T. (2006). Randomized controlled trial of telephone case management in Hispanics of Mexican origin with heart failure. *Journal of Cardiac Failure, 12*(3), 211–219.

Ries, A. L., Kaplan, R. M., Myers, R., & Prewitt, L. M. (2003). Maintenance after pulmonary rehabilitation in chronic lung disease: A randomized trial. *American Journal of Respiratory and Critical Care Medicine, 167*(6), 880–888.

Ritterband, L. M., Cox, D. J., Walker, L. S., Kovatchev, B., McKnight, L., Patel, K., et al. (2003). An Internet intervention as adjunctive therapy for pediatric encopresis. *Journal of Consulting and Clinical Psychology, 71*(5), 910–917.

Rodrigue, J. R., Baz, M. A., Widows, M. R., & Ehlers, S. L. (2005). A randomized evaluation of quality-of-life therapy with patients awaiting lung transplantation. *American Journal of Transplantation, 5*(10), 2425–2432.

Rollman, B. L., Belnap, B. H., Mazumdar, S., Houck, P. R., Zhu, F., Gardner, W., et al. (2005). A randomized trial to improve the quality of treatment for panic and generalized anxiety disorders in primary care. *Archives of General Psychiatry, 62*(12), 1332–1341.

Rotheram-Borus, M. J., Swendeman, D., Comulada, W. S., Weiss, R. E., Lee, M., & Lightfoot, M. (2004). Prevention for substance-using HIV-positive young people: Telephone and in-person delivery. *Journal of Acquired Immune Deficiency Syndromes, 37*(Suppl. 2), S68–77.

Scherer, M. J. (2002). *Assistive technology: Matching device and consumer for successful rehabilitation.* Washington, DC: American Psychological Association.

Simon, G. E., Ludman, E. J., Tutty, S., Operskalski, B., & Korff, M. V. (2004). Telephone psychotherapy and telephone care management for primary care patients starting antidepressant treatment: A randomized controlled trial. *Journal of the American Medical Association, 292*(8), 935–942.

Sisk, J. E., Hebert, P. L., Horowitz, C. R., McLaughlin, M. A., Wang, J. J., & Chassin, M. R. (2006). Effects of nurse management on the quality of heart failure care in minority communities: A randomized trial. *Annals of Internal Medicine, 145*(4), 273–283.

Smeulders, E. S., van Haastregt, J. C., van Hoef, E. F., van Eijk, J. T., & Kempen, G. I. (2006). Evaluation of a self-management programme for congestive heart failure patients: Design of a randomised controlled trial. *BMC Health Services Research, 6,* 91.

Southard, B. H., Southard, D. R., & Nuckolls, J. (2003). Clinical trial of an Internet-based case management system for secondary prevention of heart disease. *Journal of Cardiopulmonary Rehabilitation, 23*(5), 341–348.

Stoy, D. B., Curtis, R. C., Dameworth, K. S., Dowdy, A. A., Hegland, J., Levin, J. A., et al. (1995). The successful recruitment of elderly black subjects in a clinical trial: The crisp experience. Cholesterol reduction in seniors program. *Journal of the National Medical Association, 87*(4), 280–287.

Street, R. L. (2003). Mediated consumer-provider communication in cancer care: The empowering potential of new technologies. *Patient Education and Counseling, 50*(1), 99–104.

Strong, L. L., Von Korff, M., Saunders, K., & Moore, J. E. (2006). Cost-effectiveness of two self-care interventions to reduce disability associated with back pain. *Spine, 31*(15), 1639–1645.

Stuifbergen, A. K., Becker, H., Blozis, S., Timmerman, G., & Kullberg, V. (2003). A randomized clinical trial of a wellness intervention for women with multiple sclerosis. *Archives of Physical Medicine and Rehabilitation, 84*(4), 467–476.

Sue, D. W., & Sue, D. (1999). *Counseling the culturally different: Theory and practice* (3rd ed.). New York: J. Wiley & Sons.

Tatti, P., & Lehmann, E. D. (2003). A prospective randomised-controlled pilot study for evaluating the teaching utility of interactive educational diabetes simulators. *Diabetes, Nutrition & Metabolism, 16*(1), 7–23.

Thomas, R. J., King, M., Lui, K., Oldridge, N., Pina, I. L., Spertus, J., et al. (2007). AACVPR/ACC/AHA 2007 performance measures on cardiac rehabilitation for referral to and delivery of cardiac rehabilitation/secondary prevention services. *Journal of the American College of Cardiology, 50*(14), 1400–1433.

Thorpe, K. E. (2006). Factors accounting for the rise in health-care spending in the United States: The role of rising disease prevalence and treatment intensity. *Public Health, 120*(11), 1002–1007.

Tranmer, J. E., & Parry, M. J. E. (2004). Enhancing postoperative recovery of cardiac surgery patients: A randomized clinical trial of an advanced practice nursing intervention. *Western Journal of Nursing Research, 26*(5), 515–532.

van den Berg, M. H., Ronday, H. K., Peeters, A. J., le Cessie, S., van der Giesen, F. J., Breedveld, F. C., et al. (2006). Using Internet technology to deliver a home-based physical activity intervention for patients with rheumatoid arthritis: A randomized controlled trial. *Arthritis and Rheumatism, 55*(6), 935–945.

Verheijden, M., Bakx, J. C., Akkermans, R., van den Hoogen, H., Godwin, N. M., Rosser, W., et al. (2004). Web-based targeted nutrition counselling and social support for patients at increased cardiovascular risk in general practice: Randomized controlled trial. *Journal of Medical Internet Research, 6*, e44. Retrieved July 16, 2008, from http://www.jmir.org/2004/4/e44/

Vidrine, D. J., Arduino, R. C., Lazev, A. B., & Gritz, E. R. (2006). A randomized trial of a proactive cellular telephone intervention for smokers living with HIV/AIDS. *AIDS, 20*(2), 253–260.

Wagner, B., Knaevelsrud, C., & Maercker, A. (2006). Internet-based cognitive-behavioral therapy for complicated grief: A randomized controlled trial. *Death Studies, 30*(5), 429–453.

Wagner, T. H., Baker, L. C., Bundorf, M. K., & Singer, S. (2004). Use of the Internet for health information by the chronically ill. *Preventing Chronic Disease, 1.* Retrieved August 14, 2008, from http://www.cdc.gov/pcd/issues/2004/oct/04_0004.htm

Walther, J. B., Pingree, S., Hawkins, R. P., & Buller, D. B. (2005). Attributes of interactive online health information systems. *Journal of Medical Internet Research, 7*(3), e33.

Whitten, P. S., Mair, F. S., Haycox, A., May, C. R., Williams, T. L., & Hellmich, S. (2002). Systematic review of cost effectiveness studies of telemedicine interventions. *British Medical Journal, 324*(7351), 1434–1437.

Williams, K., Prevost, A. T., Griffin, S., Hardeman, W., Hollingworth, W., Spiegelhalter, D., et al. (2004). The proactive trial protocol—a randomised controlled trial of the efficacy of a family-based, domiciliary intervention programme to increase physical activity among individuals at high risk of diabetes [isrctn61323766]. *BMC Public Health, 4,* 48.

Wilson, P. M., & Mayor, V. (2006). Long-term conditions. 2: Supporting and enabling self-care. *British Journal of Community Nursing, 11*(1), 6–10.

Winzelberg, A. J., Classen, C., Alpers, G. W., Roberts, H., Koopman, C., Adams, R. E., et al. (2003). Evaluation of an Internet support group for women with primary breast cancer. *Cancer, 97*(5), 1164–1173.

Woolf, S. H., Chan, E. C. Y., Harris, R., Sheridan, S. L., Braddock, C. H., III, Kaplan, R. M., et al. (2005). Promoting informed choice: Transforming health care to dispense knowledge for decision making. *Annals of Internal Medicine, 143*(4), 293–300.

Woollard, J., Burke, V., Beilin, L. J., Verheijden, M., & Bulsara, M. K. (2003). Effects of a general practice-based intervention on diet, body mass index and blood lipids in patients at cardiovascular risk. *Journal of Cardiovascular Risk, 10*(1), 31–40.

Yates, B.C., Anderson, T., Hertzog, M., Ott, C., & Williams, J. (2005). Effectiveness of follow-up booster sessions in improving physical status after cardiac rehabilitation: Health, behavioral, and clinical outcomes. *Applied Nursing Research, 18*(1), 59–62.

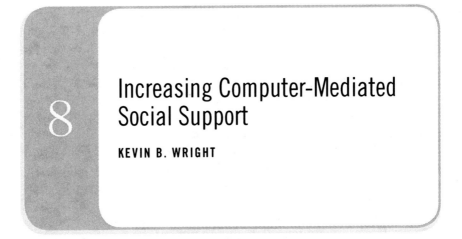

Increasing Computer-Mediated Social Support

8

KEVIN B. WRIGHT

The rapid adoption of the Internet by many segments of society over the past 15 years has spurred the growth of various Web sites and on-line communities for people seeking social support for health concerns (Wright, 2000; Wright & Bell, 2003). The Internet provides many options for individuals with health concerns who seek to supplement or replace traditional (face-to-face) sources of social support. The Internet appears to facilitate the maintenance of supportive relationships among people who know one another from face-to-face contexts (such as family members and friends) as well as the development of new relationships online (e.g., individuals who "meet" in computer-mediated contexts, such as online support communities).

This phenomenon has attracted the attention of social scientists and medical researchers who are interested in the benefits of computer-mediated social support for people with health concerns, including important outcomes such as reduced stress and increased coping skills (King & Moreggi, 1998; Preece & Ghozati, 2001; Wright, 2000). With annual health care costs in the United States soaring above $1 trillion a year (U.S. Census Bureau, 2001), researchers have become increasingly interested in ways that computer-mediated social support can be used by patients as a low-cost means of maintaining health and coping with illness as well as for prevention of disease. Despite over a decade of research in the area of computer-mediated social support, it remains a fertile context for researchers interested in the impact of new technologies for health care.

This chapter explores the various ways in which the Internet and related new technologies may increase social support for people coping with a variety of health concerns. Toward that end, the chapter explores the various types of social support available online, the link between social support and health outcomes, relational dilemmas surrounding the provision of social support, and advantages and disadvantages of online support groups/communities. In addition, it focuses on several theoretical frameworks that have been useful in past research in terms of understanding the nature of computer-mediated social support and provides suggestions for future researchers and practitioners who are interested in understanding computer-mediated social support and how this knowledge can be applied to potentially improve the lives of individuals dealing with health concerns.

SOURCES OF SOCIAL SUPPORT ON THE INTERNET

The Internet provides a surprisingly vast array of potential sources of social support for people seeking informational, emotional, and even tangible support online. However, the majority of studies have focused on support within online support groups and communities, largely ignoring the use of Internet as a means of facilitating traditional supportive relationships, such as those with family members and friends. This section will briefly explore potential sources of computer-mediated social support.

As stated above, most researchers have explored online support groups and communities as sources of online support. This is not surprising, given the rapid growth of these groups in recent years. For example, a brief search of support groups and communities on Yahoo yields thousands of health-related groups dealing with almost every possible physical and mental health issue. Early research dealing with support provision within these groups tended to understand the various types of support that are provided within these groups/communities (Alexander, Peterson, & Hollingshead, 2003; Braithwaite, Waldron, & Finn, 1999; Weinberg, Schmale, Uken, & Wessel, 1995), and several researchers were concerned with whether more complex types of support, such as emotional support, could be adequately provided by group/community members (Campbell & Wright, 2002; Galinski, Schopler, & Abell, 1997; Preece & Ghozati, 2001). This research found that many types of social support are provided within these groups/communities, including informational support, emotional support, and validation, and they sometimes helped to facilitate tangible support (when participants later met face-to-face). In addition, findings from several of these studies suggest that the constraints of the medium do not appear to inhibit the provision of emotional support.

Few studies have examined the use of health-related Web sites as a source of informational support, despite the fact that several studies have found that health information is one of the most popular topics that individuals research on the Internet (Fox & Ranie, 2000; Harris Interactive, 2001). Among communication researchers, the lack of research interest in these Web sites as sources of social support is most likely due to their largely non-interactive nature. However, while Web sites such as those sponsored by the Centers for Disease Control and Prevention, the National Institutes of Health, the National Cancer Institute, and WebMD certainly provide links to support groups/communities and Web chats, their main purpose is to provide individuals with information about a wide variety of health concerns, including cancer, HIV, hypertension, pregnancy, allergies, diet and exercise, and mental health issues. Moreover, these Web sites appear to be important sources of informational support (Bass, 2003; Eng, 2001; Wright, 2007). In addition, information from these online sources appears to spur increased interaction between patients and providers within health care settings (Aspden & Katz, 2001; Bass, 2003; Napoli, 2001).

Much less is known about family members and friends as sources of online social support. However, in our increasingly mobile society, the Internet appears to be an important resource for maintaining relationships among family members and friends, especially in cases where people are geographically separated from these traditional sources of social support. Yet the Internet may facilitate supportive interactions among family members and friends who are part of a person's daily face-to-face support network. For example, many people use the Internet (through e-mail and chat applications) and cell phone texting to conveniently send and receive messages from members of their face-to-face support network while they are engaged in other activities (e.g., work and school). Social network sites such as MySpace and Facebook appear to help people maintain supportive relationships with family members and friends even though they often overlap with traditional face-to-face support networks (Dwyer, 2007; Ellison, Stein-field, & Lampe, 2007; Snyder, Carpenter, & Slauson, 2006). Future research in computer-mediated social support would benefit by exam-ining the use of e-mail, chat applications, and social network sites as potential resources for obtaining health-related social support from family members and friends.

SOCIAL SUPPORT AND HEALTH OUTCOMES

Social support researchers have devoted a great deal of attention to the link between adequate social support provision to important physical and psychological health outcomes. Studies from a variety of disciplines have consistently linked traditional sources of social support to morbid-ity and mortality rates (Berkman & Symes, 1979; Bruunk, 1990; Cohen, 1988; House, Landis, & Umberson, 1988; Uchino, Cacioppo, & Kiecolt-Glaser, 1996). Prolonged exposure to stress has been found to impair immune system response; increase risk for hypertension, heart disease, and stroke; and lead to increases in depression, tension, and nervousness (Ballieux & Heijen, 1989; Clow, 2001; Kohn, 1996).

Researchers have identified two distinct ways in which social sup-port appears to influence health outcomes. The buffering model of social support (Cohen & Wills, 1985; Dean & Lin, 1977) posits that an individ-ual's social network helps to shield him or her from stress or reduce the amount of stress he or she may experience when he or she encounters both major crises and everyday sources of stress. The social capital and other resources associated with one's support network can help buffer or offset stressors, including those related to health concerns. The main effects model of social support asserts that there is a direct relation-ship between social support and health outcomes (Aneshensel & Stone, 1982). Positive interactions with one's support network in everyday rela-tionships appear to elevate mood, reduce stress, and make people more resilient to stressful situations (Berkman & Syme, 1979; Cohen, 1988).

Of course, there are many mediating variables that influence the relationship between social support and health outcomes, including an individual's coping abilities (Edwards & Trimble, 1992; Kohn, 1996) and perceptions of the support provider and type of support offered (Al-brecht & Goldsmith, 2003; Burleson, 1994). For example, informational support is sometimes perceived as unwanted advice, individuals can dis-miss certain problems when offering support, the timing of support may be inappropriate, and there are a number of other relational concerns that can undermine the potential benefits of social support. This following section discusses some of these relational concerns in greater detail.

RELATIONAL CONCERNS WHEN PEOPLE SEEK/PROVIDE SUPPORT

The process of seeking support within relationships can be a difficult process for many individuals facing illness, who must coordinate meeting their needs with attempting to manage relational concerns (Albrecht & Goldsmith, 2003). According to these Albrecht and Goldsmith, partners must cope not only with a stressor but also with the relational strains created by the stressor and the difficulties inherent in coordinating their individual coping attempts. The practice of seeking support can involve a complicated process of managing difficult individual coping needs while simultaneously attempting to manage delicate relational concerns. Findings from a variety of research programs suggest that many individuals find it difficult to obtain appropriate support from friends and family since they may feel their closer ties lack experience or have limited information about certain problems (see Albrecht, Burleson, & Goldsmith, 1994; Barbee, Derlega, Sherburne, & Grimshaw, 1998; Brashers, Neidig, & Goldsmith, 2004; Pakenham, 1998). Furthermore, many people may feel uncomfortable discussing their problems with their strong ties for a variety of other reasons, such as a desire to avoid feeling stigmatized or patronized or being judged when discussing sensitive topics.

Other complicating relational concerns in social support situations may include reluctance to receive inappropriate support, or not wanting to appear vulnerable or incapable of handling one's own problems. In addition there are complications associated with role obligations and reciprocity issues in many relationships (Albrecht & Goldsmith, 2003; Chesler & Barbarin, 1984; Cline, 1999; LaGaipa, 1990). Role obligations refer to the idea that we sometimes feel obligated to support our loved ones even during times when we may not necessarily want to help them due to our own concerns. Role obligations in supportive encounters have been found to lead to resentment in some cases (Rook, 1995). Reciprocity issues in supportive encounters include problems that occur when one relational partner is under-benefited (i.e., gives more support than he or she receives), and when a partner is over-benefited (i.e., receives more support than he or she can give in return). People with health problems often find themselves in a position where they are over-benefited as people in their social network attempt to support them during their time of need. However, the inability to help others in such situations has been found to lead to feelings of inadequacy, helplessness, and demoralization in some cases (Bakas, Lewis, & Parson, 2001).

RESEARCH ON COMPUTER-MEDIATED SUPPORT GROUPS

Nearly 25 million Americans are estimated to be members of some type of health-related support group (Kessler, Mickelson, & Zhao, 1997), and they are the most common way that individuals in this country attempt to change health behaviors (Davison, Pennebaker, & Dickerson, 2000). Support groups have a long history in the United States, arising from a variety of grassroots efforts in which people bypass professional health care institutions and structures to form communities based on their collective experience of facing similar illnesses and medical conditions (Katz, 1993; Katz & Bender, 1976; Yalom, 1995). In recent years, there has been a substantial increase in the number of computer-mediated social support groups and communities (Walther & Boyd, 2002; Wright & Bell, 2003). Several researchers have identified a number of advantages associated with computer-mediated support groups/communities for participants as well as many disadvantages. The following sections will discuss these.

Advantages of Computer-Mediated Support Groups/Communities

While relatively few studies have examined computer-mediated support groups/communities, researchers in the last decade have identified a number of advantages for those who use them (Braithwaite et al., 1999; Galinski et al., 1997; Query & Wright, 2003; Wright, 2000, 2002). One primary advantage is convenient access to the group/community 24 hours a day from different locations. Many online support groups/communities feature both asynchronous communication (e.g., bulletin boards, e-mail) and synchronous communication (e.g., chat rooms or chat applications) capabilities so that participants can obtain support from others in real time or post messages to the group. This provides people with access to support when they are facing immediate concerns (although the number of people using synchronous applications tends to be relatively small) and allows them to make comments or pose questions to the larger group/community by posting comments via bulletin board or mass e-mail.

These online groups/communities also offer individuals increased anonymity compared to traditional face-to-face sources of social support (including support groups). This can lead users to feel less stigmatized about visible health conditions (as well as conditions that are not readily apparent), reduce communication apprehension in terms of initiating communication with others, and enable users to self-disclose sensitive information in a less risky environment.

Computer-mediated support groups/communities offer participants access to an extended support network capable of providing informational, emotional, and (in some cases) instrumental support. The medium facilitates communication among a concentrated number of individuals sharing similar health concerns. By comparison, suppose a person who has recently been diagnosed with pancreatic cancer decides to seek support within his or her face-to-face community. Even with great effort, it is unlikely that he or she would be able to find a large network of individuals living with pancreatic cancer who would be willing to provide support. However, on the Internet, the ability of the medium to bring together people who are geographically dispersed (yet share common interests) can lead to a substantially larger network of potential support providers than would be possible face-to-face. This also allows for a larger number of perspectives about the health issue around which the group/community is centered.

In addition to the sheer number of people to whom Internet support groups/communities can provide, these groups/communities also introduce individuals to a more diverse social network than they are typically able to access face-to-face. In most face-to-face networks, individuals tend to seek support from family members and close friends. These individuals tend to be somewhat homogenous in terms of demographics, attitudes, and backgrounds. By contrast, online support groups/communities tend to help people transcend these similarities and introduce them to a more heterogeneous network of individuals (despite the fact that they share a common health concern). Many potential supportive relationships in the face-to-face world are thwarted due to perceptions that others are dissimilar.

For example, in the face-to-face world, individuals tend to rely heavily on in-group/out-group differences (Giles, Mulac, Bradac, & Johnson, 1987) when comparing themselves to people who appear to be members of a different social group (e.g., based on sex, race, age, background). In the computer-mediated environment, many of these social cues are unavailable due to the reduced nonverbal information available in most contexts. People may be more likely to judge individuals on the quality of their verbal messages (i.e., postings) than to make snap judgments based on visible social cues. As a result, participants can often receive more unique and novel viewpoints about the health issue they are facing than what they are able to obtain in traditional face-to-face support networks. This provides individuals with more opportunities for social comparisons with other individuals facing similar health concerns. This may help shatter perceptions of uniqueness when it comes to coping with health issues (e.g., feelings of "Why me?") and allow individuals to examine their own health problems vis-à-vis the issues other group/community members are facing.

Other advantages that these groups/communities offer include the ability for people to both receive and provide social support to others in a convenient way. This phenomenon has been labeled the "helper principle," and it is a common feature in both face-to-face and online support groups (Cline, 1999; Yalom, 1995). Essentially, the ability to help others may circumvent some of the reciprocity issues discussed earlier in this chapter. In other words, the ability to help others by providing informational and emotional support online in addition to receiving support may offset feelings of inadequacy and helplessness.

Moreover, researchers have also found that the act of expressing one's thoughts in written form (which is typically the means by which people communicate in online support groups/communities as they post messages, chat, or send e-mails to each other) has therapeutic value (Diamond, 2000; Weinberg et al., 1995). Expressing thoughts in e-mails, on bulletin boards, and in chat applications appears to allow psychological distance between a person and his or her thoughts. This provides opportunities for individuals to reflect on their thoughts, reexamine them, and rearticulate them prior to sending messages to the group. Moreover, recent research suggests that the act of sending affectionate messages in supportive exchanges (both in face-to-face and computer-mediated contexts) is related to reduced total cholesterol levels and cortisol levels (Floyd, Mikkelson, Hesse, & Pauley, 2007). Both cholesterol and cortisol are physiological products of stress, and both have been linked to heart disease and stroke among individuals facing long-term stressful situations. This research provides an important empirical link between supportive communication and physical health outcomes. However, future research would benefit from examining the relationship between supportive writing and cholesterol/cortisol levels among individuals who use computer-mediated support groups.

Disadvantages of Computer-Mediated Support Groups/Communities

Computer-mediated support groups/communities may also have a number of disadvantages. Wright (2000, 2002), in a survey of many types of health-related online support groups, identified several. One problem is the relatively short period of membership that is seen in health-related groups. Participants often join online groups/communities when they are initially worried about a health problem or when then they have been recently diagnosed with an illness. However, members appear to stop using these groups/communities after a few weeks. It seems that once some people feel that their initial concerns about a health issue have been addressed by the group, they decide to stop affiliating with the group and (presumably) seek support elsewhere. Such short-term membership may lead to several problems, including difficulty locating specific members and fewer old-timers, or individuals who have been using the group/community to deal with an illness/ health concern for a long period of time. Such individuals often have a unique perspective in terms of how to cope with the health issue. For example, in Alcoholics Anonymous, long-term members play a crucial role in terms of mentoring newly recovering alcoholics. Researchers have found that long-term members play similar roles in other types of health-related support groups (Rosenberg, 1984; Spiegel, Bloom, & Yalom, 1981).

In addition, despite greater access to individuals who share similar health concerns in online support groups/communities, participants often find the lack of immediacy (associated with reduced social presence) in communicating with others frustrating. Wright (2002) also found that online support group members missed the ability to engage in haptic communication (i.e. hugs and other expressions of supportive touch) with fellow participants.

Other disadvantages of computer-mediated support groups include off-topic remarks from participants, spam, privateers (people who try to use the group/community for their own selfish purposes), and flaming (i.e., antisocial behavior). These behaviors tend to increase negative perceptions of the group/community, and they may curtail membership if they occur frequently. For example, the author of this chapter witnessed mass postings of Jenny Craig diet products while he was studying online support groups for women with anorexia and bulimia. In other words, these privateers found the eating disorder support groups a convenient place to pitch diet products to women who were concerned about their weight. Early computer-mediated communication researchers posited that the reduced social cues associated with the medium may encourage antisocial behaviors due to the lack of physical presence of other participants (Walther, 1996; Walther & Burgoon, 1992). In other words, it is much easier to be disruptive online since a person is in little danger of physical retaliation from other members.

Moreover, the medium may facilitate deceptive practices. The anonymity associated with online support groups/communities makes it difficult to assess with whom one is really communicating. In some cases, individuals may misrepresent themselves or pretend to have an illness in order to receive attention from others, or they may be using the group/community for a variety of other reasons unrelated to the purpose of the group/community.

Finally, some members of society may have difficulty accessing or using these groups due to financial and educational issues. For example, while the cost of computers and Internet access has dropped considerably in the past decade, some social groups (i.e., older individuals and people living below the poverty level) may not have the means to access computer-mediated support resources. Literacy issues may also make it difficult for many people to participate given the necessity to possess reading, writing, and computer skills in order to use these groups.

THEORETICAL APPROACHES TO THE STUDY OF COMPUTER-MEDIATED SUPPORT GROUPS/COMMUNITIES

This section presents several theoretical frameworks that have been used to understand computer-mediated support groups/communities in prior research. These perspectives provide important insight into the processes associated with computer-mediated social support. Specifically, these theories help provide explanations as to why several features of computer-mediated support groups/communities appeal to participants.

Social Information Processing Theory

Social information processing theory argues that in computer-mediated communication, message senders portray themselves in a socially favorable manner to draw the attention of message receivers and foster anticipation of future interactions (Fulk, Steinfield, Schmitz, & Power, 1987; Walther, 1992). Message receivers, in turn, tend to develop an idealized image of the sender by placing too much value on minimal text-based cues. In addition, the asynchronous format of most computer-mediated interactions (and to some extent in synchronous formats, such as chat rooms) gives the sender and the receiver more time to edit their communication, making computer-mediated interactions more controllable and less stressful than the immediate feedback loop inherent in face-to-face interactions. Idealized perceptions and optimal self-presentation in the computer-mediated communication process tend to intensify in the feedback loop, and this can lead to what Walther (1996) labeled "hyperpersonal interaction," or a more intimate and socially desirable exchange than face-to-face interactions.

Hyperpersonal interaction is enhanced when no face-to-face relationship exists, so that users construct impressions and present themselves "without the interference of environmental reality" (Walther, 1996, p.33). Hyperpersonal interaction has been found to skew perceptions of relational partners in positive ways, and in some cases, computer-mediated relationships may exceed face-to-face interactions in terms of intensity; this can occur within online support groups (King & Moreggi, 1998; Walther, 1996; Wright & Bell, 2003).

Theory of Weak Tie Social Networks

One theoretical framework that has been used to explain many advantages of face-to-face and computer-mediated support networks is Granovetter's (1973, 1979, 1982, 1983) theory of weak ties (Adelman et al., 1987; Walther & Boyd, 2002; Wright & Bell, 2003). According to Adelman and associates (1979), "weak ties" refers to a "wide range of potential supporters who lie beyond our circle of family and friends" (p. 136). These relationships often lack the frequency of interaction and intimacy associated with closer ties (i.e., close friends and family members) and may include individuals such as neighbors, clergy, retail service providers, counselors, face-to-face support group members, and people who interact within Internet communities. Despite less frequent interaction and lower levels of intimacy, weak ties can often be important sources of social support (Adelman et al., 1987; Granovetter, 1982, 1983), especially in contexts such as the Internet (Walther & Boyd, 2002; Wright & Bell, 2003). Researchers have found that there are advantages and disadvantages associated with seeking support in weak tie networks, depending upon the support needs and goals of the individual.

According to Granovetter (1983), "whether one uses weak or strong ties for various purposes depends not only on the number of ties one has at various levels of tie strength but also on the utility of ties of different strengths" (p. 209). The utility of the particular social network an individual chooses to use when disclosing problems and seeking social support is influenced by a number of factors, including the type of stressful situation he or she is facing, the degree of stigma or potential for embarrassment surrounding the problem, the need for emotionally meaningful relationships, desire for new or novel information, the perceived understanding and competencies of potential support providers in the network, judgments about role obligations, and the perceived resources and social capital of social network members.

One reason why individuals may opt for a weak tie over a strong tie support network is that weak ties often provide access to diverse points of view and information that tend not to be available within more intimate relationships (Adelman et al., 1987). Typically, many individuals form close relationships with others who are similar to them in terms of demographics, attitudes, and backgrounds (Botwin, Buss, & Shackelford, 1997; Thiessen & Gregg, 1980). This homogeneous preference can limit the diversity of information and viewpoints obtained about topics, including health concerns.

Access to more diverse viewpoints about health problems can provide individuals with more varied informational support about health issues, and interacting with different types of people increases the number of social comparisons a person can make about his or her health condition vis-à-vis others (Adelman et al., 1987). The opportunity for more social comparisons has been found to be an integral component of support groups (Helgeson & Gottlieb, 2000), and they often help individuals manage uncertainty about their health conditions. Individuals facing difficult health concerns may often obtain more useful information by moving beyond their traditional strong tie support network. Using a weak tie network such as a support group whose members may also have the disease can offer perspectives from others who are likely to share similar feelings about their condition, even if they are dissimilar in terms of demographics, attitudes, and/or background. Furthermore, interacting with multiple individuals in a support group setting allows users to make assessments about how one is coping with a problem compared to others, further helping to reduce uncertainty and anxiety.

For a variety of reasons, strong tie support networks can be perceived as inadequate or incapable of providing satisfactory support, and a range of factors, both practical and psychological, have been shown to influence an individual's decision to pursue weak tie support networks as an alternative. This appears to particularly be the case when it comes to seeking support for health issues. Health concerns are often difficult topics for people to discuss, especially when one is communicating with a close loved one. Researchers have found that family members and friends often minimize the concerns of those close to them who are seeking support related to difficult health problems. In many cases, it is not uncommon for close ties to steer conversational topics away from emotional talk about problems, refrain from engaging in in-depth discussion of such topics, or avoid consequent interaction altogether (Cline, 1987; Dakof & Taylor, 1990; Dunkel-Schetter & Wortman, 1982; Helgeson, Cohen, Shultz, & Yasko, 2000).

In addition, studies have found that role obligations and related reciprocity issues in close ties can lead to problems with the provision of social support. Support for a loved one who is ill can lead to increased conflict, resentment, and negative feelings for both parties involved due to reluctance to form new complicated role obligations on one hand, and feelings of guilt and shame stemming from the perceived inability to reciprocate, on the other (Albrecht & Goldsmith, 2003; Chesler & Barbarin, 1984; LaGaipa, 1990; Pitula & Daugherty, 1995). Although a person may care deeply for those he or she is close to, he or she may easily feel overburdened if a loved one becomes ill and needs a great amount of support, and the stress experienced can lead to conflict. At the same time, many individuals who receive support from family members and friends may feel uncomfortable and reluctant to accept the support when they do not have (or perceive that they do not have) the ability to reciprocate (Chesler & Barbarin, 1984). This discomfort is based on a sense of inequity that may lead individuals receiving support to feel over-benefited if they cannot help or return the favor to their friends in a similar manner. According to LaGaipa (1990), these "social obligations may override the positive effect of companionship and social support. Such constraints may have a negative effect on a person's mental well-being that may not make up for the beneficial aspects of personal relationships" (p. 126).

In contrast, since they tend to be less emotionally attached, weak tie network members may be more willing to talk about difficult and/or unpleasant health concerns. Moreover, many diseases and medical conditions have been found to carry a social stigma (Mathieson, Logan-Smith, Phillips, MacPhee, & Attia, 1996; Sullivan & Reardon, 1985), and this dehumanizing process can negatively affect the provision of social support (Bloom & Spiegel, 1984). Because members of weak tie networks do not typically share an intimate relational history, they have been found to be less likely to judge one another and frequently encourage one another to share concerns and feelings about living with various stigmatized health problems.

Because other group members may also be contending with similar health concerns, the similarity between members in terms of health concerns increases empathy and understanding of the situation and fosters opportunities for other types of emotional support such as affirmation and validation. In addition, because of their reduced emotional attachment, weak tie network members are far more adept at providing objective, disimpassioned feedback about health problems and are generally more willing to discuss risky topics than strong tie networks of family and friends (Adelman et al., 1987).

Social Comparison Theory

Social comparison theory (Festinger, 1954) is another potentially useful framework for understanding how perceptions of others within computer-mediated networks may provide individuals dealing with health-related issues with relevant information that may influence their health decision-making processes. According to social comparison theory, individuals make assessments about their own health and coping mechanisms by comparing them to those of others in their social networks (Helgeson & Gottlieb, 2000).

Helgeson and Gottlieb (2000) argue that lateral comparisons, comparisons to similar others, may normalize people's experiences and reduce uncertainty and stress among those dealing with health concerns. Lateral comparisons appear to validate people's experiences (e.g., interactions with providers, fears, frustrations) and reduce their sense of social isolation when they are coping with health concerns. However, comparing oneself to others in these environments often leads to positive or negative self-assessments. For example, if a person with cancer feels that he or she is coping with problems less effectively than others in the online support network, this may create upward comparisons, which could produce feelings of frustration, or it could serve as a source of inspiration to the person to cope more effectively by emulating the successful behaviors of those other members. Conversely, downward comparisons to others in the network, such as when an individual feels that he or she is coping better than other members, can lead to positive self-assessments and/or to negative feelings about others if interactions with the other members are perceived as being unhelpful.

In terms of computer-mediated supportive environments, online support groups, support communities, and even social network sites (e.g., MySpace) may facilitate access to a larger network of individuals facing similar health concerns and increase the number of social comparisons a person can make.

Optimal Matching Model

The optimal matching model posits that an optimal match between the needs of support seekers and the resources/abilities of support providers is important in terms of coping with the many relational challenges associated with communicating social support (Cutrona & Russell, 1990; Goldsmith, 2004). For example, if an individual is seeking emotional support and validation for an eating disorder and he or she perceives that members of his or her support network have competently listened, expressed empathy, and acknowledged the severity of the issue, then this would be considered an example of an optimal match between the support seeker and support providers. Conversely, if an individual desires emotional support, and members of his or her support network provide unwanted advice (a negative form of informational support), then this would be considered a bad (or less-than-optimal) match.

Goldsmith (2004) contends that optimal matches in supportive episodes may lead to more positive perceptions of relational partners and the type of support that is being offered, and this, in turn, may ultimately influence positive health outcomes. However, research drawing from this perspective has also found evidence that optimal support network patterns are dynamic and may change when an individual is coping with a non-life-threatening illness or a life-threatening illness (Carstensen & Fredrickson, 1998; Lockenhoff & Carstensen, 2004).

Moreover, these network patterns may also differ depending upon whether a person is in the early stages or the late stages of an illness. This framework may be helpful in terms of understanding why people facing health concerns may be drawn to computer-mediated social support, particularly when members of their traditional support network are no longer able to adequately meet their needs following the diagnosis of an illness or when encountering other health problems. It may also be the case that many of the advantages of computer-mediated support groups/communities (described above) meet individuals' support needs (e.g., the desire for anonymity, multiple perspectives, convenience), and this influences usage patterns. While this model has been applied to a variety of face-to-face supportive contexts (see Goldsmith, 2004), relatively few researchers have used this framework to investigate computer-mediated support (Turner, Grube, & Meyers, 2001; Wright & Muhtaseb, 2005). Yet this perspective may help to provide important insights into the supportive needs of individuals who seek computer-mediated support.

WAYS TO INCREASE COMPUTER-MEDIATED SOCIAL SUPPORT

Computer-mediated social support is still a relatively new area of research, and additional studies are needed to understand the strengths and limitations of these groups in terms of their ability to offer people facing health concerns adequate support. More research needs to assess the potential long-term health benefits of these groups. Most studies of computer-mediated support have been cross-sectional, and longitudinal designs are needed to assess the impact of this type of support on physical and mental health outcomes. In addition, all the current studies reviewed in this chapter relied on either surveys or content analyses of computer-mediated support groups/communities. The limitations of such approaches are well known, particularly in terms of their inability to adequately control for extraneous variables or to build a compelling case for causal relationships among variables. Future research would benefit from controlled randomized studies that compare the impact of computer-mediated social support with traditional face-to-face sources. This section briefly explores these and other limitations of the current research in this area. In addition, it highlights several areas of research that scholars should consider in the future that may help increase our understanding of the nature and usefulness of computer-mediated support for individuals dealing with health concerns.

There is a strong need to raise awareness of the potential of computer-mediated networks to increase access to traditional sources of social support, including family members and friends. E-mail, chat applications, and social network sites provide multiple opportunities for individuals to engage in supportive communication with family and friends throughout the day. These online resources may help individuals maintain relationships with important sources of social support. Given recent research (Floyd et al., 2007) that suggests that affectionate writing (including supportive communication) may be linked to important physical health outcomes (such as reduced cholesterol and cortisol levels), future researchers should continue to examine computer-mediated support among traditional support network ties.

However, given the difficulties that individuals encounter with traditional close ties, such as greater interpersonal risk in disclosing information, homogeneity of information, and role obligations, future researchers should continue to examine the advantages and disadvantages of online support groups and support communities for people facing health concerns. While earlier research on these groups/communities has identified a number of potential advantages for people seeking social support (e.g., multiple perspectives, less risk, fewer role obligations, the therapeutic value of expressing thoughts in written form), and they have advanced theories about possible underlying processes (e.g., weak tie network theory, social comparison theory), relatively few studies have linked these advantages to physical health outcomes in controlled longitudinal studies (see Shaw, Hawkins, McTavish, Pingree, & Gustafson, 2006, for exceptions). These types of research efforts typically require funding from organizations such as the National Institutes of Health and the Centers for Disease Control and Prevention, which may explain why so few of them have been conducted. However, such research is necessary in order to assess the viability of these groups for improving the health of participants.

Future research efforts should also consider designing interventions that will help increase access to computer-mediated social support, particularly among underserved populations (i.e., lower-socioeconomic-status groups, minorities, and individuals with low literacy levels). Such initiatives should focus on increasing computer access and computer literacy training among members of these populations. One particular underserved population is older adults, particularly female caregivers and older people facing health concerns (especially those individuals who have not had opportunities to learn about the Internet and computer-mediated communication). Given the rapid growth of this population in recent years and the lack of opportunities many individuals in this demographic group have had to learn computer skills (e.g., many members of the oldest cohort of older adults, such as people in their late 1980s and 1990s, retired from the workplace before the use of computers and the Internet became widespread), and the relatively high correlation between aging and health problems, older adults are a challenging and important group to target when one is designing interventions centered around computer-mediated social support.

There is also a need to educate individuals who are facing specific health concerns (such as various types of cancer) about the strengths and limitations of computer-mediated support groups/communities. Many people who currently use these groups may be unaware of the potential health benefits associated with them or problems that can occur. Health professionals and other researchers would benefit from conducting studies of currently available groups and identifying groups that may best meet the needs of patients/interested parties. At this point in time, anyone can create an online support group/community, and there is little data regarding the quality of these groups. An alarming statistic from one study is that between 30% and 40% of health information regarding cancer on the Internet (including information disseminated in online support groups/communities) was found to be inaccurate (Bierman, Golladay, & Baker, 1999). This, of course, raises questions about the accuracy of information surrounding other diseases and health issues. There is a great need to assess the quality and credibility of information that individuals receive in support groups/communities. In addition, it would be helpful to identify groups/communities that have a history of spam, privateers, conflicts, and other negative elements that may undermine the health benefits of participating in such groups.

Finally, potential group users should be educated about the relationship between social support and health outcomes, social support processes, and the nature of computer-mediated social support. Despite the fact that there is over a decade of research on computer-mediated social support, there have been few efforts to disseminate the findings to lay populations or to increase health literacy regarding these groups. Future interventions and research efforts should find ways to raise awareness of the benefits and limitations of these groups (in terms of health benefits) among online support group/community participants (the most important stakeholders).

CONCLUSION

Computer-mediated social support is an important health communication area to study in the new media landscape. Most of the previous research suggests that online support has potential health benefits for those individuals who use computer-mediated support groups/communities or who engage in other types of online support. However, despite some of the advantages of using these resources, there are also problems associated with them. The use of the Internet as a vehicle for obtaining social support from traditional sources (i.e., family and friends) remains an important area for future research. In addition, future research should continue to focus on the relationship between computer-mediated support and health outcomes, and researchers should attempt to disseminate findings to potential users and health care professionals in an effort to increase education about these sources of social support.

REFERENCES

Adelman, M. B., Parks, M. R., & Albrecht, T. L. (1987). Beyond close relationships: Support in weak ties. In T. L. Albrecht & M. B. Adelman (Eds.), *Communicating social support* (pp. 126–147). Newbury Park, CA: Sage.

Albrecht, T. L., & Goldsmith, D. J. (2003). Social support, social networks, and health. In T. L. Thompson, A. M. Dorsey, K. I. Miller, & R. Parrott (Eds.), *Handbook of health communication* (pp. 263–284). Mahwah, NJ: Erlbaum.

Alexander, S. C., Peterson, J. L., & Hollingshead, A. B. (2003). Help is at your keyboard: Support groups on the Internet. In L. R. Frey (Ed.), *Group communication in context: Studies of bona fide groups* (2nd ed., pp. 309–334). Mahwah, NJ: Erlbaum.

Aneshensel, C. S., & Stone, J. D. (1982). Stress and depression: A test of the buffering model of social support. *Archives of General Psychiatry, 39,* 1392–1396.

Aspden, P., & Katz, J. E. (2001). Assessments of the quality of health care information and referrals to physicians: A nationwide survey. In R. E. Rice & J. E. Katz (Eds.), *The Internet and health communication: Experiences and expectations* (pp. 107–119), Thousand Oaks, CA: Sage.

Ballieux, R. E., & Heijen, C. J. (1989). Stress and the immune response. In H. Weiner, I. Floring, R. Murison, & D. Hellhammer (Eds.), *Frontiers of stress research,* (pp. 51–55). Toronto, Canada: Huber.

Bass, S. B. (2003). How will Internet use affect the patient? A review of computer network and closed Internet-based system studies and the implications in understanding how the use of the Internet affects patient populations. *Journal of Health Psychology, 8*, 25–38.

Berkman, L. F., & Syme, L. S. (1979). Social networks, host resistance, and mortality: A nine-year follow-up study of Alameda County resident. *Journal of Epidemiology, 109*, 186–204.

Bierman, J. S., Golladay, G., & Baker, J. (1999). Evaluation of cancer information on the Internet. *Cancer, 86*, 381–390.

Binik, Y. M., Cantor, J., Ochs, E., & Meana, M. (1997). From the couch to the keyboard: Psychotherapy in cyberspace. In S. Kiesler (Ed.), *Culture of the Internet* (pp. 71—100). Mahwah, NJ: Erlbaum.

Bloom, J. R. (1982). Social support, accommodation to stress and adjustment to breast cancer. *Social Science Medicine, 16*, 1329–1338.

Bloom, J. R., & Spiegel, D. (1984). The relationship of two dimensions of social support to the psychological well-being and social functioning of women with advanced breast cancer. *Social Science Medicine, 19*, 831–837.

Botwin, M.D., Buss, D.M., & Shackelford, T.K. (1997). Personality and mate preferences: Five factors in mate selection and marital satisfaction. *Journal of Personality, 65*, 107–136.

Brashers, D. E., Neidig, J. L., & Goldsmith, D. J. (2004). Social support and the management of people living with HIV or AIDS. *Health Communication, 16*, 305–331.

Burleson, B. R. (1994). Comforting messages: Significance, approaches, and effects. In B. R. Burleson, T. L. Albrecht, & I. G. Sarason (Eds.), *Communication of social support: Messages, interactions, relationships and community.* Newbury Park, CA: Sage.

Burleson, B. B., & Goldsmith, D. J. (1998). How the comforting process works: Alleviating emotional distress through conversationally induced reappraisals. In P. A. Andersen & L. K. Guerrero (Eds.), *Handbook of communication and emotion: Research, theory, applications, and contexts* (pp. 245–280). San Diego: Academic Press.

Braithwaite, D. O., Waldron, V. R., & Finn, J. (1999). Communication of social support in computer-mediated groups for people with disabilities. *Health Communication, 11*, 123–151.

Bruunk, B. (1990). Affiliation and helping interactions within organizations: A critical analysis of the role of social support with regard to occupational stress. In W. Stroebe & M. Hewstone (Eds.), *European review of social psychology* (Vol. 1, pp. 293–322). Chichester, UK: Wiley.

Campbell, K., & Wright, K. B. (2002). On-line support groups: An investigation of relationships among source credibility, dimensions of relational communication, and perceptions of emotional support. *Communication Research Reports, 19*, 183–193.

Chesler, M. A., & Barbarin, O. A. (1984). Difficulties of providing help in a crisis: Relationships between parents of children with cancer and their friends. *Journal of Social Issues, 40*, 113–134.

Cline, R. J. (1999). Communication within social support groups. In L. R. Frey (Ed.), D. S. Gouran, & M. S. Poole (Assoc. Eds.), *The handbook of group communication theory and research* (pp. 516–538). Thousand Oaks, CA: Sage.

Clow, C. (2001). The physiology of stress. In F. Jones & J. Bright (Eds.), *Stress: Myth, theory, and research* (pp. 47–61). Harlow, UK: Prentice-Hall.

Cohen, S. (1988). Psychosocial models of the role of support in the etiology of physical disease. *Health Psychology, 7,* 269–297.

Cohen, S., & Wills, T. A. (1985). Stress, social support, and the buffering hypothesis. *Psychological Bulletin, 98,* 310–357.

Davison, K. P., Pennebaker, J. W., & Dickerson, S. S. (2000). Who talks? The social psychology of illness support groups. *American Psychologist, 55,* 205–217.

Dean, A., & Lin, N. (1977). The stress buffering role of social support: Problems and prospects for systematic investigation. *Journal of Health and Social Behavior, 32,* 321–341.

Diamond, J. (2000). *Narrative means to sober ends: Treating addiction and its aftermath.* New York: Guilford Press.

Dwyer, C. (2007). *Digital relationships in the "MySpace" generation: Results from a qualitative study.* Paper presented at the 40th Hawaii International Conference on System Sciences, Waikoloa, HI. Retrieved August 20, 2007, from http://www.danah.org/SNSResearch.html

Ellison, N. B., Steinfield, C., & Lampe, C. (2007). The benefits of Facebook "friends": Social capital and college students' use of online social network sites. *Journal of Computer-Mediated Communication, 12*(4). Retrieved August 20, 2007, from http://jcmc.indiana.edu/vol12/issue4/ellison.html

Festinger, L. (1954). A theory of social comparison processes. *Human Relations, 7,* 117–140.

Floyd, K., Mikkelson, A. C., Hesse, C., & Pauley, P.M. (2007). Affectionate writing reduces total cholesterol: Two randomized, controlled trials. *Human Communication Research, 33,* 119–142.

Fox, S., & Rainie, L. (2000). The online health care revolution: How the Web helps Americans take better care of themselves. A Pew Internet and American Life Project Online Report. Retrieved January 2, 2004, from http://www.pewinternet.org

Fulk, J., Steinfeld, C. W., Schmitz, J., & Power, G. J. (1987). A social information processing model of media use in organizations. *Communication Research, 14,* 41–52.

Giles, H., Mulac, A., Bradac, J. J., & Johnson, P. (1987). Speech accommodation theory: The next decade and beyond. *Communication Yearbook 10,* 13–48.

Goldsmith, D. J. (2004). *Communicating social support.* New York: Cambridge.

Granovetter, M. (1973). The strength of weak ties. *American Journal of Sociology, 78,* 1360–1380.

Granovetter, M. S. (1982). The strength of weak ties: A network theory revisited. In P. V. Marsden, & N. Lin (Eds.), *Social structure and network analysis* (pp. 105–130). Newbury Park, CA: Sage.

Granovetter, M. (1983). The strength of weak ties: A network theory revisited. *Sociological Theory, 1,* 201–233.

Harris Interactive. (2001). The increasing impact of eHealth on consumer behavior. *Health Care News, 21,* 1–9.

Helgeson, V. S., & Gottlieb, B. H. (2000). Support groups. In S. Cohen, L. G. Underwood, & B. H. Gottlieb (Eds.), *Social support measurement and intervention* (pp. 221–245). New York: Oxford University Press.

House, J., Landis, K. R., & Umberson, D. (1988). Social relationships and health. *Science, 241,* 540–545.

King, S. A., & Moreggi, D. (1998). Internet therapy and self-help groups: The pros and cons. In J. Gakenbach (Ed.), *Psychology and the Internet: Intrapersonal, interpersonal, and transpersonal implications* (pp. 77–109). San Diego, CA: Academic Press.

Kohn, P.M. (1996). On coping adaptively with daily hassles. In M. Zeidner & N. S. Endler (Eds.), *Handbook of coping* (pp. 181–201). New York: John Wiley & Sons.

La Gaipa, J. J. (1990). The negative effects of informal support systems. In S. Duck & R. C. Silver (Eds.), *Personal relationships and social support* (pp. 122–139). Newbury Park, CA: Sage.

Lockenhoff, C. E., & Carstensen, L. L. (2004). Socioemotional selectivity theory, aging, and health: The increasingly delicate balance between regulating emotions and making tough choices. *Journal of Personality, 72,* 1395–1423.

Neuhauser, L., & Kreps, G. L. (2003). Rethinking communication in the e-health era. *Journal of Health Psychology, 8,* 7–23.

Pakenham, K. I. (1998). Specification of social support behaviors and network dimensions along the HIV continuum for gay men. *Patient Education and Counseling 34,* 147–157.

Preece, J. J., & Ghozati, K. (2001). Experiencing empathy on-line. In R. E. Rice & J. E. Katz (Eds.), *The Internet and health communication: Experiences and expectations* (pp. 237–260). Thousand Oaks, CA: Sage.

Shaw, B. R., Hawkins, R., McTavish, F., Pingree, S., & Gustafson, D. H. (2006). Effects of insightful disclosure within computer mediated support groups on women with breast cancer. *Health Communication, 19,* 133–142.

Snyder, J., Carpenter, D., & Slauson, G. J. (2006). *Myspace.com: A social networking site and social contract theory.* Dallas, TX: ISECON 23.

Spiegel, D. (1992). Effects of psychosocial support on patients with metastatic breast cancer. *Journal of Psychosocial Oncology, 10,* 113–121.

Spiegel, D., & Bloom, J. R. (1983). Pain in metastatic breast cancer. *Cancer, 52,* 149–153.

Spiegel, D., Bloom, J. R., & Yalom, I. (1981). Group support for patients with metastatic cancer: A randomized prospective outcome study. *Archives of General Psychiatry, 38,* 527–533.

Sullivan, C. F. (2003). Gendered cybersupport: A thematic analysis of two on-line cancer support groups. *Journal of Health Psychology, 8,* 83–103.

Sullivan, C. F., & Reardon, K. K. (1985). Social support satisfaction and health locus of control: Discriminators of breast cancer patients' style of coping. In M. L. McLaughlin (Ed.), *Communication yearbook* (Vol. 9, pp. 707–722). Beverly Hills, CA: Sage.

Thiessen, D. D., & Gregg, B. (1980). Human assortative mating and genetic equilibrium: An evolutionary perspective. *Ethdogy and Sociobiology, 1,* 111–140.

Turner, J. W., Grube, J. A., & Meyers, J. (2001). Developing an optimal match within on-line communities: An exploration of CMC support communities and traditional support. *Journal of Communication,* 231–251.

Uchino, B. N., Cacioppo, J. T., & Kiecolt-Glaser, J. K. (1996). The relationship between social support and physiological processes: A review with emphasis on underlying mechanisms and implications for health. *Psychological Bulletin, 119,* 488–531.

U.S. Census Bureau. (2001). *Press release.* Retrieved January 15, 2004, from http://www.census.gov/Press-Release/www/2003/cb03–08.html

Walsh-Burke, K. (1992). Family communication and coping with cancer. Impact of the We Can Weekend. *Journal of Psychosocial Oncology, 10,* 63–81.

Walther, J. B., & Burgoon, J. (1992). Relational communication in computer-mediated interaction. *Human Communication Research, 19,* 50–88.

Walther, J. B., & Boyd, S. (2002). Attraction to computer-mediated social support. In C. A. Lin & D. Atkin (Eds.), *Communication technology and society: Audience adoption and uses* (pp. 153–188). Cresskill, NJ: Hampton Press.

Weinberg, N., Schmale, J. D., Uken, J., & Wessel, K. (1995). Computer-mediated support groups. *Social Work with Groups, 17,* 43–55.

Wills, T. A. (1985). Supportive functions of interpersonal relationships. In S. Cohen & S. L. Syme (Eds.), *Social support and health* (pp. 61–82). New York: Academic Press.

Wortman, C., & Dunkel-Schetter, C. (1979). Interpersonal relationships and cancer. *Journal of Social Issues, 35,* 120–155.

Wright, K. B. (2000). Computer-mediated social support, older adults, and coping. *Journal of Communication, 50,* 100–118.

Wright, K. B. (2002). Social support within an on-line cancer community: An assessment of emotional support, perceptions of advantages and disadvantages, and motives for using the community. *Journal of Applied Communication Research, 3,* 195–209.

Wright, K. B. (2007). New technologies and health communication. In K. B. Wright & S. C. Moore (Eds.), *Applied health communication: A sourcebook.* Cresskill, NJ: Hampton Press.

Wright, K. B., & Bell, S. B. (2003). Health-related support groups on the Internet: Linking empirical findings to social support and computer-mediated communication theory. *Journal of Health Psychology, 8,* 37–52.

Wright, K. B., & Muhtaseb, A. (2005, May). *Perceptions of on-line support in health-related computer-mediated support groups.* Paper presented at the annual International Communication Association Convention, New York.

Yalom, I. (1995). *The theory and practice of group psychotherapy.* New York: Basic Books.

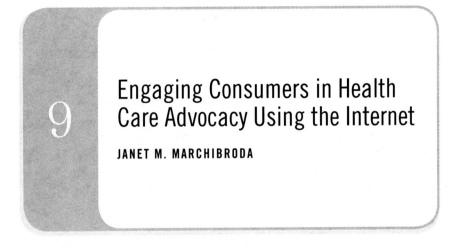

Engaging Consumers in Health Care Advocacy Using the Internet

9

JANET M. MARCHIBRODA

Increasingly, individuals are turning to the Internet and other digital applications to help them manage their health and health care. The digital environment provides ready access to general health information, social networks for sharing experiences, and, increasingly, access to health care information that has traditionally resided only within the health records of the health care provider or the health plan.

At the same time, the Internet is increasingly being leveraged to expand advocacy-related efforts targeting policy makers, enabling a wider and more diverse number of individuals to influence the public policy process.

While there is a great deal of advocacy conducted related to health care issues today, the number and amount of resources devoted by patient groups to advocacy on health care–related issues is small compared to efforts conducted by other stakeholders in the health care system—including those who deliver, support, pay for, and manage health care.

The convergence of the use of the Internet and related electronic tools to support patients in managing their health and health care and the use of the Internet for advocacy offer an opportunity to engage the voice of the consumer more fully in accelerating health care policy change.

THE NEED FOR HEALTH CARE ADVOCACY

Rising health care costs, the rising number of uninsured, and issues related to both the quality and cost of health care are areas of great concern within the U.S. health care system.

Health care spending in the United States is expected to increase from 16% of the gross domestic product (or $2 trillion) to 20% of the GDP (or $4 trillion) by the 2016 Centers for Medicare and Medicaid Services (2007). U.S. health care spending is much higher than in other industrialized countries. According to the Organisation for Economic Co-operation and Development (OECD), health care spending per capita in Switzerland—the next most costly OECD country—is only 68% of that in the United States. In Canada, it is only 57%, and in the median OECD country it is less than 44% of the U.S. level (Reinhardt, 2004).

High health care costs are having an impact on out-of-pocket costs for those who have health insurance. According to a recent survey conducted by the Kaiser Family Foundation (2006), 21% of employers reported that it is "very likely" and 28% reported that it was "somewhat likely" that they would increase the amount that employees pay for health insurance in the coming year. Health insurance premiums for workers and their employees have skyrocketed by 87% since 2000, the survey found, while workers' earnings have risen by only 20% over the same time period.

Quality is also an issue of concern for policy makers and health care leaders. According to a study published in the *New England Journal of Medicine,* U.S. adults receive about half of recommended health care services (McGlynn, 2003). And poor quality translates into higher costs. According to the Commonwealth Fund–sponsored U.S. Scorecard on Health System Performance, the current gap between national average rates of diabetes and blood pressure control and rates achieved by the top 10% of health plans translates into an estimated 20,000 to 40,000 preventable deaths and $1 to $2 billion in avoidable medical costs (Commonwealth Fund, 2006).

The number of Americans with chronic disease is also having an impact on cost. More than 125 million Americans had at least one chronic care condition in 2000, and this number is expected to grow to 157 million by the year 2020 (Wu, 2000). People with chronic conditions absorb the majority of health care spending in the United States, accounting for 78% of all health care spending in 1998 (Agency for Healthcare Research and Quality, 1998). As baby boomers continue to age, the number of individuals living with chronic conditions will continue to grow. While 12.7% of the population during the year 2000 was age 65 or older, this number is expected to grow to 20% by the year 2030 (U.S. Bureau of the Census, 2000). Finally, according to the U.S. Census Bureau, the number of uninsured Americans rose by 2.2 million in 2006 to 47 million in 2007—the largest 1-year increase since 2002.

As a result of the recognition of these health care challenges, a number of policy makers within the federal government, in Congress, and at the state level have introduced a wide range of policies related to financing, access, and the use of health information technology to address these issues.

Consumers are also recognizing the challenges of the current health care system. According to a 2006 Kaiser Family Foundation survey, over half (54%) of American adults were dissatisfied with the quality of health care, and almost a third (31%) were very dissatisfied. In addition, over 81% of Americans were dissatisfied with the cost of health care in the United States, and the majority (56%) was very dissatisfied.

The Commonwealth Fund (2006) recently conducted a survey of consumer views about key health care issues. According to that research, 38% of consumers had very serious or somewhat serious problems paying for their family's medical bills and paying for their family's medical insurance. Forty-eight percent of those surveyed were somewhat worried or very worried that they would not be able to pay medical bills in the event of a serious illness.

At the same time, 47% of consumers surveyed indicated that they were very worried or somewhat worried that they would not get high-quality care when they needed it (Commonwealth Fund, 2006). Twenty-five percent of those surveyed reported that they had experienced recommendations for unnecessary care or treatments over the past 2 years, and 17% reported having experienced over the past 2 years either the ordering of a test that had already been done or a medical, surgical, medication, or laboratory test error (Commonwealth Fund, 2006).

According to a Kaiser (2007) Health Tracking Poll related to the 2008 presidential election conducted in December 2007, health care ranks second behind Iraq as the top issue that the public wanted the presidential candidates to talk about, with 35% of respondents citing Iraq as the top issue and 30% citing health care as the top issue.

CONSUMER USE OF THE INTERNET TO SUPPORT HEALTH CARE NEEDS

Increasingly, consumers are using the Internet to support them with the management of their health and health care. Consumer interest in using the Internet to search for health information has continued to grow, along with interest in accessing information related to health care delivery. According to a Pew Internet & American Life research study, 79% of Internet users (95 million American adults) have searched online for information on at least one major health topic (Fox, 2005). According to the survey, specific diseases and treatments continue to be the most popular topics, but the greatest growth is in the number of people seeking information about doctors and hospitals, experimental treatments, health insurance, medicines, fitness, and nutrition (Fox, 2005).

A more recent Pew survey indicates that adults living with a disability or chronic disease are less likely than others to go online, but once they are online, they are more likely to look for health information. According to the survey, 51% of those living with a disability or chronic disease go online, compared to 74% of those who report no chronic conditions (Fox, 2007). The research findings further support the fact that those with chronic conditions are more likely than other e-patients to report that their online searches affected their treatment decisions, their interactions with their doctors, their ability to cope with their condition, and their dieting and fitness regimen, as noted below.

- Seventy-five percent of e-patients with chronic conditions said the information they found in their last search affected a decision about how to treat an illness or condition, compared with 55% of e-patients who reported no disability or illness.
- Sixty-nine percent of e-patients with chronic conditions said the information led them to ask a doctor new questions or to get a second opinion from another doctor, compared with 52% of other e-patients.
- Fifty-seven percent of e-patients with chronic conditions said the information changed the way they cope with a chronic condition or manage pain, compared with 36% of other e-patients.
- Fifty-six percent of e-patients with chronic conditions said the information changed the way they think about diet, exercise, or stress management, compared with 42% of other e-patients (Fox, 2007).

Research also points to consumer interest in having greater electronic access to health information. According to an October 2005 research report supported by the Markle Foundation, 60% of Americans support the creation of a secure online "personal health record" service that would allow consumers to:

- Check and refill prescriptions.
- Get results over the Internet.
- Check for mistakes in the medical record.
- Conduct secure and private e-mail communication with their doctors (Fox, 2007).

The same research report cites strong evidence that Americans would actually use an online personal health record service to:

- Check for mistakes in their medical record (69%).
- Check and refill prescriptions (68%).
- Conduct secure and private e-mail communications with their doctors (57%).
- Get results over the Internet (58%).

A more recent report released by the Markle Foundation in December 2006 offered similar insights. According to the National Survey on Electronic Personal Health Records, the public feels that access to electronic personal health records would have the following personal benefits:

- Enable them to see what their doctors write down (91%).
- Enable them to check for mistakes (84%).
- Reduce the number of repeated tests and procedures they undergo (88%).

According to research conducted by Public Opinion Strategies, and supported by the eHealth Initiative Foundation in June 2006, 70% of Americans in the Gulf Coast following Hurricanes Katrina and Rita favor the creation of secure electronic health information exchange to give both patients and clinicians access to important medical information to support their health and health care, which "with their consent[,] . . . would be protected and exchanged under current medical privacy and confidentiality standard procedures" (eHealth Initiative Foundation, 2006).

Over the past year, there has been a considerable increase in interest in "personal health records" as several health plans, employers, and commercial vendors have announced new projects. In addition, policies related to personal health records are also emerging, most notably from groups such as those sponsored by the Markle Foundation (2008). A personal health record is often defined as an electronic record on a patient's health, which is controlled by the patient, who may take it from doctor to doctor or have it available online in the event of an emergency (Dolan, 2007). Personal health records ordinarily enable patients to log their own data into a system and are also designed to offer patients better access to their own health care data from other data sources, including their providers and health plans. Personal health records are being developed and offered by a wide and diverse range of organizations, including start-up companies, hospitals, and other provider organizations, clinicians, health plans, patient communities, and even large organizations such as Google, Microsoft, and WebMD.

Personal health records are also being developed by those who have experienced difficulties with the current system. For example, FollowMe was developed by a mother who was frustrated with current methods for managing the records of her son, who was diagnosed with hydrocephalus, or excess accumulation of fluid in the brain (Gearon, 2005). This application is now being used by migrant workers in California to break down language barriers and support continuity of care (Jackson, 2004).

In addition, the number of online or virtual communities focused on health care is continuing to rise. Virtual communities are social networks formed or facilitated through electronic media (Wellman, 1997). These online communities are often called "electronic peer to peer community networks," where people with common interests gather "virtually" to share experiences, ask questions, or provide emotional support and self-help. As of January 2008, Yahoo!Groups listed more than 61,000 electronic support groups in their health and wellness section.

Examples of virtual communities include Patients Like Me and Braintalk Communities. Patients Like Me is an online platform for collecting and sharing real-world patient data, currently focusing on ALS (Lou Gehrig's disease), multiple sclerosis, Parkinson's disease, and HIV/AIDS. Patients log their symptoms, treatments, and outcomes, and the site aggregates the data to help patients with these life-changing diseases compare their experiences with symptoms, treatments, and outcomes tracked at the population level (PatientsLikeMe, 2008). As of January 2008, there were at least 5,664 patients using the site. Braintalk Communities is an online patient support group for neurology, which was established in 1993, with 19,518 members as of January 2008, 15,841 of whom were active (Braintalk Communities, 2008).

Anecdotal evidence shows that electronic peer-to-peer self-help groups might provide beneficial interventions. Tom Ferguson (1999) released the results of his survey of 191 respondents to an online service for people with chronic and serious illnesses. According to the survey results, those who responded rated online support communities as more helpful than either specialists or primary care physicians in 10 of 12 dimensions of care.

TRADITIONAL APPROACHES TO ADVOCATING FOR POLICY

Advocacy efforts conducted by interest groups play a strong role in shaping public policy in the United States. According to research, more than $2.6 billion is now spent in the United States in support of lobbying or advocacy activities (Center for Responsive Politics, 2007). In 1994, it was estimated that there were as many as 25,000 recognized interest groups, with many more small local and regional groups, both formal and informal (Rauch, 1994). An interest group is an organized body of individuals or organizations that attempts to influence public policy (Rubin, 1997).

Interest groups are increasingly the mechanism of choice for individuals and organizations who want to make their voices heard on public policy issues, in that they allow those who, individually, may have comparatively little at stake to aggregate their stakes with others, thereby making it economically and politically feasible to attempt to influence policy (Rubin, 1997).

The formation of groups and associations to influence public policy through advocacy goes back to the beginning of the United States. According to David Gergen, "the whole argument in *The Federalist Papers* in favor of the Constitution, was that, inevitably, the country would have factions—associations—and that the best way to have a safe, sound, healthy republic with a boisterous democracy would be to give them free voice, and they would compete against each other. Faction would be pitted against faction. From that contest would come a better, stronger republic (Farnham, 2005)."

Successful advocacy efforts engage in an issue early; effectively identify and persuade their targets, which may include Congress, the executive branch, the state governments, and even the corporate sector; effectively understand and influence public opinion; use information for persuasion; engage the media; effectively build and manage coalitions; mobilize grassroots support; and effectively persuade decision makers (Rubin, 1997).

According to some leaders in the field and experts in the area of advocacy, well-run advocacy efforts typically share the following attributes to ensure their success:

- They think creatively, differentiating the association or the issue to ensure that messages get heard.
- They leverage the organization's assets, which may include the knowledge and expertise of the organization's members or leaders.
- They apply campaign strategies, which involve defining the issue, developing consistent key messages, promoting local involvement, and "winning with the facts."
- They cultivate a wide group of allies, with other organizations and stakeholders.
- They define the issues by their societal benefits.
- They treat opponents with dignity and respect (Shapiro, 2003).

In addition, successful advocacy campaigns ordinarily engage organizations that represent different interests—often through coalitions—to carry a common message. A coalition is an "alliance, usually limited in time and purpose, between organizations with different agendas, working together for a common policy advocacy goal" (Rubin, 2000, p. 132.).

HEALTH CARE ADVOCACY

Nearly every stakeholder group within health care is represented by a wide range of associations and nonprofit organizations, including clinicians, community health centers, employers, health plans, hospitals and other providers, laboratories, medical device manufacturers, pharmacies, pharmaceutical organizations, public health agencies, research organizations, and even patients and consumers. In fact, of all industries, health care spends the most on lobbying activities (Center for Responsive Politics, 2007).

In addition, a large number of nonprofit organizations, think tanks, and foundations have been instrumental in influencing policy change by providing educational background and papers describing the issues.

Some consumer groups have been highly effective in driving health care policy change. The AARP is one example. The AARP, a leading nonprofit, nonpartisan organization with more than 39 million members who are age 50 and over, has been very effective over the years in driving health care policy change, including its efforts to advance a drug benefit for seniors. Its most recent health care campaign is entitled Divided We Fail; it is a collaborative effort involving the AARP, the Business Roundtable, the Service Employees Union, and the National Federation of Independent Businesses, which are engaging a variety of individuals and organizations to find bipartisan solutions to ensure affordable, quality health care and long-term financial security for everyone (AARP, 2008).

Another group that has been effective in health care advocacy is the National Partnership for Women and Families (2008). Their Americans for Quality Health Care Campaign, supported by the Robert Wood Johnson Foundation, is raising public awareness and demand for quality health care information and advocating the development and public reporting of performance measures related to quality, safety, patient experience, and cost, and incentives that will reward quality care.

INCREASE IN THE USE OF THE INTERNET FOR ADVOCACY

Across the board, over the last few years, advocacy efforts have been significantly enhanced by the use of the Internet, enabling more rapid communication of the issues to a broader set of audiences to engage their support, using Web sites, blogs, and e-mail alerts. In addition, the introduction of the Internet has enabled organizations to rapidly scale their outreach efforts to policy makers through the use of e-mail and electronic applications that make it easier to reach out to policy makers by providing contact information, key messages, and templates for communications.

For the first time, the Internet was a key force in politics in the 2004 presidential election. According to a study conducted by the Pew Internet & American Life Project, 75 million Americans—or 37% of the adult population and 61% of online Americans—used the Internet to get political news and information, discuss candidates and debate issues in e-mails, or participate directly in the political process by volunteering or giving contributions to candidates (Rainie, 2005).

According to a January 2008 Pew Research Center report, the Internet was a major source for news about the 2008 presidential campaign. The proportion of Americans who say they regularly learned about the campaign from the Internet more than doubled since 2000—from 9% to 24%. In addition, the Internet became a leading source of campaign news for young people, and the role of social networking sites such as MySpace and Facebook is a notable part of the story. Forty-two percent of those ages 18 to 29 say they regularly learned about the campaign from the Internet, the highest percentage for any news source (Kohut, 2008).

USING THE INTERNET FOR HEALTH CARE ADVOCACY

While many consumer groups have been effective in driving health care policy change, we have not yet seen very many patient-focused initiatives or sites that focus primarily on improving health and health care for the individual incorporate advocacy-related activities into their menu of services.

With the increase in the use of the Internet and electronic health information by consumers to assist in the navigation of their health and health care, and the increase in the use of the Internet for advocacy to enable broader reach and involvement by individuals, there is an opportunity for alignment of these areas, giving consumers and patients more of a voice on health care policy issues. The following describes a set of steps that can be taken to engage patients and consumers using the Internet in advocacy activities for a particular health care policy issue.

1. Clearly define the health care policy issue and develop clear and consistent key messages. Policy makers and the public have multiple issues competing for their attention, and therefore a successful advocacy campaign must carefully articulate, manage, and communicate its key messages. Clearly defining the issue and describing why it is important and the actions that must be taken is critical to success.

2. Develop a clear call to action. While many health care interest groups are well aware of and do a good job of articulating the challenges that need to be addressed, many are not as effective

when it comes to communicating a clear call to action, defining the steps they would like the members of their interest group to take to address the challenges. Action can take a variety of forms, including writing members of Congress or state legislators, signing a letter of support, or making a donation.

3. Identify consumer and patient groups that have an interest in and can help advance the health care issue through advocacy. There are thousands of consumer and patient interest groups in the United States, which vary in focus and size, and it is difficult to engage all these groups in an advocacy campaign. An analysis of the different groups can be performed to identify those whose interests are most aligned with the health care policy issue and assess which of those have the operational capabilities and resources to take on the actions required for the advocacy effort.

4. Translate the health care policy issue into messages that resonate with patients and consumers. Consumers and patients are concerned about health care, yet they are not always active in the health care policy debate. This is likely related to the general lack of public involvement in policy, lack of awareness of the issues, and skepticism about how their voice might have an impact. In addition, many of the issues related to health care policy are complex and make them difficult to understand, including the underlying reasons for current challenges related to health care quality, safety, costs, and access, which make it difficult for individuals who do not focus on health care policy issues to understand. Real stories of patients who have been affected by the challenges in the current health care system can be highly effective in communicating with individuals—in terms they understand—why policy change is needed. Health care policy issues, and the actions required, need to be translated into language that average Americans can understand. There is a wide range of consumer and patient groups in the United States, including those focused on particularly populations, such as the elderly (e.g., AARP or the National Council for the Aging), those that are disease specific (e.g., American Heart Association, the National Breast Cancer Coalition, and National Association for the Mentally Ill), and those that focus on specific issues (e.g., Friends for Cancer Research). Some of these organizations lack the resources and ability to take on issues that are not within their primary area of focus, and therefore it is critical

to translate the health care policy issue into messages that resonate for the particular consumer or patient group's interests.

5. Help to build support within consumer or patient groups by
engaging informal or formal leaders within the interest groups
as "champions." Research indicates that members of groups—
whether formal or informal—trust their peers more than those
outside the interest group. Virtual patient networks such as Patients Like Me build their model on patients sharing information
with each other, offering a framework and an environment to
facilitate that sharing. To help build support, one should seek
out—and engage—both formal and informal leaders to carry the
importance of the message to the broader group.

6. Develop an online advocacy strategy that can easily be implemented by interest groups comprised of patients and consumers. The vast majority of groups representing either patients or
consumers are under-resourced and do not have the ability to
undertake the steps required for a broad advocacy campaign. On
the other hand, their strength is often in the number of volun-
teers and participants in their organization or effort. The Internet
offers not only a lower-cost alternative to traditional advocacy efforts; it also enables a broader number of individuals to engage
in the advocacy process more efficiently than they are able to
in traditional advocacy efforts. The online advocacy strategy can
incorporate one or more of the following key elements:

   A. Web site content that includes the following:
      - A description of the issue and why it is important (in
        language that is understandable for interest group
        members).
      - Key facts—credible and statistically valid facts about the
        issue.
      - Stories—examples of real-life stories that bring life to
        the issue.
      - A call for action—the key steps that individuals can take
        to address the issue.

   B. An online networking mechanism, which enables the shar-
      ing of information among interest group members—this
      can take the form of a blog or Listserv.

   C. Online newsletters that provide updates or alerts high-
      lighting the status of the issue and calls for immediate ac-
      tion when necessary.

D.   An online resource that includes lists of e-mail and phone contact information for policy makers, as well as standard messages and templates for communications, to assist individuals in conducting outreach to policy makers and the other organizations they are trying to influence.

E.   Mechanisms to enable individuals to donate to advocacy-related activities for the health care policy issue.

7.   Develop and implement methods to measure success. Ultimately the measure of success for any advocacy campaign is whether the goal was achieved—whether legislation was passed to address the issue or impending legislation was stopped. Other interim metrics could include the following:

- How many groups (and individuals) were engaged in the issue?
- How many consumers or patients completed the call to action?
- How many policy makers took on the issue as a result of the advocacy effort?
- Did the amount of media coverage on the issue significantly increase?

There are some early examples of how patient-centered Web sites have begun to use the Internet to engage patients in the public policy process. One example is WebMD, a Web site that offers health information and tools to consumers and patients. In January 2008, WebMD launched Election 2008: Health Matters, an online health center offering a comparison of candidates' platforms on many health care issues, and providing an election message board that allowed visitors to tell their health stories and weigh in on the candidates (WebMD, n.d.).

SUMMARY AND AREAS FOR FURTHER RESEARCH

In summary, given an increasing online society, new opportunities emerge for significantly increasing the engagement of patients and consumers in advocacy efforts on health care policy issues.

Increasingly, individuals are turning to the Internet and other electronic applications to help manage their health and health care. Over the last few years there has been a significant increase in both consumer-directed applications related to health care using the Internet and the number of online communities of patients who are sharing information to improve their health and health care.

At the same time, and as indicated by early reviews of activities related to the 2008 presidential election, the Internet is being used more and more to educate, inform, and engage the public's support for policy changes and the candidates who support them. The Internet is increasingly being leveraged to expand and intensify advocacy-related efforts targeting policy makers by enabling a wider and more diverse number of individuals to engage in the public policy process.

Today's health care challenges, including those related to quality, safety, efficiency, and access, and the actions that must be taken to address these challenges, would benefit considerably from more consumer engagement and activation—to help drive changes in health care policy related to these issues.

There is a near-term opportunity to expand much-needed consumer involvement in driving health care policy change that will begin to address the challenges of the U.S. health care system by engaging individuals who currently participate either in online health communities or in other online health offerings. Traditional advocacy strategies, including clearly defining the issue, developing key messages, and creating a call to action, can also be applied in an online environment. Online communities and patient and consumer interest groups that already have an online presence are in a strong position to extend their current activities and services by also supporting advocacy-related efforts that leverage the Internet.

More research is needed to explore whether those individuals who visit patient-focused Web sites or participate in online communities primarily to inform and improve their health and health care are likely to engage in advocacy activities promoted by these health-related Web sites. More research is also needed to evaluate whether advocacy strategies that use the Internet are more effective than traditional approaches.

REFERENCES

AARP. (2008). *Divided we fail campaign.* Retrieved January 2008, from http://www.aarp.org/issues/dividedwefail/about_us/

Agency for Healthcare Research and Quality. (1998). *Medical Expenditure Panel Survey.* Retrieved August 13, 2008, from http://www.meps.ahrq.gov/mepsweb/data_stats/download_data_files_results.jsp?buttonYearandDataType=Search&cboDataYear=1998

Braintalk Communities. (2008). Retrieved January 2008, from http://brain.hastypastry.net/forums/

Center for Responsive Politics. (2007). Retrieved August 14, 2008, from http://www. opensecrets.org/lobbyists/index.asp

Commonwealth Fund. (2006). *Why not the best? Results from a national scorecard on U.S. health system performance.* New York: Author.

Dolan, P. L. (2007). *PHR: Pretty half-hearted reception.* Chicago: AMNews.

eHealth Initiative Foundation. (2007). *A Majority of Consumers Favor Electronic Health Information Exchange: Attitude and Opinion Research.* Retrieved August 13, 2008, from http://toolkit.ehealthinitiative.org/communication_and_outreach/common_ principles.mspx

WebMD. (n.d.). *Election 2008: Health matters.* Retrieved January 2008, from http:// www.webmd.com/election2008/default.htm

Eysenbach, G., Powell, J., Englesakis, M., Rizo, C., & Stern, A. (2004). Health related virtual communities and electronic support groups: Systematic review of the effects of online peer to peer interactions. *British Medical Journal, 328,* 1166.

Ferguson, T. (1999, March). E-patients prefer eGroups to doctors for 10 of 12 aspects of health care. *Ferguson Report, 1.* Retrieved August 13, 2008, from http://www. fergusonreport.com/archives/idx9903.htm

Fox, S. (2005, May 17). *Health information online.* Washington, DC: Pew Internet & American Life Project.

Fox, S. (2007). *E-patients with a disability or chronic disease.* Washington, DC: Pew Internet & American Life Project.

Gearon, C. J. (2005, March 15). A personal record: While Feds delay, some digitize their own medical records. *The Washington Post,* p. HE01.

Farnham, P. (2005, June). *A conversation with David Gergen.* Executive Update. Retrieved August 13, 2008, from http://www.asaecenter.org/PublicationsResources/ EUArticle.cfm?ItemNumber=11456

Henry J. Kaiser Family Foundation/Health Research and Educational Trust. (2006). *Employer health benefits 2006 annual survey.* Retrieved August 13, 2008, from http://www.kff.org/insurance/7527/index.cfm

Henry J. Kaiser Family Foundation. (2007, December 20). *Kaiser Health Tracking Poll: Election 2008.* Retrieved August 14, 2008, from http://www.kff.org/kaiserpolls/h08_ pomr122007pkg.cfm

Jackson, K. (2004). Medical records on the go. *For the Record, 16*(3), 30.

Kaiser Family Foundation. (2006). *Health Care in America 2006 Survey.* Retrieved August 13, 2008, from http://www.kff.org/kaiserpolls/7572.cfm

Kohut, A., Keeter, S., Doherty, C., & Dimock, M. (2008). *Social networking and online videos take off: Internet's broader role in campaign 2008.* Washington, DC: Pew Research Center.

Markle Foundation. (2008). *Markle Foundation Web Site.* Retrieved January 2008, from http://www.markle.org/markle_programs/healthcare/index.php

McGlynn, E. A., Asch, S. M., Adams, J., Keesey, J., Hicks, J., DeCristofaro, A., et al. (2003). The quality of health care delivered to adults in the United States. *New England Journal of Medicine, 348,* 2635–2645.

National Partnership for Women and Families. (2008). *Americans for quality health care program.* Retrieved January 2008, from http://www.nationalpartnership.org/site/ PageServer?pagename = qcn_index

National Survey on Electronic Personal Health Records. (2006, November). Conducted by Lake Research Partners and American Viewpoint, Markle Foundation.

PatientsLikeMe. (2008). *PatientsLikeMe Web site*. Retrieved January 2008, from http://www.patientslikeme.org

Rainie, L., Cornfield, M., & Horrigan, J. (2005). *The Internet and campaign 2004*. Pew Internet & American Life Project. Washington, DC.

Rauch, J. (1994). *Demosclerosis*. New York: Times Books.

Reinhardt, U. E., Hussey, P. S., & Anderson, G. F. (2004). U.S. health care spending in an international context. *Health Affairs, 23*(3), 10–25.

Rubin, B. (1997). *A citizen's guide to politics in America*. Armonk, NY: M. E. Sharp.

Rubin, B. (2000). *A citizen's guide to politics in America: How the system works and how to work the system* (2nd ed.). Armonk, NY: M. E. Sharp.

Shapiro, G. (2003). An effective advocate. *Association Management, 55*(6), 54–58.

U.S. Bureau of the Census. (2000). *Projections of the total resident population by 5-year age groups and sex with special age categories: Middle series, 1999 to 2100* (NP-T3). Washington, DC: Author.

Wellman B. (1997). An electronic group is virtually a social network. In S. Kiesler (Ed.), *Cultures of the Internet* (pp. 170–205). Mahwah, NJ: Erlbaum.

Wu, S., & Green, A. (2000). *Projection of chronic illness prevalence and cost inflation*. Santa Monica, CA: Rand.

10

Improving Physician–Patient Communication

PETYA ECKLER, GREGORY M. WORSOWICZ, AND KATHERINE DOWNEY

Physician–patient communication is the backbone of medical care and has been shown to influence both patient satisfaction and health outcomes (Stewart, 1995). Research in the area began in the mid-1960s and has gained momentum in the past decades as this interaction continues to evolve in terms of participants, complexity, and diversity. "Clear, candid, accurate, culturally and linguistically competent provider–patient communication is essential for the prevention, diagnosis, treatment, and management of health concerns," according to *Healthy People 2010*. Indeed, one of the objectives listed in the report is to improve the dialogue between physicians and patients (U.S. Department of Health and Human Services, 2000).

Communication between physician and patient involves two primary tasks: information exchange and relationship building, also referred to, respectively, as cure and care. Information exchange, or the cure dimension, supports the compiling of medical history, describing the problem to reach a diagnosis, and understanding treatment (Cegala, McGee, & McNeilis, 1996; van den Brink-Muinen, van Dulmen, Jung, & Bensing, 2007). It is influenced by the racial concordance between patient and doctor; the physician's use of jargon; and the patient's age, education, income, dialect, and attitudes toward illness (Gordon, Street, Sharf, & Souchek, 2006; Shuy, 1993; Siminoff, Graham, & Gordon, 2006).

The affective side of communication, or the care dimension, relates to physician friendliness, empathy, reassurance, and understanding of patient expectations and concerns; patients have found this aspect quite unsatisfactory (Myerscough & Ford, 1996; van den Brink-Muinen et al., 2007). Relationship building correlates positively with patient satisfaction and, to a lesser extent, with treatment compliance (Cegala et al., 1996). To address these distinct and sometimes conflicting aspects of communication, medical schools have developed programs for both communication and interpersonal skills (Duffy, Gordon, Whelan, Cole-Kelly, & Frankel, 2004).

Based on levels of control over the exchange, Stewart and Roter's (1989) theoretical model distinguishes several types of relationships. A paternalistic relationship has high physician control and low patient control, while a consumerist relationship has high patient and low physician control. In a mutual relationship, both parties exercise strong control. The authors state that patients may adopt a passive role by default, unaware of alternatives or unable to negotiate a more active stance. In particular, older, less educated patients are more likely to be in a paternalistic relationship, while younger, more educated, and more skeptical patients are more likely to exact a relationship with high patient control. This relationship is not a constant, however, and may change depending on the needs and circumstances of the participants, so neither model is forever appropriate or inappropriate (Stewart & Roter, 1989).

Traditionally, communication has been discussed in terms of the medical encounter and mainly the medical interview. The very structure of the interview, however, affects its content and consequences: it is unlike a regular conversation because of the imbalance in participation of the two parties. On average doctors talk for 60% of the time (range 51%–77%) and patients talk for 40% (range 23%–49%). The question-and-answer format itself has been found to correlate negatively with patient compliance and recall (Roter, 1989). Because patients rarely use this format in everyday live, it makes them uneasy and unable to share their experiences (Shuy, 1993). Information giving, on the other hand, relates strongly to satisfaction, compliance, and recall (Roter, 1989) but takes a very small share of the exchange. Even when physicians engage in information giving, they can only be effective when a positive relationship already exists and if they understand patients' attitudes to the illness (Myerscough & Ford, 1996).

While the medical interview is still considered the main communication avenue, the increasing prevalence of chronic disease and the shift from inpatient to ambulatory treatment are changing the time continuum. The exchange now starts before and continues after the actual medical encounter. New media facilitate this pre-, during, and post-visit continuum and present an opportunity to improve communication by offering access, convenience, and consistency. But technological advancements also present new challenges such as the lack of standardized guidelines, problems of reimbursement, and legal and ethical questions. This chapter discusses these issues and their implications for the future of physician–patient communication.

CURRENT STATE OF PHYSICIAN–PATIENT COMMUNICATION

After decades of scientific inquiry into physician–patient communication, findings both encourage and alarm. Communication has definitely improved, according to Stoeckle's (1982) historical perspective of patient load in Massachusetts General Hospital. In the 1900s to the 1920s, 30 patients were seen in 2 hours, while in the 1920s through the 1940s the number dropped to 15. Since the 1950s, between 6 and 9 patients have been seen in 3 hours, with an average visit time of 20 minutes. Nationwide, the average visit time in 2004 was 18.7 minutes, according to the National Ambulatory Medical Care Survey (Hing, Cherry, & Woodwell, 2006), up from 16.3 minutes in 1989 (Mechanic, McAlpine, & Rosenthal, 2001). However, some are skeptical of these data, which are based on physician self-report, because direct observation has shown significantly shorter visit duration (Gilchrist, Stange, Flocke, McCord, & Bourguet, 2004; Gottschalk & Flocke, 2005).

In addition, Stoeckle (1982) reported that the space in doctors' offices has become smaller and more intimate, hence more inviting, and waiting times for appointments, tests, and test results have decreased. Studies have demonstrated high (80%–90%) patient satisfaction with medical visit duration and other aspects of doctors' visits except for cost and waiting time (Gross, Zyzanski, Borawski, Cebul, & Stange, 1998; Stoeckle, 1982). However, Sitzia and Wood (1997) noted that although many patient satisfaction surveys report highly positive results because of their methodological and conceptual approaches, the scientific community has accepted that "substantial dissatisfaction exists with specific components of care, notably waiting times and communication in primary care."

Despite these encouraging findings, causes for concern still exist. Myerscough and Ford (1996) noted that communication is the most common cause for complaint from patients and an apparent weak point among doctors. Research has shown that half of psychosocial and psychiatric problems are missed during medical consultations, that physicians interrupt an average of 18 seconds into patients' descriptions of their problems, that half of patient problems and concerns are neither elicited by the physician nor disclosed by the patient, that patients and physicians do not agree on the main presenting problem in half of the visits, and that patients are dissatisfied with the information provided by physicians (Stewart, 1995). Physicians sometimes share uninvited personal information, which distracts the patient and interrupts the flow of the conversation (McDaniel et al., 2007). When discussing side effects of therapeutic drugs, patients usually initiate the talk and doctors are more likely to deny than affirm the possibility, even for patients who are likely to develop side effects and even when the described symptoms of possible side effects have a strong literature support to be connected to the drug (Golomb, McGraw, Evans, & Dimsdale, 2007).

While scholars generally agree that communication needs to improve, it is worth discussing how it can benefit patients and physicians. For patients, better dialogue has led to higher satisfaction; lower stress, anxiety, and pain; increased compliance; better understanding of treatment risks; less frequent use of therapeutic drugs; better-controlled hemoglobin and blood pressure; fewer emergency visits; and shorter hospital stays. For physicians, improved communication has caused higher satisfaction and fewer medical errors and malpractice lawsuits (Bull et al., 2002; Golomb et al., 2007; Greenfield, Kaplan, Ware, Yano, & Frank, 1998; Shaw, Zaia, Pransky, Winters, & Patterson, 2005; Sutcliffe, Lewton, & Rosenthal, 2004; Travaline, Ruchinskas, & D'Alonzo, 2005).

RECENT DEVELOPMENTS IN PHYSICIAN–PATIENT COMMUNICATION

In view of the recognized importance of communication for the quality of health care, a number of recent developments have aimed at improving it. These include better education and formal testing in medical schools and residency programs; the shift of the time continuum into pre-, during, and post-visit; the shift toward a patient-centered, consumerist model of communication; and the introduction of new media.

In 1978 the Society of General Internal Medicine addressed the importance of communication and started offering medical faculty an annual course on teaching effective communication skills. Communication is now in the foreground at medical schools and residency programs and the Accreditation Council for Graduate Medical Education and the Liaison Committee on Medical Education have identified these skills as core competencies. The Accreditation Council for Graduate Medical Education expects residents to create and sustain therapeutic and ethically sound relationships with patients by using effective listening, nonverbal, explanatory, questioning, and writing skills. Most (65%) medical schools in 1993 had a formal curriculum in communication skills, compared to 35% in 1978 (Kalet et al., 2004). The National Board of Medical Examiners has added a communication and interpersonal skills subcomponent to the U.S. Medical Licensing Examination, during which medical students are tested on their ability to ascertain patient expectations, feelings, and concerns; determine patient support systems and impact of illness; encourage additional questions or engage in further discussion; and make empathetic remarks about patient concerns (Guadagnino, 2006).

The time continuum of physician–patient communication has been changing due to the increasing prevalence of chronic disease, which requires continuous management, and the shift from inpatient to ambulatory treatment. Communication now starts before the medical encounter and continues afterward, and new media facilitate this pre-, during, and post-visit continuum. E-mail reminders for upcoming appointments are now commonplace, as are follow-ups with lab results. Portable media players in waiting rooms offer patients an introduction to the visit, and mobile devices in homes monitor chronic illnesses after the encounter.

In the past 30 years, the power balance has shifted from the physician to the patient, allowing the latter more control over the agenda. While the patient-centered, or consumerist, method is not necessarily recent, it is discussed here because of its continued development. We see this process in the fact that the concept of patient-centered care still lacks an agreed-upon definition, despite its widespread use. Mead and Bower (2000) consider the most comprehensive description, that of Stewart and associates (1995), who identify six interrelated components of the model: exploring both the disease and the illness experience, understanding the whole person, finding common ground regarding management, incorporating prevention and health promotion, enhancing the doctor-patient relationship, and being realistic about personal limitations and issues such as the availability of time and resources. This definition puts a clear focus on communication and holism—exploring, understanding, and negotiating both disease and illness are part of good dialogue and long-term relationship building. Mead and Bower (2000) identify five conceptual dimensions of the patient-centered approach: the biopsychosocial perspective, patient as person, sharing power and responsibility, therapeutic alliance, and doctor as person.

The last recent development is the introduction of new media. New media is a broad communication concept that can refer to any of the following:

- Emerging digital technologies and platforms—video games, virtual worlds, software, mobile devices (phones, wireless handheld devices, portable media players, electronic kiosks, interactive TV/telemedicine)
- Online communication—Internet, blogs, chat rooms, wikis, e-mail, online newsletters
- Electronic and multimedia publishing—multimedia CD-ROMs and hypertext (Hamer, 2005).

Several main characteristics differentiate new from traditional media. First is the use of multimedia applications, in which the same information can be conveyed through text, audio, video, graphics, and animation. Second is interactivity: new media are active and engaging for the user, while old media (print and broadcast) are passive. A third unique feature is customization: information is personalized to one's own needs and environment. A fourth and final characteristic is the use of hypertext: information is not presented in a linear fashion but linked with related content through hyperlinks, which allows for richer context (Pavlik, 2001).

NEW MEDIA AND PHYSICIAN–PATIENT COMMUNICATION

Internet use among American adults hit an all-time high in 2006, with 73% (147 million) going online, an increase of 7% (10 million) from the previous year. Of these users, 84 million had broadband connections at home, an increase of 25 million from 2005 (Madden, 2006). The Internet's impact on American society was also measured by how much it improved various aspects of users' lives. Users reported better ability to shop, pursue hobbies and interests, and do their jobs. Twenty percent said the Internet improved the way they got health information.

E-mail

The increasing use of new media has raised people's expectations of health care providers. In a nationally representative survey, 57%–77% of adults wanted at least one type of electronic communication with their doctor, including appointment reminders, communication of test results and consultations by e-mail, online scheduling of visits, and home monitoring devices that transmit information to the clinic. For 62% of survey respondents, their choice of a doctor would be influenced by whether he or she communicates by e-mail (Harris Interactive, 2006). Other studies have confirmed this strong interest. Eighty percent of patients at Duke Family Medicine Center were interested in e-mail communication and 42% were willing to pay a small annual fee for this service (Virji et al., 2006). In pediatric practices, 74%–80% of parents wanted e-mail communication, and 65% would choose a pediatrician based on that, but most (63%) were unwilling to pay extra (Anand, Feldman, Geller, Bisbee, & Bauchner, 2005; Kleiner, Akers, Burke, & Werner, 2002). Contrary to consumers' strong desire for electronic communication, only 2%–4% reported availability and use of such services, and another 3%–4% had access to the services but did not use them (Harris Interactive, 2006). Other studies report 5%–10% of patients e-mailing their doctors (Moyer, Stern, Dobias, Cox, & Katz, 2002; Virji et al., 2006).

Data from physicians confirm the low use of e-mail for patient communication. In a survey of Florida physicians, 17% e-mailed patients from the office but most did it rarely, and only 17% did so frequently, accounting for just 3% of the total sample. Physician e-mail users were younger, urban, non-Asian, practicing in family medicine or surgery, and working in larger practices (50 or more physicians) with high-speed Internet access (Brooks & Menachemi, 2006). A study of pediatricians in Norfolk, Virginia, revealed 79% were reluctant to e-mail patients, although 87% had access in the office, but many were open to having their staff do it (Kleiner et al., 2002). Of the Florida physicians who did not use e-mail, about half (53%) had no desire to start, and one-third (34%) were undecided. This resistance was hardly due to unease with the medium, because many e-mailed friends and family, colleagues, hospitals, and pharmaceutical companies (Brooks & Menachemi, 2006).

Physicians and patients who communicate by e-mail regularly find many advantages. Patients report e-mail is convenient for setting appointments, getting refills and referrals, and other administrative services. E-mail users are more likely to report better communication with the clinic, and many (85%) prefer it versus the telephone for non-urgent messages. E-mail also provides constant availability and 73% of messages are sent outside clinic hours (Lin, Wittevrongel, Moore, Beaty, & Ross, 2005). In another study, 58% of patient e-mails and 61% of physician e-mails were sent after hours and on weekends (Anand et al., 2005). E-mail is also more efficient for patients, as it saves them time and extra telephone calls or visits to the clinic (Leong, Gingrich, Lewis, Mauger, & George, 2005; Lin et al., 2005). E-mail communication also urges more FYI and psychosocial messages from patients, and more direct and elaborate advice from doctors (Lin et al., 2005).

Physicians experience benefits as well. Daily users report it to be a time-saving alternative to phones, as it allows patients direct access and can be maintained even when patients travel (Patt, Houston, Jenckes, Sands, & Ford, 2003). In fact, an e-mail address can provide a more reliable connection to some users than a home address or a telephone number (Virji et al., 2006). Similar to patients, most physicians (60%) see e-mail as a good way to handle administrative tasks (Moyer et al., 2002). It also allows for gathering previsit information, such as medical history and information regarding allergies and current medications, which saves time during the visit and facilitates follow-up when patients ask questions or request clarification (Patt et al., 2003).

Barriers and concerns have also been identified. Moyer and associates (2002) reported that most common among patients were preferences to speak with a real person or use the telephone and fear that the message would get lost or that the reply would take too long. Surprisingly, privacy concerns were least common. Concerns were more pronounced among nonusers than users. A patient survey by Katz, Moyer, Cox, and Stern (2003) suggested a potential conflict regarding the role of staff in e-mail exchanges. More than 75% of doctors were comfortable with staff answering patient messages, and nearly half felt patient e-mails should go to staff first. In contrast, only 32% of patients felt comfortable with staff answering e-mails to their providers, and 52% felt e-mails sent to the provider should only be read by him or her. Patient preferences regarding e-mail communication depend on the topic. E-mail is the best option for routine topics such as cholesterol results, normal PAP/PSA test results, prescription renewals, sore throat, and back pain, whereas in-person communication is preferred for sensitive issues such as breast/testicular pain, abnormal PAP/PSA test results, mental health issues, and sexually transmitted infection test results (Katz et al., 2003).

In light of the huge discrepancy between patients' desires to communicate electronically and doctors' readiness to do so (Anand et al., 2005; Brooks & Menachemi, 2006; Harris Interactive, 2006; Kleiner et al., 2002; Virji et al., 2006), physicians' concerns need to be recognized. In a survey of physicians who frequently e-mail patients, most were satisfied, but 25% said they would not recommend it to a colleague. Their most common concerns were medico-legal issues, time demands, some patients' lack of access to e-mail, patient difficulty in usage, and staff being unhappy. Most dissatisfied doctors (80%) used e-mail upon patients' request (Houston, Sands, Nash, & Ford, 2003). In another survey, 44% of physicians said e-mail would add to their workload, and half feared becoming overwhelmed. Regular e-mail users (not just with patients) had more positive attitudes than infrequent users, suggesting that concerns may result from inexperience with the medium (Moyer et al., 2002).

The topic of anxiety about time or work demands is prevalent in the literature, but no consensus exists on the actual time or effort spent on e-mail. One study reported physicians receiving one to five messages per day and spending 2 minutes responding to each, while in another, physicians estimated devoting 30 minutes daily to e-mail communication (Anand et al., 2005; Houston et al., 2003). Lin and colleagues (2005) found that e-mail diversified the format but did not increase the volume of patient messages. A study of a triage-based e-mail system, however, found that e-mail was an add-on to, not a substitute for, phone or in-person communication and did not improve overall efficiency. However, e-mail users were younger, more educated, less sick, and less likely to call or visit and until then may not have been served by other communication methods (Katz et al., 2003).

Another common concern is patients' ability to use e-mail appropriately and to distinguish between non-urgent and urgent conditions (Houston et al., 2003). Yet content analyses of e-mail messages do not substantiate these fears. White, Moyer, Stern, and Katz (2004) found no e-mails containing urgent messages, and only 5% with overly sensitive content. Most messages were formal, concise, and courteous, and directly related to medical issues, and only 43% required physician follow-up. Common topics were information updates, referral requests, appointments, prescription renewal, tests, and health questions. Anand

and associates (2005) also found relatively high levels of etiquette in e-mail communications, with no mention of urgent or acute problems and a focus on medical questions or updates, subspecialty evaluation, and administrative issues. Finally, reimbursement is also a common concern among doctors. The adage "Time is money" is particularly appropriate in this case, as doctors fear that more patient e-mails will take up more time, and hence this service should somehow be paid for (Patt et al., 2003).

Telemedicine

Although telemedicine has existed for 20 years, new media are changing it by allowing information to be transmitted online or by various digital devices, thus increasing affordability (Slack, 2001). Telemedicine offers the benefits of connecting patients and physicians over long distances and allowing underserved locations and populations access to care. It also decreases time and travel (and hence cost) of specialty consultations.

So how does telemedicine influence physician–patient communication? In a study of an Internet-based telemedicine system for emergency ophthalmologic consultation, Bar-Sela (2007) demonstrated that the approach was reliable and preferred by patients. Diagnoses by telemedicine and by the ophthalmologist were in full agreement, and 98% of patients preferred the telemedicine exam. However patient preferences seem to vary by condition. During periods of low uncertainty about their health (health maintenance) or high uncertainty (crisis situations when any physician access is appreciated), patients felt telemedicine was effective. During periods of moderate uncertainty (when medications need to be changed), they preferred face-to-face consultation (Turner et al., 2004).

Telemedicine consultations shift the locus of power between practitioners. In face-to-face encounters, the physician sets the pace, while in telemedicine the nurse does so by moving the monitor to the next person. During face-to-face interaction, the doctor can hurry the visit through nonverbal cues, but in telemedicine the nurse determines when all the questions have been resolved (Turner et al., 2004). Telemedicine changes the dynamic of the clinical encounter for the patient as well. Patients thought they approached telemedicine differently than face-to-face encounters, but a content analysis of their conversations found no significant differences. Health care providers said they treated the situations the same, but the physician was interrupted and called away during face-to-face visits, but not during telemedicine sessions (Turner et al., 2004). Liu and associates (2007) found significant differences between telemedicine and face-to-face consultations: duration was shorter, patient-centered behavior patterns (facilitation utterance, empathy utterance, and praise-utterance) were fewer, and less data were taken for the medical records via telemedicine. Still, patient attitudes toward the encounters were similar. Doctors, however, were dissatisfied with telemedicine because they thought too much time was spent on small talk, and they had difficulty asking questions and connecting with patients.

Online Health Information

Eight in 10 American Internet users (113 million) go online for health information. On a typical day in August 2006, 8 million Americans searched for health information, which makes this activity as popular as paying bills, reading blogs, and looking up a phone number or an address (Fox, 2006). Online health information benefits consumers by increasing their knowledge and involvement with their own health (Hart, Henwood, & Wyatt, 2004). Most people (51%–74%) feel reassured in their decisions, confident to raise new questions with their doctor, relieved by what they found, and eager to share their knowledge with others (Fox, 2006). However, barriers exist for a small but substantial group (10%–25%), who feel overwhelmed to make an informed decision, frustrated by lack of information or inability to find it, confused, and frightened (Fox, 2006; Hart et al., 2004). Another aspect of gathering health information online is that most consumers (75%) do not check the source or date of what they find (Fox, 2006). These findings raise doubts about consumers' confidence in their evaluation skills.

Internet use influences the physician–patient relationship when patients discuss the information they find with their physicians. When that happened, physicians said quality made all the difference: accurate, relevant information benefited, while inaccurate or irrelevant information harmed health care, health outcomes, and their relationship. However, the best predictor of a perceived deterioration in the relationship was the physicians' perception that he or she was being challenged (OR = 14.9) (Murray et al., 2003). Physicians reported patient benefits were more common than harms, but there were more problems than benefits for doctors. The main challenges were the need for longer clinical visits, patients' difficulties evaluating the information, patients' desire for new and unavailable treatments, and patients trusting the Internet more than their doctors (Potts & Wyatt, 2002).

Patient perceptions of physician authority may also be at risk. Lowrey and Anderson (2006) found that increased use of online health information was positively correlated with patients' belief that doctors are not the experts on medical knowledge. Other significant variables were income and perceptions of alternative medicine. However, this explained only 12% of the variance in perception. Other threats to physician authority, according to the authors, were the profession's specialization, popularity of alternative medicine, and the perception that doctors value power and money over patients.

The above findings suggest that online health information is mostly disadvantageous, especially for physicians, but the implementation of Web-based information prescriptions could change that. An information prescription is the prescription of "focused, evidence-based information to a patient at the right time to manage a health problem" (D'Alessandro, Kreiter, Kinzer, & Petersonet, 2004, p. 857). Such prescriptions satisfy patients' need for more knowledge in the same way as general health Web sites but also meet physicians' standards of quality, consistency, and relevance. Most patients (65%) who got them visited the Web site within a week, and after a reminder, compliance increased by 45% (Ritterband et al., 2005). Other studies confirm the high demand among patients for health information guidance (Rice & Katz, 2006; Salo et al., 2004).

Online consultations allow consumers to contact previously unknown physicians with health questions. Users most often discussed specific symptoms and requested a diagnosis or a second opinion, information on a disease, or information on a treatment or drug (Umefjord, 2006). Reasons that patients cited for choosing this option were the convenience (52%) and anonymity (36%) it offered, their own doctor was too busy (21%), they lacked time or had difficulty getting an appointment, they felt uncomfortable at a clinic, they appreciated the affordability of this option, they felt discontent with previous doctors, they felt their concerns were embarrassing, and they had a preference for written communication.

Other Digital Technologies

New media will continue to influence physician–patient communication as they penetrate the health care field. Portable media players, wireless

handheld devices, blogs, and wikis have gone mainstream and are gradually being adopted by the medical field.

Portable media players assist medical education in the University of
Michigan School of Dentistry and other universities across the country
(Boulos, Maramba, & Wheeler, 2006; Trelease, 2006). The University of
Michigan has gone one step further and introduced this technology into
physician–patient communication by giving patients iPods with video
messages that provide an orientation to the visit while they wait (Johnson, 2007). The Cleveland Clinic offers its patients online podcasts and
videocasts on various health topics.

Cell phones have also influenced communication. In some clinics
in Kansas City, Missouri, patients receive a phone message whenever
their appointment is delayed, which can decrease time spent in waiting rooms. Chin (2005) concluded that the cell phone has "promising
benefits" for the physician–patient relationship after examining patients'
postoperative calls to their surgeon. Only 17% of all calls were to the surgeon's cellular phone, and 80% of them were during business hours, and
most were urgent. But while the surgeon's cell phone was used sparingly
and mostly for emergencies, giving the number created the impression
among patients that the doctor was truly concerned with their care and
outcomes.

PRACTICAL AND OPERATIONAL CHALLENGES OF NEW MEDIA

While new media could potentially improve physician–patient communication, they also pose some practical and operational challenges for
physicians. These include the establishment of and adherence to guidelines for communication, reimbursement regulations, possible legal
ramifications, and continued adherence to prior ethical standards.

Guidelines

The American Medical Association (2002) guidelines for electronic communication state that new technologies should never replace the crucial
interpersonal contact that is the basis of the physician–patient relationship but rather enhance it. The guidelines cover communication, medical/
legal, administrative, and ethical standards. Communication guidelines
include establishing turn-around time for messages, informing patients

about privacy issues, establishing the types of transactions to be covered, informed consent, and ways to terminate an e-mail relationship. Guidelines have also been created by the eRisk Working Group, a consortium of 30 medical malpractice carriers, the AMA, and multiple national, state, and local medical societies. But while guidelines exist, they are seldom followed. Brooks and Menachemi (2006) reported that the most commonly practiced rule (48%) was printing the e-mail and placing it in the patient's chart, followed by informing patients about privacy issues (36%). Adherence to additional rules occurred in less than 25% of cases, but frequent users of e-mail were more likely to follow five or more guidelines.

Reimbursement

The Center of Medicare and Medicaid Services has developed reimbursement guidelines for telehealth and e-consults, but physicians should be aware of what can and cannot be submitted as compliant services. For example, telehealth is reimbursed by Medicaid, but the rules are different for each state. Third-party payers often mirror government payers for allowable services but may also have their own reimbursable services. In terms of medical codes for identifying, tracking, and reimbursing for telemedicine, some states use modifiers to the existing Physicians' Current Procedural Terminology codes such as "TM" and "TV." Physicians need to know each payer's rules and regulations, which adds an administrative burden and additional expenses to their practice and has the potential to increase the cost to the patient. Still, the "quiet revolution" has already begun, according to Stone (2007), and Aetna, Cigna, and others now reimburse physicians for Web consultations in Florida, California, Massachusetts, and New York.

Ethical and Legal Issues

Each new communication medium raises its own liability concerns. When telemedicine is used, visual evidence of the visit is captured for future review. If such an encounter is later seen by non-authorized individuals, the question of informed consent becomes pertinent (Flemming, 2008). Privacy and security concerns have been expressed in regards to e-mail as well (Katz et al., 2003; Moyer et al., 2002). Unsecured, delayed, or lost e-mail can be opened by outsiders. Insufficient protections can subject patients to possible embarrassment, social stigma, and discrimination (Hodge, Gostin, & Jacobson, 1999). The security breaches of databanks and the private data collection industry that collects, analyzes, and sells consumer information are additional factors for concern (Anderson, 2007). Hodge and colleagues make the following recommendations for legal reform in regards to health information privacy: (1) recognize that identifiable health information as highly sensitive, (2) provide privacy safeguards based on fair information practices, (3) empower patients with information and rights to consent to disclosure, (4) limit disclosures of health data absent consent, (5) incorporate industry-wide security protections, (6) establish a national data protection authority, and (7) provide a national minimal level of privacy protections.

IMPLICATIONS FOR THE FUTURE

In evaluating new media's impact on physician–patient communication, we are reminded of Harris (1995), who wrote, "Just as more isn't necessarily better health care, more technology is not necessarily the answer to the health care dilemma" (p. 3). We see new media not as more technology but as an opportunity to improve physician–patient communication, provided they are used with an understanding of their strengths and limitations.

The above review of the empirical literature shows that some of new media's strengths are also their weaknesses. E-mail may be a timesaver for patients but is potentially time consuming for physicians. It enables psychosocial and FYI messages from patients but gets blamed for depersonalization. Patients prefer telemedicine for some health conditions, but not for others. While these findings seem confusing at best, the key to understanding them lies in one of the unique features of new media: customization. Offering different features to different people is new media's strongest selling point. But while customization benefits the individual, it contradicts standardization and optimization in the health care industry, and this conflict may impede widespread utilization.

New media offer challenges, but the established and potential benefits may outweigh them. The expansion of communication into a pre-, during, and post-visit continuum will improve information flow and consistency of care, especially for chronic illnesses that require long-term attention. Text messages could improve compliance by reinforcing physician authority and the value of treatment after the visit when the doctor's influence begins to wane and the influences of the social environment remain strong (Pendleton, 1983). Another controversial consequence of new media, online health information, can be turned into a tool for health education. The literature has demonstrated that patients are eager for information guidance and physicians need to respond to these needs. Research has shown that contrary to physician concerns, patients do not use e-mail for urgent messages or abuse the privilege of having their doctors' cell phone number. The evidence presented earlier suggests that a major barrier lies within physicians and the industry as a whole.

The adoption of new media ultimately depends on both the industry and the individual physician. Such an adoption will create an expanding market for new services. Pre-visit services such as payment registration, scheduling, medical information/questionnaires, and real-time notification of clinic delays and post-visit services such as customized Web sites, automated disease management systems, secure messaging, and notification of results, are technologically feasible, but technology is not the major roadblock to their adoption. Instead, the creation of appropriate guidelines, regulations, and safeguards is probably the biggest determinant of whether new media successfully enter the health care industry. But while we look at the industry for direction, we should not forget about individual responsibility. One example is in the already existing comprehensive guidelines for electronic communication, which get little attention among physicians. We need to stress the inevitability of the adoption of this technology. Consumers have been using new media with the banking, hospitality, airline, information technology, and news industries, and it is natural that they would expect the same from the health care industry. Issues of privacy, confidentiality, and security are pertinent to those businesses as well and have somehow been surmounted.

Communication through new media is rapidly becoming the norm rather than the exception, and physicians and the health care industry need to adapt to these changes. We say this while acknowledging that technology is not a one-size-fits-all tool (Flemming, 2008) and patients will benefit unequally. We also agree with Slack (2001) that the idea of new media is not to replace the doctor. Instead, we see new media as a tool that will help the physician communicate better with patients in an environment of increasing time demands, workloads, and numbers of patients needing long-term care.

REFERENCES

American Medical Association. (2002). *Guidelines for physicians—patient electronic communications.* Retrieved May 15, 2007, from http://www.ama-assn.org/ama/pub/category/2386.html

Anand, S. G., Feldman, M. J., Geller, D. S., Bisbee, A., & Bauchner, H. (2005). A content analysis of e-mail communication between primary care providers and parents. *Pediatrics, 115*(5), 1283–1288.

Anderson, J. G. (2007). Social, ethical and legal barriers to e-health. *International Journal of Medical Informatics, 76*(5–6), 480–483.

Boulos, M., Maramba, I., & Wheeler, S. (2006). Wikis, blogs and podcasts: A new generation of Web-based tools for virtual collaborative clinical practice and education. *BMC Medical Education, 6*(1), 41.

Brooks, R. G., & Menachemi, N. (2006). Physicians' use of email with patients: Factors influencing electronic communication and adherence to best practices. *Journal of Medical Internet Research, 8*(1), e2.

Cegala, D. J., McGee, D. S., & McNeilis, K. S. (1996). Components of patients' and doctors' perceptions of communication competence during a primary care medical interview. *Health Communication, 8*(1), 1–27.

D'Alessandro, D. M., Kreiter, C. D., Kinzer, S. L., & Peterson, M. W. (2004). A randomized controlled trial of an information prescription for pediatric patient education on the Internet. *Archives of Pediatrics & Adolescent Medicine, 158*(9), 857–862.

Duffy, F. D., Gordon, G., Whelan, G., Cole-Kelly, K., & Frankel, R. (2004). Assessing competence in communication and interpersonal skills: The Kalamazoo II report. *Academic Medicine, 79*(6), 495–507.

Flemming, D. A. (2008). Ethical implications in the use of telehealth and telemedermatology. In H. S. Pak, K. E. Edison, & J. D. Whited (Eds.), *Teledermatology: a user's guide.* Cambridge: Cambridge University Press..

Fox, S. (2006). *Online Health Search 2006.* Washington DC: Pew Internet & American Life Project. Retrieved May 10, 2007, at http://www.pewinternet.org/pdfs/PIP_Online_Health_2006.pdf

Gilchrist, V. J., Stange, K. C., Flocke, S. A., McCord, G., & Bourguet, C. (2004). A comparison of the National Ambulatory Medical Care Survey (NAMCS) measurement approach with direct observation of outpatient visits. *Medical Care, 42*(3), 276–280.

Gordon, H. S., Street, R. L. J., Sharf, B. F., & Souchek, J. (2006). Racial differences in doctors' information-giving and patients' participation. *Cancer, 107*(6), 1313–1320.

Gottschalk, A., & Flocke, S. A. (2005). Time spent in face-to-face patient care and work outside the examination room. *Annals of Family Medicine, 3*(6), 488–493.

Greenfield, S., Kaplan, S. H., Ware, J. E. Jr., Yano, E. M., & Frank, H. J. (1988). Patients' participation in medical care: Effects on blood sugar control and quality of life in diabetes. *Journal of General Internal Medicine, 3*(5), 448–457.

Gross, D. A., Zyzanski, S. J., Borawski, E. A., Cebul, R. D., & Stange, K. C. (1998). Patient satisfaction with time spent with their physician. *Journal of Family Practice, 47*(2), 133–137.

Guadagnino, C. (2006). Physician–patient communication. *Physician's News Digest.* Retrieved May 10, 2007, from http://www.physiciansnews.com/cover/706.html

Hamer, M. (2005). New media. In B. Franklin, M. Hamer, M. Hanna, M. Kinsey, & J. Richardson (Eds.), *Key concepts in journalism studies*. London: SAGE Publications.

Harris, L. (1995). Differences that make a difference. In L. Harris (Ed.), *Health and the new media: Technologies transforming personal and public health* (p. 3). Mahwah, NJ: Lawrence Erlbaum.

Harris Interactive. (2006). Few patients use or have access to online services for communicating with their doctors, but most would like to. *WSJ Online/Harris Interactive Health-Care Poll, 5*(16), 1–7.

Hart, A., Henwood, F., & Wyatt, S. (2004). The role of the Internet in patient–practitioner relationships: Findings from a qualitative research study. *Journal of Medical Internet Research, 6*(3), e36.

Hing, E., Cherry, D.K., & Woodwell, D.A. (2006). *National Ambulatory Medical Care Survey: 2004 summary. Advance data from vital and health statistics; no 374.* Hyattsville, MD: National Center for Health Statistics.

Hodge, J. G., Gostin, L. O., & Jacobson, P. D. (1999). Legal issues concerning electronic health information: Privacy, quality, and liability. *Journal of the American Medical Association, 282*(15), 1466–1471.

Houston, T. K., Sands, D. Z., Nash, B. R., & Ford, D. E. (2003). Experiences of physicians who frequently use e-mail with patients. *Health Communication, 15*(4), 515–525.

Johnson, L. (2007, April 4). *Learning on the go at the University of Michigan.* Presentation at the Reaching and Teaching the Digital Native: The Digital Campus Institute @ Missouri. Columbia, Missouri.

Kalet, A., Pugnaire, M. P., Cole-Kelly, K., Janicik, R., Ferrara, E., Schwartz, M. D., et al. (2004). Teaching communication in clinical clerkships: Models from the Macy Initiative in Health Communications. *Academic Medicine, 79*(6), 511–520.

Katz, S. J., Moyer, C. A., Cox, D. T., & Stern, D. T. (2003). Effect of a triage-based E-mail system on clinic resource use and patient and physician satisfaction in primary care: A randomized controlled trial. *Journal of General Internal Medicine, 18*(9), 736–744.

Leong, S. L., Gingrich, D., Lewis, P. R., Mauger, D. T., & George, J. H. (2005). Enhancing doctor-patient communication using email: A pilot study. *Journal of the American Board of Family Practice, 18*(3), 180–188.

Lin, C., Wittevrongel, L., Moore, L., Beaty, B. L., & Ross, S. E. (2005). An Internet-based patient-provider communication system: Randomized controlled trial. *Journal of Medical Internet Research, 7*(4), e47.

Lowrey, W., & Anderson, W. B. (2006). The impact of Internet use on the public perception of physicians: A perspective from the sociology of professions literature. *Health Communication, 19*(2), 125–131.

Madden, M. (2006). *Internet penetration and impact: Pew Internet & American Life Project.* Retrieved May 10, 2007, from http://www.pewinternet.org/pdfs/PIP_Internet_Impact.pdf

McDaniel, S. H., Beckman, H. B., Morse, D. S., Silberman, J., Seaburn, D. B., & Epstein, R. M. (2007). Physician self-disclosure in primary care visits: Enough about you, what about me? *Archives of Internal Medicine, 167*(12), 1321–1326.

Mead, N., & Bower, P. (2000). Patient-centredness: A conceptual framework and review of the empirical literature. *Social Science & Medicine, 51*(7), 1087–1110.

Mechanic, D., McAlpine, D. D., & Rosenthal, M. (2001). Are patients' office visits with physicians getting shorter? *New England Journal of Medicine, 344*(3), 198–204.

Moyer, C. A., Stern, D. T., Dobias, K. S., Cox, D. T., & Katz, S. J. (2002). Bridging the electronic divide: Patient and provider perspectives on e-mail communication in primary care. *American Journal of Managed Care, 8*(5), 427–433.

Murray, E., Lo, B., Pollack, L., Donelan, K., Catania, J., Lee, K., et al. (2003). The impact of health information on the Internet on health care and the physician-patient relationship: National U.S. survey among 1.050 U.S. physicians. *Journal of Medical Internet Research, 5*(3), e17.

Myerscough, P. R., & Ford, M. J. (1996). *Talking with patients: Keys to good communication* (3rd ed.). Oxford: Oxford University Press.

Patt, M., R., Houston, T. K., Jenckes, M. W., Sands, D. Z., & Ford, D. E. (2003). Doctors who are using e-mail with their patients: A qualitative exploration. *Journal of Medical Internet Research, 5*(2), 9.

Pavlik, J. V. (2001). *Journalism and new media.* Columbia: University Press.

Pendleton, D. (1983). Doctor–patient communication: A review In D. Pendleton & J. Hasler (Eds.), *Doctor–patient communication* (p. 9). London: Academic Press.

Potts, H. W. W., & Wyatt, J. C. (2002). Survey of doctors' experience of patients using the Internet. *Journal of Medical Internet Research, 4*(1), e5.

Rice, R. E., & Katz, J. E. (2006). Internet use in physician practice and patient interaction. In M. Murero & R. E. Rice (Eds.), *The Internet and health care: Theory, research, and practice* (p. 48). Mahwah, NJ: Lawrence Erlbaum.

Ritterband, L. M., Borowitz, S., Cox, D. J., Kovatchev, B., Walker, L. S., Lucas, V., et al. (2005). Using the Internet to provide information prescriptions. *Pediatrics, 116*(5), e643-e647.

Roter, D. (1989). Which facets of communication have strong effects on outcome—a meta-analysis. In M. Stewart & D. Roter (Eds.), *Communicating with medical patients* (pp. 191–195). Newbury Park, CA: Sage.

Salo, D., Perez, C., Lavery, R., Malankar, A., Borenstein, M., & Bernstein, S. (2004). Patient education and the Internet: Do patients want us to provide them with medical Web sites to learn more about their medical problems? *Journal of Emergency Medicine, 26*(3), 293–300.

Shaw, W. S., Zaia, A., Pransky, G., Winters, T., & Patterson, W. B. (2005). Perceptions of provider communication and patient satisfaction for treatment of acute low back pain. *Journal of Occupational and Environmental Medicine, 47,* 1036–1043.

Shuy, R. W. (1993). Three types of interference to an effective exchange of information in the medical interview. In A. D. Todd & S. Fisher (Eds.), *The social organization of doctor-patient communication* (2nd ed.). Norwood, NJ: Ablex.

Siminoff, L. A., Graham, G. C., & Gordon, N. H. (2006). Cancer communication patterns and the influence of patient characteristics: Disparities in information-giving and affective behaviors. *Patient Education and Counseling, 62*(3), 355–360.

Sitzia, J., & Wood, N. (1997). Patient satisfaction: A review of issues and concepts. *Social Science & Medicine, 45*(12), 1829–1843.

Slack, W. V. (2001). *Cybermedicine: How computing empowers doctors and patients for better care* (2nd ed.). San Francisco: Jossey-Bass.

Stewart, M. A. (1995). Effective physician-patient communication and health outcomes: A review. *Canadian Medical Association Journal, 152*(9), 1423–1433.

Stewart, M., Brown, J., Weston, W., McWhinney, I., McWilliam, C., & Freeman, T. (1995). *Patient-centred medicine: Transforming the clinical method.* London: Sage.

Stewart, M., & Roter, D. (1989). Introduction. In M. Stewart & D. Roter (Eds.), *Communicating with medical patients* (pp. 20–21). Newbury Park, CA: Sage.

Stoeckle, J. (1982). The improvement of communication between doctor and patient. In L. Pettegrew, P. Arntson, D. Bush, & K. Zoppi (Eds.), *Explorations in provider and patient interaction* (pp. 9–15). Humana.

Stone, J. H. (2007). Communication between physicians and patients in the era of e-medicine. *New England Journal of Medicine, 356*(24), 2451–2454.

Sutcliffe, K. M., Lewton, E., & Rosenthal, M. M. (2004). Communication failures: An insidious contributor to medical mishaps. *Academic Medicine, 79*(2), 186–194.

Travaline, J. M., Ruchinskas, R., & D'Alonzo, G. E. J. (2005). Patient–physician communication: Why and how. *Journal of the American Osteopathic Association, 105*(1), 13–18.

Trelease, R. B. (2006). Diffusion of innovations: Anatomical informatics and iPods. *Anatomical Record Part B: The New Anatomist, 289B*(5), 160–168.

Umefjord, G., Hamberg, K., Malker, H., & Petersson, G. (2006). The use of an Internet-based Ask the Doctor Service involving family physicians: Evaluation by a Web survey. *Family Practice, 23*(2), 159–166.

Umefjord, G., Petersson, G., & Hamberg, K. (2003). Reasons for consulting a doctor on the Internet: Web survey of users of an Ask the Doctor Service. *Journal of Medical Internet Research, 5*(4), e26.

U.S. Department of Health and Human Services. (2000). *Healthy People 2010* (2nd ed.). Washington, DC: U.S. Government Printing Office.

van den Brink-Muinen, A., van Dulmen, A.M., Jung, H. P., & Bensing, J. M. (2007). Do our talks with patients meet their expectations? *Journal of Family Practice, 56*(7), 559–568.

Virji, A., Yarnall, K., Krause, K., Pollak, K., Scannell, M., Gradison, M., et al. (2006). Use of email in a family practice setting: Opportunities and challenges in patient- and physician-initiated communication. *BMC Medicine, 4*(1), 18.

White, C. B., Moyer, C. A., Stern, D. T., & Katz, S. J. (2004). A content analysis of e-mail communication between patients and their providers: Patients get the message. *Journal of the American Medical Informatics Association, 11*(4), 260–267.

Health Literacy in the Digital World

CHRISTINA ZARCADOOLAS AND ANDREW PLEASANT

Across the long and complex history of advances in all forms of information and communication technologies, one truth has remained—literacy is key to success. The continuing importance of literacy, despite dramatic changes in technological interfaces from the pencil to the portable computer, reveals the adaptability and generative nature of the uniquely human skill of making meaning from symbols.

Literacy skills play an important role in health as well. The recognition of health literacy, and its potential to improve health and quality of life, began slowly but is rapidly growing. Over 30 years of evidence shows that a significant portion of the U.S. adult population has difficulty accessing, understanding, and using information about health (Institute of Medicine, 2003a; Nielson-Bohman, Panzer, & Kindig, 2004; Rudd, 2002; Schwartzberg et al., 2004; Zarcadoolas, Pleasant, & Greer, 2006). A disproportionate number of members of ethnic minorities and Whites of low socioeconomic status have a higher risk of poor health and poor living environments as well as risk from environmental health hazards. This reflects the often co-occurring realities of social and environmental injustice as well as low literacy and health literacy.

The National Assessment of Adult Literacy indicates that 88% of the country—nearly 9 of 10 adults—are below the "proficient" level in health literacy (Kutner, Greenberg, Jin, & Paulsen, 2006). According to the National Assessment of Adult Literacy's evaluation scheme, this means that 12% of the participants were "proficient," meaning that they could generally (but not necessarily always):

- Find the information needed to define a medical term within a complex document
- Judge information to decide which legal document applies to a specific health care situation
- Calculate an employee's share of health insurance costs for a year using a table based on income and family size

The finding that 3% of the participants in a sample of approximately 19,000 adults could not complete the assessment in English or Spanish and were excluded from the results compounds concern (Kutner et al., 2006). Further, over 300 studies have demonstrated that most health materials are beyond the comprehension skills of most Americans (Rudd, Moeykens, & Colton, 2000). Taking that evidence base into consideration, it is clear that the so-called proficient level may be only just sufficient to successfully navigate the health care system and is not a widely shared skill level in the United States.

A variety of studies and methodologies report that individuals with low health literacy often experience poor adherence to medical regimes, poor understanding of the complex nature of their own health, lack of knowledge about medical care and conditions, little understanding of medical information, low understanding and use of preventive services, poorer self-reported health, increased hospitalization, increased health care costs, and poor health status (Nielsen-Bohlman et al., 2004; Schwartzberg, VanGeest, & Wang, 2005).

In this chapter we discuss the important intersection between health literacy and the fairly recent emergence of information and communication technologies as an access point to health information, care, and services. We introduce health literacy as a critical analytical tool to explore issues of health communication in the digital world by discussing two case examples: geographic information system maps for emergency preparedness and electronic medical records, specifically those intended for patients.

DEFINING HEALTH LITERACY

Health literacy is the wide range of skills and competencies that people develop to seek out, comprehend, evaluate, and use health information and concepts to make informed choices, reduce health risks, and increase quality of life (Zarcadoolas, Pleasant, & Greer, 2003, 2005, 2006). These skills allow individuals to use information to understand and adapt to new situations as they emerge.

Health literacy is the dynamic interplay of literacies in fundamental, scientific, civic, and cultural domains and the context those skills are used within. Thus, health literacy is a critical characteristic in professionals (e.g., the ability to communicate using health literacy skills) and the public alike.

Fundamental literacy refers to the skills and strategies involved in reading, speaking, writing, and interpreting numbers. Among adults in the United States, fundamental literacy skills are generally poor (Kirsch et al., 1993; Niels-Bohman et al., 2004). Low fundamental literacy in the United States and around the globe continues to be a critical yet often ignored social determinant of health inequities. This is equally true of accessing, understanding, evaluating, and using health information and health systems.

Differences in fundamental literacy cause a frequently encountered mismatch between the way information about health is generally presented and the abilities of many Americans to find, understand, evaluate, and use that information. For instance, health information uses unnessarily complex medical terms such as "influenza" (versus "flu"), radiology (versus "where to get an x-ray"), "sodium" (versus "salt"), and "myocardial infarction" (versus "heart attack"). Despite growing awareness of this disconnect and its importance, one all too frequently encounters written and spoken information at the 12th-grade level or higher from the health and allied professions when most Americans' skill level is at the 8th-grade level or lower (Kirsch et al., 1993; Nielsen-Bohlman et al., 2004). With adequate political will, this problem is resolvable, and that resolution will have the potential to produce cost savings, efficiency gains, and better health outcomes.

Science literacy refers to levels of competence with science and technology, including some awareness of the scientific process. This specifically includes knowledge of fundamental scientific concepts, the ability to comprehend technical complexity, and an understanding of scientific uncertainty and the fact that rapid change in the accepted science is possible. For instance, on an advanced level, it takes a solid understanding of how science works to be able to accept and understand how clinical guidelines once taken as truth, for example in regard to hormone replacement therapy, can rapidly change in the light of new findings. Improving health literacy skills involves preparing communicators to better explain this process. As a result, the public can be better prepared to understand and evaluate such changes in the underlying science without a loss of trust in the health care and health research system.

Civic literacy refers to abilities that enable citizens to become aware of public issues and to be involved in the decision-making process. This includes media literacy skills, knowledge of civic and governmental processes, and an understanding that individual health decisions can affect public health. Skills in the civic domain directly relate to an individual's capacity to effectively judge sources of information and to navigate issues of power and inequity as they manifest in daily lives. This includes an understanding that one's personal actions can influence the health of others and the community at large. At its core, civic literacy skills provide the foundation for individuals' abilities to empower themselves to play a role in society (Freire, 1980).

Cultural literacy refers to the ability to recognize and use a group's collective beliefs, customs, worldviews, and social identities in order to interpret and act on health information. For example, certain cultural groups hold physicians in particularly high esteem, and a patient questioning a doctor would be seen as disrespectful. Another example would be the culture of youth, which is often characterized by high-risk behaviors and a worldview dominated by a sense of immortality. Cultural literacy includes a recognition on the communicator's part of the importance of framing health information to accommodate such powerful cultural understandings, and skill in doing so (Kreps & Kunimoto, 1994).

Unfortunately, common misperceptions limit people's ideas of culture to notions of race and ethnicity. While race and ethnicity may reveal cultural differences, culture is more accurately understood as an important element contributing to variations in communities of practice within society. Thus, an individual may be part of several cultures at once. For instance, a surgeon is part of the culture of surgery within a hospital but may also be part of a Hispanic culture and a political culture of conservatism and a member of the culture of ballroom dance—all can indicate different cultural belief systems.

While the fundamental, scientific, civic, and cultural domains all affect health literacy, we will focus specifically on the "fundamental literacy" domain of health literacy for the remainder of this chapter. Including analysis from the other domains would exceed available space limitations so we leave that analysis for future reporting.

Understanding the mechanisms of health literacy creates a powerful opportunity to focus on both advancing the public's health literacy and tailoring communication and technologies to meet the literacy and health literacy needs of the public. Both these foci will help people help themselves make better decisions, improve health and quality of life, and reduce inequities in health. This is as true in the digital world as it is in more traditional forms of mass media and communication. Improving health literacy has the potential to influence every aspect of a person's interactions with the health care system, from interpersonal and pre-dominantly verbal interactions with a physician or nursing staff to the complex tasks of negotiating the vast sea of (often incorrect or misleading) information about health found on the Internet.

In earlier research, we clearly demonstrated the many challenges that low-literate adults face when navigating the Internet (Zarcadoolas, Blanco, Boyer, & Pleasant, 2002). In addition to the challenges posed by unfamiliar technology, the way content is presented can create further barriers related to both content and navigation. For example, much of the current Web content about health requires a relatively high level of health literacy and most users can easily recount many early difficulties in learning to navigate the Web.

MAPPING OUR WAY TO THE NEXT DISASTER? GIS, EMERGENCY PREPAREDNESS, AND HEALTH LITERACY

Following several events of national and international significance, in-cluding the 9/11 attack, and recent natural disasters such as Hurricanes Rita and Katrina, there has been a growing nationwide effort to deliver emergency preparedness information and training to residents. Accord-ingly, the New York City Office of Emergency Preparedness (2007) named the New York City Coastal Storm Plan presented to the public "Ready New York: Hurricanes and New York City Aug–Sept. 2006."

The plan's central visual is a geographic information system (GIS) data map indicating what areas of the city are designated hurricane evacuation zones, the degree of hazard in various zones, and the loca-tion of evacuation centers. The map was made available to city resi-dents on a Web site and through a mass mailing. Despite the growing popularity of GIS as a tool in public health, very little research has been done on the abilities of lay publics, including low-literacy populations, to read and use GIS data as it is presently being displayed to them. In the following section we will examine the uses of GIS, their accessibil-ity to low-literate publics, and the implications for Ready New York and other projects like it.

What Is GIS?

A geographic information system is a database system with software that can analyze and display data using digitized maps and tables for planning and decision making. A GIS can assemble, store, manipulate, and display geographically referenced data, tying these data to points, lines, and areas on a map or in a table. GIS can be used to support decisions that require knowledge about the geographic distribution of people, hospitals, schools, fire stations, roads, weather events, the impact of hazards/disasters, and so forth. Any location with a known latitude and longitude, address, or other geographic grid system can be a part of a GIS (Lauden & Lauden, 2000). GIS can include multiple layers of data (e.g., geographic information, population data, health or environmental data, construction information). The maps are frequently used as a method of constructing an argument or illustrating alternatives when communities must make a decision.

Geographic information systems can create ideal platforms for the convergence of disease-specific information and their analyses in relation to population settlements, surrounding social and health services, and the natural environment. They are highly suitable for analyzing epidemiological data, as they reveal trends and interrelationships that would be more difficult to display in tabular format. GIS allows policy makers to easily visualize problems in relation to existing health and social services and the natural environment and so more effectively target resources (Centers for Disease Control and Prevention, 2006). GIS maps have become a ubiquitous means of analyzing and presenting health and emergency information at the global, federal, and state levels (Centers for Disease Control and Prevention, 2000, 2006, 2007; Federal Emergency Management Agency, 2004; National Library of Medicine, 2006; World Health Organization, 2006). Significantly, 80%–90% of all government databases, including public health, contain geo-referenced information (Cheves & Wang, 2004).

Simultaneously, GIS maps are becoming a common way of communicating information to lay publics (Federal Emergency Management Agency, 2004; FloridaDisaster.org, 2008; New York Office of Emergency Management, 2006). GIS maps are frequently used by federal and state agencies, the media, academic communities, and community agencies working on health and environmental issues (CECHI, 2005; West Harlem Environmental Action, n.d.). The Center for Disease Control's GATHER (Geographic Analysis Tool for Health & Environmental Research) is a premier example of the provision of pertinent public health GIS information to the public health community and the general public. (More about the GATHER can be learned at http://gis.cdc.gov)

These uses of GIS require audiences to understand elements such as the distribution of risk across space and the concentration of elevated risk in particular communities. For example, GIS has been used in the Gulf states as an information tool for "identifying sources and routes of contaminants, evaluating the potential for future exposures, assessing human exposures that occurred in the immediate aftermath of the hurricanes, and assessing the immediate and longer term health impacts associated with these exposures" (National Institute of Environmental Health Sciences, n.d.).

The current trend in GIS is Web-based mapping. This capability can allow users to view an already created map, or create maps based on their own specifications, on their personal computers. "Web-based mapping is expected to widely expand the use of GIS in the workplace, in schools, and in homes" (Federal Emergency Management Agency, 2004). An example of the growing adoption of GIS technology as a teaching and community advocacy tool can be seen with West Harlem Environmental Action. This leading environmental justice organization began creating and posting GIS maps on its Web site in 1999 in order to allow residents to work with the health and pollution data that provided them with an understanding of the relationship between the two and their advocacy and policy implications (West Harlem Environmental Action, n.d.).

GIS and Ready New York

As stated earlier, New York's Office of Emergency Management developed and circulated an 8.5×11-inch printable PDF map in July of 2006 to be used by the public in the case of a hurricane-related evacuation. The plan attempts to tell New Yorkers about the level of hurricane hazard in their neighborhood and where to go if they need to evacuate. The brochure version of the plan was mailed to all residents living in designated hurricane evacuation zones in New York City. The plan includes a large fold-out map indicating what areas of the city are designated hurricane evacuation zones, degree of hazard, and where evacuation centers are located in these areas (see Figure 11.1).

The readability of this map was tested in a study conducted in East Harlem by the Mount Sinai School of Medicine (Zarcadoolas, Boyer, Krishnaswami, & Rothenberg, 2007). According to the 2000 U.S. census, close to 260,000 people with an average household income of approximately $20,000 a year reside in East and Central Harlem ($18,564 for

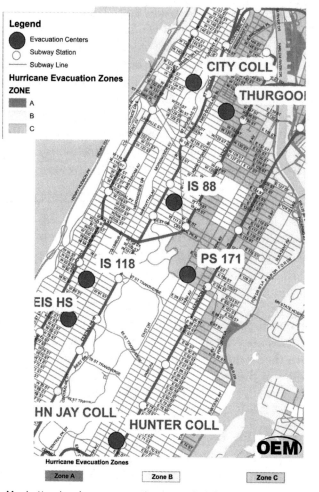

Figure 11.1 Manhattan hurricane evacuation zones (original map in color).

East Harlem and $21,508 for Central Harlem) (New York City Department of City Planning, 2001). More than a third of the residents are living in poverty.

Almost a third of residents in East Harlem (31%) and Central Harlem (22%) report being in fair or poor (versus very good or good) health (Olson, 2006). In 1996, Central Harlem had the highest crude death rate of any health district in New York City, at 14.1 per 1,000 people compared to a citywide rate of 9.1 per 1,000 (New York City Department of Health and Mental Hygiene. 2006). In 1996, there were 423.4 coronary heart disease deaths per 100,000 people, in contrast to the Healthy People 2000 goal of 115 for Blacks. There are higher rates of sexually transmitted infections, adolescent pregnancies, depressive disorders, childhood asthma, and homicides as well.

Harlem is a very diverse community with a wide range of ethnic backgrounds and languages spoken. Eighteen percent of East and Central Harlem residents are not proficient in English (New York City Department of City Planning, 2001). Of those who do not speak English, 82% speak Spanish (Healthy Harlem, 2006). Because of the high density of Hispanics, the southern portion of East Harlem is referred to as Spanish Harlem or El Barrio. Harlem also has very low literacy levels. Forty-six percent of East Harlem residents and 33.5% of Central Harlem residents have not graduated from high school (New York Department of Health and Mental Hygiene, 2006). Community residents of Harlem have a rich history of organizing to promote health and challenge environmental exposures that pose health hazards in the community but have often lacked access to the technical and informational resources to help them in their efforts to understand and prioritize health risks.

Methods

The study design was a cross-sectional survey consisting of face-to-face intercept interviews throughout the community. To be eligible, participants had to be 18 years or older. There were 178 residents in a convenience sample (134 English speaking, 44 Spanish speaking), interviewed in various locations throughout East and Central Harlem. Spanish-language interviewers were staff of the health education department, bilingual native speakers of Spanish with extensive experience in community relations. English-language interviewers were trained ethnographers supervised by a sociolinguist specializing in health literacy.

Survey questions required the respondents to refer to an enlarged version of the CSP Hurricane Evacuation Zone map. Other survey questions sought demographic information on the respondents' age, sex, educational attainment, language, and length of time living in New York City, and information on respondents' current knowledge of, attitudes toward, and preparedness for emergency situations. Surveys were administered during August and September of 2006. Of the respondents, 40% ($n = 72$) had not graduated from high school, a number very representative of the U.S. census statistics, which suggest that 39% of

East and Central Harlem adults have not graduated from high school (New York City Department of City Planning, 2006).

Findings

Findings reveal that the current map used to communicate vital information about hurricane emergencies to the public is not readable and usable by a significant portion of the Harlem community. The vast majority (73.9%) of surveyed residents who had not completed high school could not correctly determine if they lived in a hurricane evacuation zone, which zone they lived in, or the correct location of the nearest hurricane evacuation center. Furthermore, 40% of those who had not graduated from high school could not use the map to locate where they lived (see Table 11.1). After education was adjusted for, the other demographic variables (age, sex, language, and length of time living in New York City) were not significant.

Those who had completed high school were over nine times more likely than those who had not graduated from high school to correctly identify which evacuation zone they lived in. Yet even nearly half of those who had higher education (high school or some college) said they did not know how to get to the closest evacuation center.

When it comes to residents' trust in emergency preparedness officials, there is also reason for concern. Even before residents determined that the map was not clear and decipherable, 40% said that they do not ("somewhat," "a little," "not at all") trust emergency directions from city officials.

Launched in July 2003, the Office of Emergency Management's Ready New York is a preparedness campaign aimed at helping New Yorkers prepare for all types of emergencies. The ongoing campaign includes hazard specific brochures, public service announcements for radio and television, a speaker's bureau, print and outdoor advertising, and community emergency response teams. As part of Ready New York, New Yorkers have been urged to have a "Go Bag" ready. This is a collection of items residents should have packed and ready in the event of an evacuation.

In terms of overall preparedness, only 16% of all those surveyed said they have a Go Bag ready in their home. Also, many of these individuals were able to list very few items that are recommended to be included in the bag. While 69% said they would include water in a Go Bag, 64% included non-perishable food, and 44% a flashlight, only about a third said they would include medicine, and about 24% thought they were supposed to include important documents.

Table 11.1

ABILITY TO ANSWER QUESTIONS CORRECTLY WHILE LOOKING AT MAP (BASED ON EDUCATION LEVEL)

	EDUCATION STATUS	INCORRECT *n* (%)	CORRECT *n* (%)	ODDS RATIO (CONFIDENCE INTERVAL)*
Can you point to where you live?	Low education	29 (40.3)	43 (59.7)	5.65 (2.58, 12.35)
	High education	11 (10.7)	92 (89.3)	1.0
Judging from these maps, do you live in hurricane evacuation zone?	Low education	51 (73.9)	18 (26.1)	6.58 (3.32, 12.99)
	High education	31 (30.1)	72 (69.9)	1.0
What zone do you live in?	Low education	57 (82.6)	12 (17.4)	9.35 (4.44, 19.61)
	High education	34 (33.7)	67 (66.3)	1.0
Which hurricane evacuation center is closest to your home?	Low Education	46 (65.7)	24 (34.3)	5.32 (2.75, 10.31)
	High education	27 (26.5)	75 (73.5)	1.0
Do you know how to get there?	Low education	57 (82.6)	12 (17.4)	5.15 (2.46, 10.75)
	High education	47 (48.0)	51 (52.0)	1.0

Low Education = Less than High School; High Education = At least High School graduate / GED
*95% confidence interval

CASE STUDY: ELECTRONIC MEDICAL RECORDS

There is growing concern that patients need to be more involved in decisions about their own health care. This concern is only compounded in an era in which patient information is often fragmented across providers, medical institutions, and laboratories. As a result, there is a growing movement to create tools to help patients take a more proactive role in their care. Electronic medical records (EMRs) in a wide variety of forms have been adopted by provider practices, hospitals, insurers, and other health facilities in great numbers over the last few years. These records are used to track and manage patient care, improve health outcomes and decrease health care costs, especially for the management of chronic disease (Bodenheimer & Grumbach, 2003; Weingerten, Henning, Badamgarav, et al., 2002).

The Institute of Medicine has called for all physicians to use electronic prescribing tools by the year 2010, and federal authorities have stated a goal of 100% EMR use by the year 2014 (Bush, 2003; Institute of Medicine, 2003b). In 2007 the National Governors Association partnered with Health Management Associates to survey states regarding electronic health information undertakings and needs. All 42 states surveyed indicated that e-health activities were significant in their states, and almost 70% of states described e-health activities as very significant (Smith et al., 2008).

An essential companion to the physician electronic record is the patient health record (PHR/EHR). We will use the term EMR to refer to all forms of patient-accessible electronic forms of medical records. Various forms of patient health records now exist in great numbers. Smart cards, electronic patient portals, and Web-based personal health records are proliferating and attempt to bring together fragmented information from multiple sources. The number of patient-oriented EMRs that offer tailored educational materials or personal medical information is growing, and the choices offer a wide spectrum of functions for patients. These functions include accessing personal health records, sharing health records (e.g., with designated family members or caregivers), entering data into a health record, checking/filling prescriptions, checking and making appointments, checking/paying copayments, participating in support groups, accessing educational materials for health-decision support and health self-assessment tools, messaging with health providers, using diagnostic/therapeutic tools, and signing up for reminders to support self-management of care.

For example, the New York City Department of Health and Mental Hygiene, as part of a mayoral initiative to improve the quality and efficiency of health care in New York City, is supporting the adoption and use of an EMR primarily among providers who care for patients who live in the areas of New York City that have the greatest health disparities. The Department of Health and Mental Hygiene has established a primary care information project to support the adoption and use of state-of-the-art EHRs, especially among providers who care for the city's underserved and vulnerable populations (New York City, 2007).

Consumer self-management support is being designed through the insertion of tools in the eClinicalWorks EMR. Providers may be supported in implementing and documenting shared decision making, goal setting, and progress related to chronic disease and preventive self-care. An electronic or printed summary of each encounter and plan may be given immediately to the consumer. Self-management e-tools are based on paper tools developed by the Department of Health and Mental Hygiene's Clinical Systems Improvement Team in collaboration with New York City primary care providers. Consumers will be linked to the EMR through a Web portal that can be opened with a secure password; they may fill in structured information on demographics, health history, and health goals that can be accepted into a progress note. Also, current medications may be verified, and lab, radiology, and billing reports may be viewed. Consumers may be alerted to care that is due and may send and receive messages to request follow-up services or information. Health education and community resource information will be accessible via uploaded practice-specific documents or Web links.

The EMR and patient portal enhancements will build on the Department of Health and Mental Hygiene's Take Care New York initiative, which has already distributed 2 million paper patient health records ("passports") to engage patients in becoming more involved in managing their own health (New York City Department of Health and Mental Hygiene, n.d.). The initiative urges New Yorkers to get their colon, breast, and cervical cancer screenings as needed and informs them about 10 core health issues, including smoking cessation.

However, both in New York City and nationally, there is very little research on the actual usability or effectiveness of these new tools for patient self-management, especially among at-risk populations that already experience increased health disparities and, often, low health literacy. Although not explicitly from a health literacy perspective, Winkelman, Leonard, and Rossos (2005) reviewed constraints embedded in EMRs that limit their use by patients in self-directed disease management. Issues hindering access and usability of the information that they identified include the lack of prioritization or use of patient vocabularies in their structures, reflecting the fact that traditional medical records as well as EMRs have been mainly designed for physicians, not patients.

Ross and Lin (2003) reviewed studies in which patients were given access to their medical records, both paper based and electronic, and they created a framework for evaluating the resulting positive and negative outcomes for both patients and providers. In addition to problems that surfaced in many studies, they reported problems with vocabulary and meaning. However, none of the studies looked specifically at the health literacy load of the records.

HEALTH LITERACY LOAD ANALYSIS

A health literacy load analysis entails a structural and functional analysis of a text for the purpose of clarifying the likely demands of the material on health consumer/patient comprehension and use. Conducting a health literacy load analysis entails coding, categorizing, and analyzing a text in terms of health literacy assumptions and demands. The product of the load analysis is a list of elements that can be tested for usability. While the list of potential text elements is theoretically infinite, it is constrained by the function of the text, the context of use, and the intended target user of the text.

The health literacy load analysis plays an important role because it "unpacks" the text and requires the researcher to identify what linguistic, reading, and interpretation skills are likely assumed and required of the reader. Health literacy load analysis is adapted from text analysis methods designed by Zarcadoolas, Pleasant, and Greer (2004, 2006) and based on an elaborated model of health literacy.

The two examples of EMRs in Figures 11.2 and 11.3 present the reader with a range of complex comprehension and use tasks. In each, the fundamental literacy load of this information is high. The text alternately refers to science, civic, and culturally framed knowledge. Examples of health literacy skills and concepts assumed and therefore required of users are:

- Functions of a written record (fundamental literacy domain)
- Function of a laboratory test as a health indicator (science literacy domain)
- Reliability of scientific tests (science literacy domain)
- Acceptance and relevance of statistically defined notions of "normal" (cultural literacy domain)
- Knowledge and skills of how to act on the information provided (civic literacy domain)

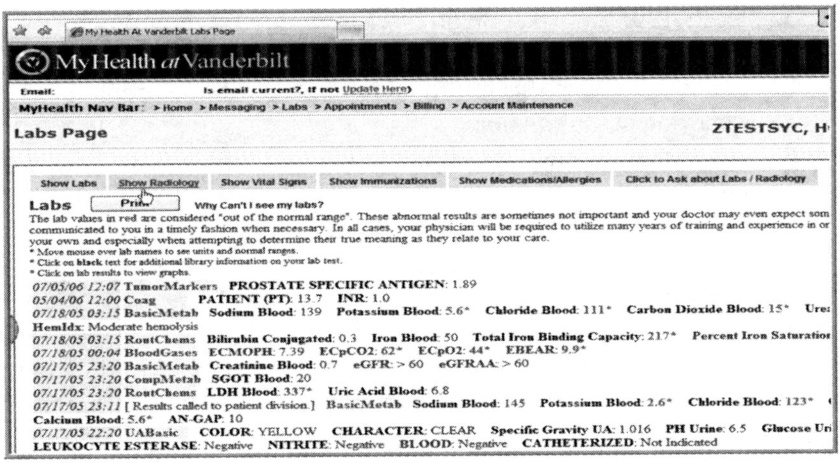

Figure 11.2 Screen shot of My Health at Vanderbilt.

LOSS OF WEIGHT[783.21]   9/6/2005
  Comment: 4/07 Patient had a significant drop in weight but then restabilized at about 105 pounds which is where he stays now excpet when his weight went up from his episode of congestive heart failure
ABNORMALITY OF GAIT[781.2]   11/29/2005
  Comment: 11/05 Patient has been having difficulty with falling and tripping. He was sent to Neurologist who thought that the most probable working Dx was foot drop and ordered EMGs and NCTs to be done mid Dec. If these confirm this suspicion then an orthotic would be in order. He suggested that MRA be done with gradient echo sequences of head and neck.
REFUSAL OF IMMUNIZATION[Z99.9]   5/30/2006
  Comment: Pneumovax, influenza
ATRIAL FIBRILLATION[427.31]   4/5/2007
  Comment: 4/07: New onset - rapid ventricular response. Sent to BIMC ER.
CONGESTIVE HEART FAILURE NOS[428.0]   4/25/2007
  Comment: 4/07 Hospitalized at BI on family practice service for congestive heart failure and fluid overload due to atrial fibrillation with rapid heart rate.

Figure 11.3 Excerpt from provider EMR after visit summary (Institute for Urban Family Health, 2007).

One of the claims that has been made for EMRs is that these records can be an aid to disease management and shared decision making between provider and patients. For instance, in the record in Figure 11.2, the provider may set a goal for lowering LDL level over a 6-month period. From a health literacy perspective, accomplishing that task would require that the patient:

1. understand the concept of LDL,
2. understand existing guidelines for "healthy" LDL both in an epidemiological sense *and* in regard to his or her personal context,

3. locate LDL information on the EMR,
4. understand how to interpret trend information,
5. understand what this information implies with respect to health behavior, and ultimately
6. put that knowledge to action to help motivate positive behavior change.

Similarly, a health literacy load analysis of the example in Figure 11.3 would predict that the average patient would have real difficulty locating, understanding, evaluating, and using the highly condensed medical language and health concept presented. Complexities include vocabulary—"atrial fibrillation," "congestive heart," "rapid ventricular response," "EMT," "NCT"—and scientific/medical concepts and information—What might the foot drop be an indicator of? What would the MRA be trying to diagnose?

The linguistic structure, informational content, and physical layout of EMRs in their present iteration do not take account the well-documented low fundamental literacy and low health literacy of the adult U.S. population.

CONCLUSION

There is growing recognition that understanding the mechanisms of health literacy in the realm of public health contexts is necessary to create a safer, healthier public (Nielsen-Bohlman et al., 2004; Pleasant & Kuruvilla, 2008; Zarcadoolas et al., 2005, 2006). Digital technologies are universally assumed to offer the latest and greatest technological fix to improve health communication, but many efforts are hampered by failures to address the core issues of health literacy. This is unfortunately not a new phenomenon, but health literacy is continuing to take its place as the primary concerns in health communication of all types.

There has been national attention given to ensuring the public has clear and understandable emergency preparedness information, but our analysis of the usability of GIS map information in the New York City coastal storm plan raises serious doubts that information in this format is effectively informing the public. As a result, it is likely that an estimated 160,000 residents of Central and East Harlem would not be able to find the evacuation center closest to their home by using these specific hurricane evacuation maps.

Improved maps can play an important role in presenting and advancing the public's understanding of and engagement in a wide range of health and safety information, from emergency preparedness information to other epidemiologic information, such as asthma rates, diabetes prevalence, and exposure to toxicants. Future research should focus on analyzing the specific text and graphic complexity of GIS maps in order to create more accessible, easy-to-read, and easy-to-use geographic information system maps. These revised tools can then be added to a suite of public health communications that may enable community members to participate in more meaningful dialogue and informed decision-making processes about public health and safety issues.

Ideally, an analysis of the health literacy load compares the health literacy burden of an informational resource to user characteristics. As demonstrated in relation to electronic medical records, even a quick analysis focusing on the fundamental domain of health literacy provides important insights into potential problems users may encounter. Our analysis is supported by others who have found that even health professionals encounter similar problems with EMRs (Crosson, Stroebel, Scott, Stella, & Crabtree, 2005). This is a process performed far too seldom, in part, we suggest, because health organizations have not sufficiently invested in the capacity to perform such analyses.

Health care communication in a digital world cannot sidestep the demands of health literacy. Rather it increases the health literacy demands placed on users. As the world moves toward personalized electronic medical records, a host of issues emerge, but the question of how understandable and accessible the digital information will be underlies each and every issue. Every effort to use emerging information and communication technologies to help people help themselves to better their health has to pass through health literacy first. Therefore, we conclude this chapter by arguing that continuing development of EMRs and patient health records as well as the entire scope of digital access to health information—without prioritizing a serious consideration of the health literacy demands—can only sadly perpetuate the already too-long history of top-down information provision that fails to meet the desired communication outcomes and increases inequities in health.

The same core issue remains, whether health information is presented via a digital or more traditional manner: do the materials as presented match the user's skills, abilities, and level of knowledge so that users can find, understand, analyze, and use that information to make better decisions about health? If developers of the digital world of health and medical information are unable to directly and completely answer that question, then the development needs to be reconsidered before these implementations are launched.

REFERENCES

Bodenheimer, T., & Grumbach, K. (2003). Electronic technology: A spark to revitalize primary care? *Journal of the American Medical Association, 290,* 259–264.

Bush, G. W. (2004, April 26). *Remarks.* American Association of Community Colleges Annual Convention. Minneapolis, MN.

CEHI, Children's Environmental Health Initiative. (2005). *Spatial Analysis and Geographic Information Systems.* Nicholas School of Environment and Earth Sciences, Duke University. Retrieved July 18, 2008, from http://www.nicholas.duke.edu/cehi/spatial.htm

Centers for Disease Control and Prevention. (2000, May 11). *Using mapping and spatial analysis technologies for health protection: A public health training network satellite broadcast.* Retrieved January 10, 2008, from http://www2.gov/phtn/gis/relatedlinks.asp

Centers for Disease Control and Prevention. (2006). *Gather: Geographic analysis tool for health & environmental research.* Retrieved February 20, 2008, from http://gis.cdc.gov

Centers for Disease Control and Prevention. (2007). *GIS and public health.* Retrieved January 10, 2008, from http://www.cdc.gov/nchs/gis.htm

Cheves, G. I., & Wang, J. T. L. (2004). *Database-driven Web-enabled Public Health GIS Using XHTML, SVG, ECMAScript, DOM and a Three-tier Architecture.* Abstract 2004, SVG Open Conference. Retrieved October 12, 2007, from http://www.svgopen.org/2004/paperAbstracts/WebEnabledPublicHealthGIS.html

Crosson, J. C., Stroebel, C., Scott, J. G., Stella, B., & Crabtree, B. F. (2005). Implementing an electronic medical record in a family medicine practice: Communication, decision making, and conflict. *Annals of Family Medicine, 3,* 307–11.

Federal Emergency Management Agency. (2004). *How FEMA uses GIS in disaster management response.* Retrieved February 8, 2008, from http://www.gismaps.fema.gov/gis04.shtm

Florida Division of Emergency Management. (2008). *Disaster preparedness maps.* Retrieved February 18, 2008, from http://floridadisaster.org/PublicMapping/index.htm

Freire, P. (1980). *Education for critical consciousness.* New York: Continuum.

Healthy Harlem. (2005). *Harlem health statistics.* Retrieved February 15, 2007, http://www.healthyharlem.org/pdfs/statistics/Demographics.pdf

Institute of Medicine. (2003a). *The future of the public's health in the 21st century.* Washington, DC: National Academic Press.

Institute of Medicine. (2003b). *Priority areas for national action: Transforming health care quality.* Washington DC: National Academy Press.

Kirsch, J. S., Junegeblut, A., Jenkins, L., & Kolstad, L. A. (1993). *Adult literacy in America: A first look at the results of the National Adult Literacy Survey (NALS).* Washington, DC: Department of Education.

Kreps, G. L., & Kunimoto, E. N. (1994). *Effective communication in multicultural health settings.* Thousand Oaks, CA: Sage.

Kutner, M., Greenberg, M., Jin, Y., & Paulsen, C. (2006). *The health literacy of America's adults: Results from the 2003 National Assessment of Adult Literacy.* Washington, DC: National Center for Education Statistics. Retrieved February 12, 2008, from http://nces.ed.gov/pubsearch/pubsinfo.asp?pubid = 2006483.

National Academy of Sciences Institute of Medicine. (2000). *Clearing the air: Asthma and indoor air exposures.* Washington, DC: National Academy Press.

National Center for Education Statistics. (2006). *National assessment of adult literacy.* Retrieved April 20, 2007, from http://nces.ed.gov/NAAL/index.asp?file = KeyFindings/Demographics/Overall.asp&PageId = 16)

National Institute of Environmental Health Sciences. (n.d.). *Hurricanes Katrina and Rita.* Retrieved July 18, 2008, from http://balata.ucsd.edu:8080/gridsphere/gridsphere

National Library of Medicine. (2007). *ToxMap.* Retrieved February 10, 2007, from http://toxmap.nlm.nih.gov/toxmap/combo/select.do;jsessionid = 3DD11C64F27D38FB97011B219AC2DDF3

New York City. (2007). *Electronic health records for the primary care provider.* Retrieved from http://www.nyc.gov/html/doh/downloads/pdf/chi/chi26–1.pdf

New York City Department of City Planning. (2001). *2000 US Census.* Retrieved January 10, 2007, from http://home2.nyc.gov/html/dcp/html/census/demo_profile.shtml

New York City Department of City Planning. (2007). *Epidemiology services: Sortable statistics.* Retrieved February 15, 2007, from http://www.nyc.gov/html/dcp/html/pub/demograp.shtml

New York City Department of Health and Mental Hygiene. (n,d.). *Take care New York.* Retrieved July 18, 2008, from http://nyc.gov/html/doh/html/tcny/index.shtml

New York City Department of Health and Mental Hygiene. (2006). *The 2006 New York City community health profiles.* Retrieved February 15, 2007, from http://www.nyc.gov/html/doh/html/stats/stats-demo.shtml.

New York City Office of Emergency Management. (2006). *New York City hazards: Hurricane evacuation zones.* Retrieved February 18, 2008, from http://home2.nyc.gov/html/oem/html/hazards/storms_evaczones.shtml

New York City Office of Emergency Preparedness. (2007). *Ready New York: Hurricanes and New York City Aug–Sept. 2006.* Retrieved June 27, 2008, from http://www.nyc.gov/html/oem/downloads/pdf/hurricane_brochure_english_06.pdf

Nielsen-Bohlman, L., Panzer, A. M., & Kindig, D. A. (Eds.). (2004). *Health literacy: A prescription to end confusion.* Washington, DC: Institute of Medicine of the National Academies. Retrieved February 20, 2008, from http://www.iom.edu/report.asp?id = 19723

Olson, E. C., Van Wye, G., Kerker, B., Thorpe, L., & Frieden, T. R. (2006). *Take care Central Harlem. NYC Community Health Profiles* (2nd ed.). New York: New York City Department of Health and Mental Hygiene.

Pastore, M. (2001). *Interest high, but Internet too costly for inner city.* Retrieved February 8, 2008, from http://www.clickz.com/showPage.html?page = 561201

Pleasant, A., & Kuruvilla, S. (2008). A tale of two health literacies? Public health and clinical approaches to health literacy. *Health Promotion International.* Retrieved February 28, 2008, from http://heapro.oxfordjournals.org/cgi/content/abstract/dan001v1.

Ross, S. E., & Lin, C.-T. (2003). The effects of promoting patient access to medical records: A review. *Journal of the American Medical Informatics Association, 10*(2), 129–138.

Rudd, R., Moeykens, B., & Colton, T. (1999). Health and literacy: A review of medical and public health literature. In J. Comings, B. Garners, & C. Smith (Eds.), *The annual review of adult learning and literacy* (pp. 158–199). San Francisco: Jossey-Bass.

Schwartzberg, J., VanGeest, J., & Wang, C. (Eds.). (2005). *Understanding health literacy: Implications for medicine and public health.* Chicago: AMA Press.

Smith, V. K., Gifford, K., S. Kramer, S., Dalton, J., MacTaggart, P., & Warner, M. L. (2008, February). State e-health activities in 2007: Findings from a state survey. *Commonwealth Fund, 86.*

Urban and Regional Information Systems Association. (2007). *GIS in public health conference.* Retrieved February 10, 2007, from http://www.urisa.org/health/workshops

U.S. Department of Health and Human Services. (2000). *Healthy people 2010 understanding and improving health.* Retrieved February 15, 2007, from http://www.healthypeople.gov/

West Harlem Environmental Action, Inc. (n.d.). *GIS maps.* Retrieved July 18, 2008, from http://old.weact.org/gis/samplemaps.html

Weingarten, S. R., Henning, J. M., Badamgarav, E., Knight, K., Hasselblad, V., Gano, A. Jr., & Ofman, J. J. (2002). Interventions used in disease management programmes for patients with chronic illness—Which ones work? *British Medical Journal, 325*(7370), 925–932.

Winkelman, W. J., Leonard, K. J., & Rossos, P. G. (2005). Patient-perceived usefulness of online electronic medical records: Employing grounded theory in the development of information and communication technologies for use by patients living with chronic illness. *Journal of the American Medical Informatics Association, 12,* 306–314.

World Health Organization. (2006a). *GIS and public health mapping.* Retrieved February 16, 2007, from http://www.who.int/health_mapping/gisandphm/en/index.html

World Health Organization. (2006b). *WHO's public health mapping program.* Retrieved July 18, 2008, from http://www.who.int/health_mapping/en/

Zarcadoolas, C. (2006, September 7). *Advancing health literacy through an expanded model.* Paper presented at Surgeon General's Workshop on Improving Health Literacy. Bethesda, MD.

Zarcadoolas, C., Blanco, M., Boyer, J., & Pleasant, A. (2002). Unweaving the Web: An exploratory study of low-literate adults' navigation skills on the World Wide Web. *Journal of Health Communication, 7,* 309–324.

Zarcadoolas, C., Pleasant, A., & Greer, D. (2003). Elaborating a definition of health literacy: A commentary. *Journal of Health Communication, 8,* 119–120.

Zarcadoolas, C., Pleasant, A., & Greer, D. (2005). Understanding health literacy: An expanded model. *Health Promotion International, 20,* 195–203.

Zarcadoolas, C., Pleasant, A., & Greer, D. (2006). *Advancing health literacy: A framework for understanding and action.* San Francisco: Jossey-Bass.

Zarcadoolas, C., Boyer, J., Krishnaswami, A., & Rothenberg, A. (2007). How usable are current GIS maps: Communicating emergency preparedness to vulnerable populations? *Journal of Homeland Security and Emergency Management, 4*(3). Retrieved July 18, 2008, from http://www.bepress.com/jhsem/vol4/iss3/16/

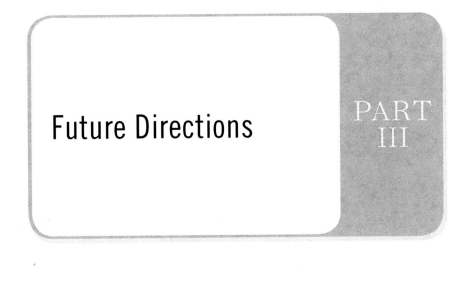

Future Directions

PART
III

12

Making the Grade: Identification of Evidence-Based Communication Messages

E. SALLY ROGERS AND MARIANNE FARKAS

We live in an information age amid growing demands for instantly accessible information that is tailored to users' needs and preferences and accessible through countless forms of media. The demand for information has burgeoned in the past few years; information about current events and consumer products, scholarly materials, and health information, to name only a few, can be accessed in the blink of an eye. Availability of health-related information in particular has grown exponentially through media outlets such as newspaper columns, magazines with health-specific cover stories, and the emergence of Web sites such as emedicine.com and healthcentral.com. Prior to the explosion of information sources, people relied primarily on physicians to address their questions and generally did not possess detailed knowledge about various health conditions. Today there is a virtual glut of health information and communication. This growth is partially demand driven, but advances in technology also expand and alter the ways in which we obtain information. These forces have combined to dramatically alter the media landscape with respect to health communication.

Preparation of this chapter was partially supported by the National Institute on Disability and Rehabilitation Research, Knowledge Dissemination and Utilization grant (Grant #H133A050006). The views expressed in this chapter do not necessarily represent the views of NIDRR and are the sole responsibility of the authors.

325

Fueling this trend is the fact that individuals increasingly rely on the Internet as a primary resource to address questions about health conditions. In fact, the Pew Internet & American Life Project (2007) reports that 86% of Internet users with a disability or chronic health condition have looked online for health information and that those individuals are "more likely than other e-patients to report that their online searches affected treatment decisions, their interactions with their doctors, and their ability to cope with their condition."

Our focus in this chapter is on communication about mental health and the use of that information by consumers, mental health organizations, practitioners, and practitioner organizations (like the United States Psychosocial Rehabilitation Services Association). We explore two fundamental problems arising from the changing landscape of health communication. The first is the question of how today's lay users evaluate the quality of health and mental health information at their disposal. Consumer availability of voluminous information that is often technical and complex means that users are primarily on their own to decipher and make use of the information they locate. Complicating this concern is the finding from the Pew Internet & American Life Project (2007) that only 14% of "e-patients" (individuals living with a disability or chronic disease who go online) report that they "always" check the source and date of health information they find on the Internet. This is a potentially worrisome finding, especially for individuals who may be in medical crisis, or who have heightened concerns and needs relative to their health and mental health.

It is important that users make meaningful discriminations about the credibility and value of health information, and to do so, they need tools. There is also concern that much of the new knowledge in mental health is not being utilized and has not filtered down to affect the lives of individuals with mental health disabilities in meaningful ways. We explore this "knowledge gap" and the growing need to examine health information for quality and for relevance to users. Finally, we describe our attempts to address these problems and the knowledge gap through an innovative federally funded project.

THE KNOWLEDGE GAP

Research funds expended over the past few decades in health and mental health have been primarily aimed at the creation of new knowledge through basic and applied research, with little attention paid to the ultimate use of that knowledge. However, as we gain a better understanding of the barriers to the use of new information, we begin to understand the need for proactive strategies to overcome them. Attempts to translate research findings into health and mental health practice have suggested that new knowledge often does not get utilized once research information is available. Some have described this failure as the "know-do" gap (World Health Organization, 2005) and the "Science-to-Service Divide" (National Institute of Mental Health, 1999). Passive approaches to addressing this gap are ineffective—resources and active planning to promote adoption of information must be developed and undertaken in order for that knowledge to be used in the real world (Grimshaw, et al., 2001; Sudsawad, 2007). The National Institutes of Health, recognizing this problem, have begun funding "translational research" as a way of bringing basic research findings to applied settings—that is, "practice informed by science" (Vernig, 2007).

One of the common reasons for knowledge gaps is the difference in perspectives that exists between individuals who generate new knowledge (such as academics and researchers) and those who use new knowledge (such as providers of services, advocates, and individuals with disabilities and their family members). Participatory action research methods and the emerging field of "knowledge translation" examine this gap, address difficulties of facilitating change through new knowledge, translate new knowledge into innovative services and practices, and promote the adoption of health and mental health practices that result from promising research (Selener, 1997; Sudsawad, 2007).

KNOWLEDGE TRANSLATION

Until recently, purveyors of knowledge and those conducting research studies were expected only to engage in "knowledge transfer," a simple linear process by which research studies were conceived, planned, executed, and then made available to users to promote change (Landry, Lamari, & Amara, 2001). In contrast, the emerging discipline of knowledge translation argues that in order to ensure the use and adoption of new information and research results, the creation of new knowledge must involve early and frequent interactions between researchers and potential users. Central to the distinction between knowledge transfer and knowledge translation is the understanding that knowledge translation is not unidirectional, simple, or linear.

The Canadian Institute of Health Research (2005) has defined knowledge translation as "the exchange, synthesis and ethically-sound application of research findings within a complex set of interactions among researchers and knowledge users. In other words, knowledge translation can be seen as an acceleration of the knowledge cycle; an acceleration of the natural transformation of knowledge into use." Within the context of health research, knowledge translation aims to "to accelerate the capture of the benefits of research . . . through improved health, more effective services and products, and a strengthened health care system" (Canadian Institute of Health Research, 2005). The World Health Organization (2005) has largely adopted this definition.

Professional journals and organizations provide traditional dissemination venues for new research knowledge. Occasionally, media outlets publicize stories of particular interest to the lay public, but researchers are expected to focus their dissemination efforts on other professionals and are rewarded for doing so. This model of dissemination is limited because it does not consider the potential needs of users, nor does it consider how the changing media landscape is providing users with direct access to information. Principles of knowledge translation suggest that individuals are more likely to make use of or adopt new information when it is presented in forms that are compatible with their needs and when the information is available when they want and need it (Sudsawad, 2007). Obstacles to the use of new information include the fact that users generally do not have the knowledge or skills to understand complicated and often contradictory scientific information and may be confused about the implications of research findings for their own health or mental health problems.

Two examples stand out as illustrations of confusing and contradictory health communications: the first was generated by the Woman's Health Initiative study, the largest trial of hormone replacement therapy conducted to date. Prior to the study, physicians frequently recommended hormone replacement therapy based on results of earlier observational studies. But the initial and highly publicized negative results of the study caused many women to abruptly terminate hormone replacement therapy. Since then, more nuanced analyses of the Woman's Health Initiative results have caused great confusion and have also forced physicians and women to reconsider the value of hormone replacement therapy (Mendelson & Karas, 2007).

Similarly confusing have been reports about exposure to sunlight and ultraviolet rays. For decades, physicians strongly urged patients to protect themselves at all costs from sunlight, but newer research studies are describing the potential benefits of exposure to sunlight to generate Vitamin D (Holick, 2007). These studies, often highly publicized in the mainstream media, leave consumers confused and skeptical about health communications.

NEED FOR KNOWLEDGE TRANSLATION AND EVIDENCE-BASED PRACTICES

The large volumes of information available, the complex and seemingly contradictory health messages, and the fact that much of our research knowledge has not filtered down to users or translated into changes in day-to-day health practices have led the National Institute on Disability and Rehabilitation Research (2005) to invest heavily in programs of knowledge translation after decades of funding disability-related research. The Center for Psychiatric Rehabilitation has been funded to examine disability research for quality and relevance to users and then to convert that research information into usable, accessible information for individuals with disabilities, their advocates, service providers, and family members.

Coupled with this recent focus on knowledge translation is the growing emphasis on evidence-based practices. This parallel trend calls for medical practices to be derived from an evidence base or a body of research that informs health and mental health practices (Sackett et al., 1996; Stout & Hayes, 2005). Entire health and mental health systems are being refocused to deliver services that have an evidence base. The underlying premise of evidence-based practice is that there is valuable research information and expert opinion that can be brought to bear in a systematic way to provide better services and treatment, and that health systems should only invest their resources in treatments that can be demonstrated to work based on research studies. It is clear, however, that we need methods with which to systematically examine the quality of the health information that emanates from research studies. Both the push toward evidence-based practices and the emerging principles of knowledge translation have implications for the communication of health and mental health information.

RATING THE QUALITY OF RESEARCH

Standards for determining the quality of research in health care began taking hold about 2 to 3 decades ago. Driven by the need for protocols to guide medical care, health care providers often did not have a systematic set of decision rules to guide their treatment. Without best practice or treatment protocols grounded in current research, individuals presenting for health care with similar disorders can receive vastly different treatments, some of which may be inferior to others (Goodman, 2003). Studies indicated that the vast majority of health care treatments and procedures were not based in evidence (Goodman, 2003). At the same time, large bodies of research on the same health topic were accumulating, thus leading to a systematic process of synthesizing research (Starr & Chalmers, 2003). With the evidence-based practices movement there was growing awareness of the importance combing the research literature, synthesizing research that met a defined level of quality, having medical experts agree on the meaning and conclusions of these syntheses, and developing treatment guidelines from them.

As a result of this emphasis, we have witnessed in the past 2 decades growing efforts to review and rate the quality of health research so that the findings of rigorous and credible research studies in specific areas can be synthesized. The proliferation of systems for rating the quality of research prompted the federal Agency for Healthcare Research and Quality (2002) to undertake an examination of these rating systems. The agency concluded that three major criteria should be used to evaluate new knowledge or research: quality, quantity, and consistency.

Quality in a research study suggests that the study was designed and conducted, and the results were analyzed, in such a way to minimize potentially misleading findings. While this may appear to be a straightforward concept, researchers frequently disagree about the methods and procedures that must be used to ensure the quality of research studies.

The second criterion, quantity, has to do with the number of studies conducted on a particular topic and the number of individuals involved in those studies. The quantity of research studies is important since, except in rare cases, one would not want to change a health practice based on one or two studies with small numbers of participants. Having multiple studies with large numbers of participants increases confidence in the findings.

The last criterion is consistency—the extent to which similar findings are reported from multiple studies. A common complaint among users is that different conclusions on the same topic are often reached (e.g., the hormone replacement therapy study), leading to confusion about which findings are accurate or credible. The more consistent the findings across several studies are, the more confident one can be in those findings and the changes in treatment that those findings suggest.

Most systems that rate the quality of research rely ultimately (after judging individual indicators of quality) on a rating hierarchy. Examples of those ratings include scales ranging from "strong evidence" to "moderate evidence" to "some evidence" to "no evidence," and grades such as A, B, C, D, with A representing excellent evidence. With these summary scores, professionals and laypersons can receive evidence-based health messages and a means by which to judge whether the prevailing evidence for a health practice is excellent, good, fair, or poor. An example of how this can be useful exists in the treatment of breast cancer. Research on the use of mastectomies, lumpectomies, and other treatments for breast cancer is available to assist both professionals and consumers needing that health information. Both professionals and laypersons can examine the quality of research information available for each of these treatment modalities through research syntheses and can use that information to make informed decisions about treatments. The growing need to ground new treatments in the existing evidence and the need to rate the quality of that evidence means that health communications can be based in high-quality research with consistent findings.

INITIATIVES TO RATE AND SYNTHESIZE HEALTH CARE RESEARCH

The Cochrane Collaborative (www.cochrane.org) was developed in response to this growing need to examine health research for quality and then synthesize it. It is now the largest initiative evaluating health care research in the world (Starr & Chalmers, 2007). To date, the Cochrane Collaborative has conducted hundreds of systematic reviews of research studies on a host of topics ranging from use of acetaminophen for migraines and the use of caffeine to treat asthma to the use of zinc supplementation. The collaborative has grown exponentially in the past 10 years and now is a major source of information for health care workers, researchers, and the public, providing "plain language" summaries. Largely a volunteer endeavor, the Cochrane Collaborative's goal is to compile and periodically update critical reviews of all relevant randomized clinical trials in various health topics. In each case, the research literature is scoured and experts rate and synthesize the findings, which in turn facilitates the development of practice recommendations. Cochrane Collaboration reviews are highly regarded because of their comprehensiveness and completeness.

Systems for grading and synthesizing research in areas other than health care have developed as well. These include the Campbell Collaborative (www.campbellcollaboration.org), a spinoff of the Cochrane Collaborative that focuses on education and social and behavioral sciences. In addition, there is the federally funded National Registry of Evidence-Based Programs and Practices, which evaluates the quality of mental health and substance abuse interventions and disseminates that information through a Web site. The What Works Clearinghouse, sponsored by the U.S. Department of Education, evaluates research on educational curricula.

KNOWLEDGE TRANSLATION AND THE DISABILITY RIGHT TO KNOW CLEARINGHOUSE

The Cochrane and Campbell collaboratives have largely focused their efforts on synthesizing research based on clinical trials and have not focused intensively on disability-related research. Clinical trials require individuals in a study to be randomly assigned to get the active intervention, to get a placebo, or to receive a less desirable intervention. However, because of the complexity of people's disabilities and the interventions needed to address them, it is often not possible to conduct randomized clinical trials in disability research. Thus, disability researchers often rely on studies that are not randomized and are non-experimental, observational, or correlational in nature. Such studies are often hypothesis-generating studies rather than studies that test the effectiveness of one intervention or drug over another (that is, hypothesis-testing studies). While some researchers consider non-experimental research to be inferior in quality to randomized clinical trials, such studies often can be quite informative for the field and for users and providers of services.

Because there are few systems to grade or evaluate such non-experimental research, we developed such standards as part of our knowledge translation efforts. We will apply these standards to specifically chosen topics in the mental health disability area, rate the research using these standards, synthesize the findings, and use that information to develop information products for our users and to populate our Web site (the Disability Right to Know). Most importantly, we are being guided by the principles and practices of knowledge translation to create evidence-based health messages that are targeted to the needs of individuals with disabilities, their providers, advocates, and family members.

BEYOND RESEARCH QUALITY

Beyond the issue of the quality of health information is the issue of its relevance to users. There are few services or products for which consumers are unable to ascertain the value of what they purchase; health care, unfortunately is often one. The difficulty of placing a value on particular health care interventions has resulted in calls for the assessment of consumers' perceptions of value. Recently, physicians and other health care providers have turned their attention to "value-based practices," which requires the perceived value of a particular practice or intervention, as well as its quality or effectiveness, to be taken into account (Brown, Brown, & Sharma, 2005). Brown and colleagues contend that value-based practices will lead to higher-quality health care because they require a calculation of the importance of an intervention to an individual compared to its presumed benefit—in essence, a personal cost-benefit analysis. Similarly, in the disability and mental health fields, to transform systems so they are "consumer-centric," it is essential to take into account how consumers value various services in addition to the effectiveness of those services (Anthony, 2005; Farkas & Anthony, 2006).

The principles of knowledge translation also suggest that to promote the utilization of new knowledge we must examine not only its quality, but also its potential value to those who are expected to use it (Lavis, Robertson, Woodside, McLeod, & Abelson, 2003). Not all research is meaningful to people or generates a "take home" message. Research may have no apparent relevance or application to consumers or providers and thus may fail to achieve the expected utilization or hoped-for impact (Stryer, Tunis, Hubbard, & Clancy, 2000). Without a clear sense of the implications of research findings for their day-to-day functioning and quality of life, users may not find relevance or meaning in them (Ratzan, 2004). As noted earlier, simply making information available (i.e., focusing on knowledge transfer versus knowledge translation) will not necessarily result in utilization of that information (Farkas, Jette, Tennstedt, Haley, & Quinn, 2003).

The notion that perceived value to the user is an important consideration leads to the question of whether there are systematic methods for assessing the value, meaning, or relevance of new information or research findings. In fact, there are few such standards even in general medicine (Gold, Siegal, Russell, & Weinstein, 1996). The lack of standard approaches to assess value contributes to the problem of providing target audiences with useful evidence-based health communications and, in turn, promoting the adoption of new research findings.

In general medicine, cost-utility formulas have been developed as one way of calculating perceived value to the consumer and weighing various health practices (Brown et al., 2005). These formulas attempt to assign metrics (e.g., time lost or gained, money spent or saved, quality-of-life measures) to interventions that have been found to be scientifically effective. In the disability and mental health fields, such formulas may be overly restrictive, not applicable, or just difficult to apply. While some cost-utility variables can be easily translated, other dimensions are difficult to quantify.

In our knowledge translation grant, in addition to the scale for rating research quality described earlier, we have developed a "meaning scale" with assistance from users and consumers of mental health services. The scale will allow users of information to review research findings relative to their own perceptions of its relevance or value. Since the perception of what is or is not valuable is subjective, we focused on three overarching factors from which meaning or value may be derived.

The first criterion by which we rate perceived meaning or value is whether the research findings are, or can be, translated into relevant information for day-to-day functioning so that they have personal implications for the user. This means that researchers must extend their typical interpretations of findings so that they have implications for people's day-to-day activities or roles. Without such interpretation it may be difficult for users to understand the value of the information to his or her situation or interests.

The second criterion for rating perceived relevance to users has to do with involvement of individuals with disabilities in the design, conduct, or interpretation of the research. Participatory approaches to the conduct of research (Greenwood & Whyte, 1993) have been growing in application and are now seen as having strategic purpose and value beyond the studies themselves for utilization of the findings (Selener, 1997). Research that has been developed with the active input of a community of individuals has a greater likelihood of producing information that is useful or meaningful to that community.

Finally, in terms of assessing meaning or relevance to the user, research findings in the absence of tools with which the new information can be used are less relevant to users. Research information may have implications for new services or interventions, but researchers often do not provide practical tools for implementation. For example, treatment guidelines and protocols serve to support the application of new information in the real world. Research studies that provide readers with links to such tools are perceived as more immediately valuable or meaningful to users than is research information that leaves its readers to create their own mechanisms for implementation or use.

Understanding the meaning or perceived value of research information to users, while difficult to measure, is critical to ensure that research findings make their way to the public. Our attempts to develop a tool that can be used to assess meaning are intended to increase the utilization and reach of disability-related research information.

PROMOTING KNOWLEDGE TRANSLATION OF HEALTH AND MENTAL HEALTH INFORMATION

Several important considerations come to mind regarding the promotion of the translation of research-based information for persons with disabilities in today's electronic digital environment. First and foremost is the need to understand the access barriers to the Internet and other electronic media confronted by individuals with disabilities. The Pew Internet & American Life Project (2007) found that only about half of those living with a disability or chronic disease go online, compared to 74% of those without a disability. Similarly, in an analysis using nationally representative survey data, Dobransky and Hargittai (2006) found that people with disabilities are less likely to live in households with computers, are less likely to use computers, and are less likely to go online. However, when socioeconomic factors were taken into account, they concluded that at least some individuals with disabilities (for example, individuals with hearing impairments) are not less likely to use the Internet than the general population (Dobransky & Hargittai, 2006). Furthermore, individuals with disabilities are unemployed in greater numbers than the general population, meaning that they have less capacity to purchase both computers and Internet access. Because of their higher rates of unemployment, they also report that they have less Internet access through their work (University of Montana, 2006). Taken together, these data suggest that the socioeconomic and employment status of individuals with disabilities must be considered in the promotion of health communication and knowledge translation using electronic media and the Internet.

In addition, physical and cognitive impairments may create access barriers for this population. Individuals with disabilities may have special requirements for using computers and related technologies; this is especially true of individuals who are visually impaired or hard of hearing or who have limited use of their upper extremities due to conditions such as quadriplegia or rheumatoid arthritis. Individuals with disabilities may have needs for assistive technologies that make the Internet more accessible to them (World Wide Web Consortium, 2005). Making these assistive technologies more affordable and available is one way to increase Internet access for individuals with disabilities and to further close the so-called digital divide (University of Montana, 2006).

In addition to considering issues of access, we can promote the meaningful use of health information by finding meaningful ways to involve users in knowledge translation efforts, beginning with the planning stages of projects that are intended to culminate in transfer of knowledge. The dictates of participatory action research cited earlier (cf. Selener, 1997) provide guidance on how consumers with disabilities can help shape the research agenda; in a similar fashion, consumers can help shape knowledge translation agendas. Modalities ideally suited to increasing the involvement of persons with disabilities in knowledge translation in this digital environment are the increasingly popular online communities of user groups with a common focus (Kim, 2000; Pew Internet & American Life Project, 2001). Such communities could be constructed specifically to provide a vehicle for input into knowledge translation efforts.

The widespread availability of disability-accessible information and assistive technologies means that individuals with disabilities can independently access information without relying on human assistance such as that of a personal assistant or reader. Furthermore, individuals with psychiatric disabilities who want to conceal their disabilities because of stigma can peruse and use the Internet anonymously and without revealing their condition to others (Cook, Fitzgibbon, Batteiger, Grey, Caras, Dansky, & Priester, 2005). Because of this ready and anonymous access, the Internet has the potential to be a great equalizer and therefore to be enormously liberating for many individuals with disabilities. The Web and other electronic media can level the playing field by giving them access to information that heretofore has only been available to medical professionals and other privileged individuals.

However, vetting the voluminous health information remains a challenge (Bernstam, Walji, Sagaram, Sagaram, Johnson, & Meric-Bernstam, 2008). Individuals promulgating health information are considering different ways of rating Internet information for accuracy. However, the extent to which the existing systems can rate the content of Web sites for accuracy remains a question (Bernstram et al., 2008), as they tend to focus on objective and factual questions that do not necessarily account for accuracy (for example, quality criteria rating factors such as display of authorship and date of creation).

This approach to rating health information accuracy can and should be taken further to include a "seal of approval" approach, perhaps similar to the "Bobbie Approved" approach that is used to endorse Web sites that reach an acceptable level of accessibility. Such a method for evaluating health and mental health information that has reached a certain standard of quality or rigor would mean that consumers with disabilities could rely more heavily on that information in their health decision making. The Medical Library Association (www.mlanet.org) provides another model of how to assist health consumers locate quality information by providing detailed guides especially for lay consumers, including references to the top 10 most useful health Web sites and the top 10 cancer, diabetes, and healthy heart Web sites. Such guides can go a long way toward assisting consumers who must sort through volumes of often questionable health information.

SUMMARY AND CONCLUSIONS

Health information is voluminous and is accessible in a wide variety of formats, those formats having expanded with the explosion of digitally based communication. Often, however, health and mental health information is complex and not easily evaluated for quality by the general public and consumers of health services. To improve health and mental health communications, there is a need for new knowledge to be developed with utilization needs in mind, to be rated for quality and synthesized, and to be assertively promulgated to users. Promulgation can be enhanced by use of the Web and other digital common systems and devices. The recent emphasis on knowledge translation and the movement toward evidence-based practices in health and mental health care have both influenced the focus on quality research and the understanding of how to promote utilization of research results. Health and mental health professionals are more attentive to the need for providing evidence-based practices and for utilizing quality research to guide their treatments.

Systems for rating research have been developed over the past 20 years, as have large-scale initiatives to review and summarize research findings. These syntheses can and should serve as the basis for accurate health communications. Disability researchers can learn from these directions in the medical world and health care arena. That is, disability research should be evaluated for quality and synthesized, and its utilization should be assertively promoted. This will help advance the National Institute on Disability and Rehabilitation Research (2008) mission, which is "to generate, disseminate and promote new knowledge to improve the options available to disabled persons." Our knowledge translation grant and activities are designed to help achieve this mission.

REFERENCES

Agency for Health Care Research and Quality. (2002). *Systems to rate the strength of scientific evidence* (No. Evidence Report 47). Rockville, MD: U.S. Department of Health and Human Services.

Anthony, W. (2005). Value based practices. *Psychiatric Rehabilitation Journal, 28*(3), 205–206.

Brown, M., Brown, G., & Sharma, S. (2005). *Evidence-based to value-based medicine.* Washington, DC: American Medical Association Press.

Canadian Institutes of Health Research. (2005). *About knowledge translation.* Retrieved September 9, 2006, from http://www.cihr-irsc.gc.ca/e/29418.html

Cook, J. A., Fitzgibbon, G., Batteiger, D., Grey, D. D., Caras, S., Dansky, H., & Priester, F. (2005). Information technology attitudes and behaviors among individuals with psychiatric disabilities who use the Internet: Results of a Web-based survey. *Disability Studies Quarterly, 25*(2). Retrieved January 11, 2008, from http://www.dsq-sds.org/_articles_html/2005/spring/cook_etal.asp

Dobransky, K., & Hargittai, E. (2006). The disability divide in Internet access and use. *Information, Communication and Society, 9*(3), 313–334.

Farkas, M., Jette, A., Tennstedt, S., Haley, S., & Quinn, V. (2003). Knowledge dissemination and utilization in gerontology: An organizing framework. *The Gerontologist, 43*,1, 47–56.

Farkas, M., & Anthony, W. A. (2006). Systems transformation through best practices. *Psychiatric Rehabilitation Journal,* 87–88.

Gold, M. R., Siegal, J. E., Russell, L. B., & Weinstein, M. C. (1996). Cost effectiveness in health and medicine. *Journal of American Medical Association, 276,* 1172–1177.

Goodman, K. (2003). *Ethics and evidence-based medicine: Fallibility and responsibility in clinical science.* New York: Cambridge University Press.

Greenwood, D. J., & Whyte, W. (1993). Participatory action research as a process and as a goal. *Human Relations, 46*(2), 175–192.

Grimshaw, J., Shirran, L., Thomas, R., Mowatt, G., Fraser, C., Bero, L., et al. (2001). Changing provider behavior: An overview of systematic reviews of interventions. *Medical Care, 39*(Suppl. 2), 112–145.

Holick, M. F. (2007). Vitamin D deficiency. *New England Journal of Medicine, 357*(3), 266–281.

Kim, J. (2000). *Community building on the Web: Secret strategies for successful online communities.* Berkeley, CA: Peachpit Press.

Landry, R., Amara, N., & Lamari, M. (2001). Utilization of social science research knowledge in Canada. *Research Policy, 30*(2), 333–349.

Lavis, J. N., Robertson, D., Woodside, J. M., McLeod, C. B., & Abelson, J. (2003). How can research organizations more effectively transfer research knowledge to decision makers? *Milbank Quarterly, 81*(2), 221.

Mendelsohn, M. E., & Karas, R. H. (2007). HRT and the young at heart. *New England Journal of Medicine, 356*(25), 2639–2641.

National Center for the Dissemination of Disability Research. (n. d.) *NIDRR brochure and mission.* Retrieved January, 2, 2008, http://www.ncddr.org/new/announcements/nidrr_brochure.html

National Institute on Disability and Rehabilitation Research. (2005). *Long-range plan for fiscal years 2005–2009.* Retrieved January 2, 2008, from http://www.ed.gov/legislation/FedRegister/other/20061/021506d.pdf

National Institute on Mental Health Advisory Council. (1999). *Clinical treatment and services research workgroup: Bridging science and services.* Rockville, MD: National Institute of Mental Health.

Pew Internet & American Life Project. (2001). *Internet and the American Life project: Online communities: Networks that nurture long-distance relationships and local ties.* Retrieved January 15, 2008, from http://www.pewinternet.org/report_display.asp?r = 47

Pew Internet & American Life Project. (2007). *Pew Foundation, Pew Internet and the American Life Project, E-patients with a disability or chronic disease.* Retrieved January 31, 2008, from http://www.pewinternet.org/pdfs/EPatients_Chronic_Conditions_2007.pdf

Ratzan, S. C. (2004). A realistic goal? Health information for all by 2015. *Journal of Health Communication, 9,* 487–489.

Sackett, D. L., Rosenberg, W. M. C., Muir Gray, J. A., Haynes, R. B., & Richardson, W. S. (1996). Evidence based medicine: What it is and what it isn't. *British Medical Journal, 312,* 71–72.

Selener, D. (1997). *Participatory action research and social change* (2nd ed.). Ithaca, NY: Cornell University Press.

Starr, M., & Chalmers, I. (2003). *The evolution of the Cochrane Library, 1988–2003.* Retrieved January 11, 2008, from http://www.update-software.com/history/clibhist.htm

Stout, C., & Hayes, R. (2005). *The evidence-based practice: Methods, models, and tools for mental health professionals.* New Jersey Hoboken: John Wiley and Sons.

Stryer, D., Tunis, S., Hubbard, H., & Clancy, C. (2000). The outcomes of outcomes and effectiveness research: Impacts and lessons from the first decade. *Health Services Research, 35,* 977–993.

Sudsawad, P. (2007). *Knowledge translation: Introduction to models, strategies, and measures.* Austin, TX: Southwest Educational Development Laboratory, National Center for the Dissemination of Disability Research.

University of Montana, Research and Training Center on Disability in Rural Communities. (2006, June). *Disability and the digital divide: Comparing surveys with disability data.* Retrieved January 31, 2007, from http://rtc.ruralinstitute.umt.edu/TelCom/Divide.htm

Vernig, P. (2007). From science to practice: Bridging the gap with translational research. *Association for Psychological Science Observer, 20.* Retrieved January 1, 2008, from http://www.psychologicalscience.org/observer

World Health Organization. (2005). *Bridging the "know-do" gap: Meeting on knowledge translation in global health*. Retrieved September 25, 2006, from http://www.who.int/kms/WHO_EIP_KMS_2006_2.pdf.

World Wide Web Consortium. (2004). *How people with disabilities use the Web*. W3C Working Draft, World Wide Web Consortium.

13

New Strategies of Knowledge Translation: A Knowledge Value Mapping Framework

JUAN D. ROGERS

The new media landscape is part and parcel of the emergence of knowledge societies. Knowledge with social, economic, and political implications is created at increasing rates by an increasing number of sources and is the object of market transactions, management concerns, and policy agendas (David & Foray, 2002; Steinmuller, 2002). The flow of increased volumes of knowledge through media, especially new information and communication technologies, not only makes more knowledge available in more places and in more formats but also challenges the stability of the meaning of the enormous volume of knowledge content that is circulating (Steinmuller, 2002). The institutional arrangements that have developed over time to create, validate, distribute, and apply knowledge are being pushed to the limit. In many areas there seem to be difficulties in ensuring that either existing knowledge or the best knowledge is available when, where, and for whom it is needed. Health care is one area in which the knowledge society has an enormous impact—both with benefits, since many new ways to treat disease are created continuously, and difficulties, since there is a growing consensus that the flow of knowledge is not as smooth and stable as one might wish (Choi, 2003; Davis et al., 2003).

Other chapters in this volume have addressed these issues from the point of view of developing new media approaches to facilitate the flow of information and knowledge. In this chapter, we will address them from the point of view of the alternative representations of knowledge that may be necessary given the various communities of creators and users of health care knowledge and how they relate to each other.

Specifically, we will focus on the notion of knowledge translation that has been suggested in various parts of the international health care community. Our purpose is twofold. First, we will give an interpretation and assessment of the current discourse on knowledge translation. Then, we will provide a basic framework for new strategies in knowledge translation on the basis of our assessment. In this chapter, we will first outline current discussions of knowledge translation. The second section will identify the social groups and communities that must communicate. The third section analyzes what we know about knowledge flow and how its relation to the values of the communities previously identified affects knowledge translation. The fourth section develops the notion of knowledge value mapping for capturing specific configurations of knowledge and value within which knowledge flows of interest could or do take place. On this basis, a framework for developing knowledge translation strategies is proposed.

KNOWLEDGE TRANSLATION AND THE DEFINITION OF A COMMUNICATION AGENDA

There are several definitions of knowledge translation in the literature and in health care policy documents. The Canadian Institutes of Health Research's definition of knowledge translation is one of the best known:

> [Knowledge translation] is the iterative, timely and effective process of integrating best evidence into the routine practices of patients, practitioners, health care teams and systems in order to effect to optimal health-care outcomes and to optimize health care and health care systems. (cited in National Center for the Dissemination of Disability Research, 2005, p. 2)

The definition adopted by the National Institute for Disability and Rehabilitation Research of the U.S. Department of Education is:

> The collaborative and systematic review, assessment, identification, aggregation, and practical application of high-quality disability and rehabilitation research by key stakeholders (i.e., consumers, researchers, practitioners, and policymakers) for the purpose of improving lives of individuals with

disabilities. (National Center for the Dissemination of Disability Research, 2005, p. 2)

As our subject pertains to the process and conditions of the creation of scientific knowledge and its fate in terms of validation, dissemination, use, and amplification in the larger societal context, it is critical to identify the role these definitions play. There are two main possibilities. First, the definitions could be indicating an entity, category, or property pertaining to phenomena observed in the world. This is the typical use of definitions in the research mode, and knowledge translation would be either a label for an observed entity in the social world (such as an organization, for instance) or a construct that serves to explain social phenomena (such as social class, for example).

Alternatively, the definitions could be indicating an abstract entity or set of conditions that does not exist but could come into existence if certain actions are taken. This is the typical use of definitions in the policy- and decision-making realms. Clearly, these two definitions of knowledge translation, with their similarities and differences, belong in the second class. They are not labels used in the process of describing an observed reality. Rather, they are labels used to define an agenda of action so that a certain envisioned state of affairs becomes reality.

In other words, knowledge translation has not been "discovered" in the process of research. It is part of a policy proposal to achieve certain goals. It may be the case that in the process of arguing for this course of action, certain actions taken by relevant groups are identified as a case of knowledge translation, and their outcome noted as an example of what is desired. Therefore, the argument would say, if more such actions are taken under the conditions specified by the definition, more desirable outcomes of the same sort should happen (Canadian Institutes of Health Research, 2006).

The discussion that the definitions generate depends greatly on this distinction. If they were part of the research process, then we would discuss whether the knowledge claims associated with the identification of knowledge translation in the real world are valid based on the evidence that was collected, whether that evidence is in fact what the researchers say it is and how it relates to prior knowledge about related phenomena, and so forth.

Since these definitions belong in the agenda-setting class, their discussion has the format typical of deliberations on decision making, which include the justification of goals, the selection of proper means toward their achievement, and the assessment of the feasibility and sustainability of their implementation, among other things. In other words, knowledge translation must be made to happen with policy instruments. The outcomes should then be assessed in order to establish whether the desired goals were realized (Choi, 2005; Grimshaw et al., 2004; Grimshaw, Santesso, Cumpston, Mayhew, & McGowan, 2006; Lavis, 2006; Lavis, Robertson, Woodside, McLeod, & Abelson, 2003; National Institute for Disability and Rehabilitation Research, 2005; Nutley & Davies, 2000; Sudsawad, 2007; van Kammen, de Savigny, & Sewankambo, 2006; Zwarenstein & Reeves, 2006). The two forms of discussion of knowledge translation are related, since the proposed interventions in the world must match up with what we know about the phenomena that the proposals intend to control or affect. Still, each one has its specific purpose.

Point of Departure: A Gap

In general terms, the attention paid to knowledge translation comes in response to a growing consensus that there is "a gap between what we know and what we do" (Canadian Institutes of Health Research, 2004, p. 2) in health care. The evidence for this gap comes from various fields of clinical practice in which too much variation in the application of certain treatments occurs in spite of the existence of evidence recommending one approach over the others (Davis et al., 2003; Kerner, Rimer, & Emmons, 2005b). However, there are several different underlying reasons given for this gap in the literature. In some cases the gap has to do with the large volume of knowledge being produced and the limited ability of users, including clinical practitioners, to absorb it (Choi, 2005; Graham, Logan, Harrison, Straus, Tetroe, Caswell, & Robinson, 2006). This is the information glut gap. Others see a gap between the complexity of the knowledge produced and the ability of the users to understand it completely and use it (Choi, 2003, 2005; Kerner, 2006). This is the knowledge complexity gap. Still others see a gap between the knowledge produced by research and the criteria used by policy makers and administrators to make decisions. The reason for this gap has to do with at least two factors, one related to the policy process, and the other to the peculiarities of the research community. On one hand, the institutionalization of policy processes may include policy legacies, peculiar time frames, and varying levels of authorization for consideration of policy priorities leading to difficulties in the timely application of research knowledge in policy deliberations (Lavis, Ross, Hurley, Hohendadel, Stoddart, Woodward, & Abelson, 2002). On the other hand, the specific focus of research topics, often perceived to be removed from pressing issues of practice and full of jargon in its mode of communication, is difficult to align with the interests and mode of information acquisition of policy makers (Choi, 2003). This is the "two-communities theory" of knowledge utilization (Caplan, 1979, p. 459). For this reason, the policy-making realm appears resistant to changes suggested by research find-ings. So we have a relevance-criteria gap.

The detection of the symptoms of a gap between available knowledge and current practice motivates the implementation of initiatives to rem-edy the situation. Most of the evidence brought to bear on the proposals has to do with the nature of these symptoms rather than the nature of the underlying causes. An exception is the study by Lavis and colleagues (2002) that explored the use of health services research knowledge in health policy making in Canada. But in general, very little empirical and analytical work has been directed at elucidating the underlying nature of the perceived problem. Furthermore, even in this exceptional study, the interpretation of results assumes that the nature of the problem of applying research in various areas, such as clinical practice, policy mak-ing, and consumer choice, is essentially the same for all fields of knowl-edge. This particular study invoked Caplan's two-communities theory as background. But it failed to recognize that Caplan was articulating the specific problem of the use of social science knowledge in policy making, for which the relationship between research knowledge claims about social actors and the policy focus is often direct. There is less overlap between the medical knowledge about the clinical benefits of treatments for disease, on one hand, and the knowledge of reasons and circumstances under which social actors may or may not choose to use them, on the other. Therefore, the knowledge flow problem identified as a gap between available knowledge and current practice has not been fully articulated, leading to a key assumption of knowledge translation proposals, namely, that knowledge flow problems are essentially uniform or invariant across diverse fields of knowledge and, therefore, indepen-dent of knowledge content.

Intended Effects: Health Care Outcomes via Behavior Modification

The desired outcomes of the implementation of knowledge translation are health benefits for the target population. These are expected to occur as a result of utilization of the highest-quality research knowledge, as determined by its grounding in evidence, and generally assumed to be already available. The gaps discussed above represent interruptions or obstacles to this process. In all cases described in the literature, there is a group or community of mediating stakeholders in the chain from research to outcomes via utilization that has not aligned its practices with the implications of the available certified knowledge. Knowledge translation strategies in the form of interventions aimed at behavior modification are suggested to remedy the situation (Canadian Institutes of Health Research, 2004; Grimshaw et al., 2001).

Each one of the gaps mentioned earlier suggests a core strategy that fits the problem. The remedy for an information glut, for example, is to summarize the enormous volume of information in ways that maintain the integrity and validity of the original sources while significantly reducing the volume. Users are then expected to use the information. A knowledge complexity gap requires another type of simplification that also preserves the ultimate validity of its substance but makes it better suited to the knowledge absorption means at users' disposal. Once again, users are then expected to apply the knowledge provided in the simplified format. A relevance-criteria gap is similar to the other two in that a reformulation of the content that is closer to the regular mode of knowledge acquisition and use by the target groups is needed. In this case, the new format must show how the original content is relevant to the user's agenda even though it didn't appear so in its original formulation. In all these versions of the gap, the new form of the same substantive content naturally suggests the analogy of a translation. The original meaning of the content must remain the same while it is expressed in the language of the target group.

According to this view, once the content of the knowledge is put in terms amenable to acquisition by intended users, it should have an effect on them so that the implications of the knowledge can be realized through the actions of users who adopt it. The ultimate measure of the success of a knowledge translation strategy is not the reformulated knowledge product in the form of a systematic review, a new set of guidelines for medical decisions, or a redesigned continuing education program, for example. Rather, it is the observable and measured change in behavior by the user group of interest in line with what knowledge producers believe are the implications of the knowledge they created. Much of the literature on knowledge translation strategies and interventions uses the language of "behavior modification" very generally as the desired result of the process (Choi, 2005; Davis et al., 2003; Grimshaw et al., 2001, 2004; International Development Research Center,

2005, Lavis, 2006; National Health Service, 1999). Except for the end users, namely the patients or persons with disabilities who are the ultimate beneficiaries of the application of health knowledge, whose level of education and expertise is not a condition for receiving the benefits of knowledge use, the other communities of users are highly educated professionals and decision makers who have a degree of autonomy in their work environment. Therefore, framing the measurable results of knowledge translation as behavior modification begs for scrutiny, which will be brought later in this chapter.

Knowledge Translation as a Communication Problem

This summary review of knowledge translation suffices to conclude that at its core it is a communication problem. It is possible to view both the gap diagnoses and the proposed remedies as communication failures and new communication strategies, respectively. In all articulations of the problem there is a need to convey meaningful content to a target audience. As a matter of fact, the very notion of translation, taking something expressed in an original language and expressing it in another, is one of the classical communication problems, one that has been studied from multiple disciplinary perspectives for centuries (Gertzler, 2001).

This analogy with linguistic translation is obviously intentional in the formulations of knowledge translation but is not meant to be adopted as a complete theoretical model. The reasons for using this analogy are important, though. Since knowledge translation definitions are agenda-setting statements or normative definitions, there are aspects of linguistic translation that illuminate its key priorities. Central among these is the idea of taking substantive content formulated in the context of one community using its own language and rephrasing it in terms of the habitual communication patterns of another so that the original meaning is preserved. In spite of the fact that the definitions expand on this simple notion with statements describing the process as "iterative, timely and effective" or "collaborative and systematic," and with an established goal such as "to effect optimal health care outcomes" or "improving the lives of individuals," ultimately the priority of preservation of meaning is an explicit expectation of those who engage in knowledge translation. They assume that when the reformulation of content with preservation of meaning (i.e., translation) works properly, the realization of the potential impact will be observed in terms of those circumstances and objectives. In other words, when the users are able to understand the meaning of the knowledge in question, after participating in the process described in the clarifying statements, they will use it and its benefits will be realized.

The conceptualization of problems related to the creation, dissemination, and use of knowledge as communication problems is standard (Rogers, 1995). Many of the existing analyses of knowledge translation–related issues are presented in terms of communication. The strategies to address diagnosed problems are communications strategies (e.g., guideline formulation and dissemination, systematic reviews for specific audiences, design of curricula for continuing education, use of media strategies to make content in these efforts available). The assumptions of the presentation of knowledge translation as a communication problem need to be explored in detail.

COMMUNITIES OF PRODUCER-USERS IN NEED OF TRANSLATION

The challenge of knowledge translation starts with the recognition that there are at least two communities, producers and users, for whom the core meaning of some knowledge content is relevant but who, for various reasons, do not have the same material or cognitive means of accessing it. Devising alternative means of access has been one of the main objects of attention for knowledge translation (Canadian Institutes of Health Research, 2004, 2006; van Kamen et al., 2006). In doing so, the diversity of uses of knowledge and of user contexts have been the first phenomenological observations that knowledge translation analysts have made (Jacobson, Butternill, & Goering, 2003; Landry, Lamari, & Amara, 2001, 2003; Lavis, 2006; van Kerkhoff & Szlezak, 2006).

Closer scrutiny of knowledge utilization reveals that the original intuitive formulation of two sides, producers and users, with two distinctive and mutually exclusive roles to play in the dynamics of knowledge is too simplistic to be of any analytical value. In most contemporary conditions, knowledge is created or produced in complex networks of teams of researchers affiliated with various sorts of organizations, such as universities, industry laboratories, and government institutes (Zwarenstein & Reeves, 2006). They interact in varying degrees with decision makers, some having oversight responsibilities within their own organizations and others related to funding agencies and policy institutions that affect their work. There are also growing interactions with business persons, with clinicians and practitioners in the case of health research, and often with end users, patients, or advocates for people who have some stake in what researchers work on. The strategic design for knowledge translation in the Canadian public health system actually aims at increasing these sorts of interactions (Canadian Institutes of Health Research, 2004).

All the individuals, groups, and organizations not doing research work we mentioned above are potential users of research in some form (Sudsawad, 2007). To these we might add other sets of people who may not interact directly with researchers or the entities they work in but may pick up knowledge they create from publications or press releases.

Two important points must be made about this situation. First, the content of knowledge as it moves through the link between any two nodes may change in important ways. For example, researchers constantly consider their understanding of priorities and needs of decision makers and users' experiences in the reformulation of their research work. So there are multiple paths for knowledge to flow toward the creators that impinge on the very content of their research. Second, the outcome of this complex network of interactions in a particular field is a pattern of knowledge flow that can follow any path through the links in the network. The content and meaning of knowledge is not completely determined by those who hold the label of creators or producers. As a matter of fact, the actual attributions of meaning of the knowledge that flows between any two points in the network, either in direct contact with each other or indirectly connected through another producer-user, cannot be assumed to remain constant. The actual meaning attributions at each point must be determined empirically. In sum, the two roles of producer and user of knowledge are not clear cut and mutually exclusive. In every instance of use there is a degree of transformation of the knowledge, unless the use is limited to a verbatim repetition of a linguistic formulation without further impact (Bozeman & Rogers, 2002; Rogers & Bozeman, 2001).

The multiplicity of paths of knowledge flow in the process of knowledge creation and use has been widely recognized and built into models of the process of innovation (Forrest, 1991; Kline & Rosenberg, 1986). More importantly, though, from the point of view of knowledge translation, what is not often recognized analytically is that creation and use are intertwined and that most instances of use are actually use and transformation. Furthermore, the specifics of how meaning is created in the process of use and transformation for each set of users is crucial for understanding the flow of knowledge (Bozeman & Rogers, 2001).

There are numerous common examples of these phenomena to illustrate the point. We often think of uses of science as the application of research results to problem solving. This is the case, for example, when research on disability provides the foundation for developing assistive technologies to enhance the quality of life of persons who are affected by those disabilities. A slightly different and highly public instance of the use of scientific knowledge occurs in the case of environmental science. Research results are used to attribute responsibilities for its preservation and design regulations with legal force either to prevent more damage or to reverse some of the changes. These are not, strictly speaking, problem-solving applications. Moving still further away from the first case scenario, we can see a reverse flow in the case of the development of drugs to treat certain diseases that may draw on the experience of patients who suffer side effects to do research on new ones that do not produce side effects. A fourth example comes from the use of theories in one field to inspire the study of completely different phenomena in another field. A case in point is the application of evolutionary theory from biology to economic phenomena to develop evolutionary economics (Nelson & Winter, 1982). In the process of technological innovation, this transformation of knowledge as it is used is also recognized (Savory, 2006).

These four examples actually involve different patterns of knowledge flow through different sorts of networks of people and organizations. But what they all have in common is that at the point where research knowledge is used, a specific sort of knowledge creation must happen for the application to go forward. First, the general results from research that are brought to bear on the point of use must be matched to the problems. So the results must be interpreted and the problems articulated so that they are embedded in a common meaning frame. Second, in most realistic situations the problems are not trivial; thus misalignments and difficulties arise. Solutions to these new problems must be developed or called for.

A key component of the original translation analogy is undermined by these findings. The content to be translated is no longer completely predefined and stable or under the control of one set of participants in this process. It is no longer just a matter of putting one linguistic formulation of research results into another linguistic formulation that is accessible to a target audience. It is necessary to understand how the reformulations of knowledge that occur at every node of interest in the network take shape. In the debate over evidence-based medicine, a key element of the articulation of knowledge translation in the literature (Estabrooks, Thompson, Lovely, & Hofmeyer, 2006), this shifting of the meaning of knowledge content at different points of the producer-user network has been noted. Buetow (2002) suggests that a "medicine of meaning" must inform the framework for establishing fruitful relations for production and use of health knowledge. A key aspect of this framework is the inclusion of relevant users in the definition of what counts as evidence in evidence-based medicine because otherwise the very practice of medicine loses much of its meaning.

Any useful understanding of knowledge translation must account for these processes and the phenomena that are associated with them. This leads us to a triple agenda for the development of knowledge translation approaches. In the first place, we have a phenomenological dimension, which must address all the empirical aspects of knowledge flow processes relevant to knowledge translation. This section has begun to anticipate what is involved by describing the network of relations and diversity of producer-user roles that any such process necessarily involves.

Second, we have a policy dimension that stems from the normative point of departure for knowledge translation given in its definitions. There are goals in specific fields of knowledge, such as health care systems or disability and rehabilitation research, that must be realized. From the definitions of knowledge translation we have "to effect optimal health care outcomes and to optimize health care and health care systems," and "the purpose of improving lives of individuals with disabilities." Therefore, our investigation of knowledge flows and their consequences will be guided by the question of which processes lead to outcomes aligned with these goals.

Finally, we have a communication dimension, given by the nature of the knowledge flow processes that the goals of knowledge translation define. Most of the challenges are essentially about the creation of meaning in the context of social relations, which lies squarely in contemporary understandings of communication phenomena (Fiske, 1990). Furthermore they arise in the context of new communication phenomena, and many of the actions to be taken will have significant communication elements. These are communication challenges created in part by the emergence of a new media landscape that demands analysis and approaches suited to these new realities. The challenges of knowledge translation do not represent a typical "old" problem that can now be solved with "new" media. Rather, they are problems created by a new set of circumstances in the status of science and its role in contemporary society, which require new understanding in order to inform appropriate strategies in the new knowledge society.

CONTENT AND VALUE IN KNOWLEDGE FLOWS

Observed Content–Value Interaction in Knowledge Utilization

The next step is to explore the knowledge flows under the purview of knowledge translation in order to understand how they occur and what factors impinge on the use-and-transformation instances of relevant producer-users. There are several implications from the discussion so far that can be summarized as follows:

- Users of knowledge are likely to be different from each other.
- Most users of knowledge are also creators of knowledge, and vice versa.
- There are multiple paths of knowledge flow with no a priori priority.
- Interacting groups of producer-users are likely to have different modes of internal communication.
- Interacting groups of producer-users are likely to have different criteria to assess validity and utility of knowledge.

The interactions of researchers and policy makers in the health care field, one of the three perceived gaps that motivate knowledge translation, have been studied by knowledge translation researchers (Amara, Ouimet, & Landry, 2004; Lavis, 2006; Lavis, Posada, Haines, & Osei, 2004). They observe that health research knowledge as it comes from clinical research is not sufficient for developing health policies. For example, policy makers often need cost-benefit analyses of implementation proposals and comparisons of their potential impact with competing or existing policies and regulations, which clinical research results do not include and, furthermore, clinical researchers are ill equipped to do (Grimshaw et al., 2004). This example points us in an important direction, namely, that the priorities and values of a specific producer-user community creates specific demands on the shape of the knowledge content at stake. As a result, knowledge will be adapted, extended, or refined or will undergo other sorts of transformations in the very act of its use. Alternatively, if the transformation process does not occur under current circumstances, the knowledge flow will be impeded and it will not be used.

Amara and associates (2004) studied several types of knowledge use by policy makers in government agencies and point out that in order to increase knowledge use of all types and in all policy areas, the users had to interact more with the researchers and provide them with additional incentives and guidelines for adapting their work to the needs of policy and public management. In other words, it is knowledge flow in the reverse path that is needed in order to increase the utilization down the primary path. These conclusions implicitly recognize the production role of the users.

Welch and Dawson (2006) studied the implementation of evidence-based practice in the field of occupational therapy. Practitioners in this field are embedded in a hierarchy of health care organizations and government health agencies. Health policies in the United Kingdom, where the study was conducted, demand that the implementation of evidence-based practice be demonstrated throughout occupational therapy practice under the National Health Service. Their study reveals that most of the onus of practice change is put on individual occupational therapy practitioners without significant organizational support. They detect numerous obstacles to the success of this process, including perceived labor unfairness, misalignment of the evidence-based practice materials with their form of knowledge acquisition and application in the field, lack of ownership of the content of evidence-based practice presented to them, and a lack of structures of mutual support for engaging in learning new practice guidelines. A very significant constellation of values underlying the conclusions drawn by this study is at stake. There are labor and professional values related to distribution of effort, relations with colleagues, and the assessment of demands within their work and professional hierarchy. There are also epistemic values at stake related to the selection and application of knowledge content in their field of practice.

Studies of knowledge use, especially those directed at sponsors or managers of research who are evaluators of the process rather than the direct producers or users under their responsibility in the field, clearly state that goals or objectives of the use of knowledge must be established first so that the outcomes of knowledge utilization can be assessed (Conner, 1980). The analytical process of assessing utilization involves paying close attention to the priorities and modes of communication of the target users to detect the factors that facilitate or hinder the use of the knowledge in question. In the words of a group of researchers working on the application of research to rehabilitation practice, bringing research to clinical practice always "requires a learning framework that focuses on the intended users of research as the most critical element of the process" (Farkas, Jette, Tennstedt, Haley, & Quinn, 2003, p. 48).

In a recent review of knowledge translation, Sudsawad (2007) found that numerous approaches and measures have been developed in different fields of knowledge to conceptualize and measure its use. The very diversity of possibilities seems to be the most striking lesson drawn from that exercise. If we set it against the background of the variety of communities of producer-users that are relevant in most important cases of knowledge flow, that result is not so surprising. Among other things, most approaches to knowledge utilization assume, often unwittingly, an inadequate model of communication. They use the "process model" of communication that originated with the study of technical communication problems (Fiske, 1990). The knowledge to be utilized is analogous to the message exchanged between a sender and a receiver through a channel of communication that links them. Most of these studies attempt to measure whether the "message," namely, the knowledge content of interest, has actually been received by the intended receiver. The examples of empirical research we have reviewed so far indicate that the stability of the roles of producer and user, analogous to the sender and receiver in this model, cannot be assumed. Therefore, in approaching knowledge translation as a problem of understanding and participating in knowledge flows in complex social networks, it is necessary to adopt a communication model that allows for the creation of meaning in the communication process (Fiske, 1990). For this, it is necessary to directly account for the content–value combinations that are present in the knowledge flows of interest.

The definitions of knowledge translation that identify normatively the problems of interest point to the complexity and interactivity that should be expected in the process. However, by retaining control over all the details of knowledge content and passing down in the form of evidence-based medicine or evidence-based practice a predetermined fixed set of meanings, they do not recognize, in a full analytical sense, the set of social and communication phenomena within which knowledge translation processes are embedded. As a result, the development of strategies for achieving the desired outcomes becomes a fragmented and frustrating exercise of fitting abstract procedures in realms that seem either unprepared or indifferent or hostile to their implementation (Ball, Wadley, & Roenker, 2003).

In sum, knowledge translation processes do not merely involve the two languages of the producer and the user. Nor do they refer simply to a single field of knowledge content. There are as many translation challenges as there are distinct content–value interactions affecting the knowledge flow.

Articulation of Content–Value Combinations in Different Contexts

The knowledge translation agenda includes the objective of implementing evidence-based medicine and evidence-based practice (Davis et al., 2003; Estabrooks et al., 2006; Lavis, 2006; Zwarenstein & Reeves, 2006). Therefore, a brief consideration of the sources and nature of evidence in the process of knowledge creation and validation is in order and made necessary by the assertion in the previous sections that the meaning of knowledge content in most knowledge flows of interest is not completely predetermined and stable.

A fairly standard view in the philosophy of science today is that evidence acquires meaning in relation to some theory for which it is evidence. Furthermore, what is discussed today is not whether evidence can stand alone but rather to what extent data gathered with the purpose of assessing a theory is sufficient to confirm it or disconfirm it, or provide the basis for a definitive choice between rival theories (Dawid, 2006; Mayo, 1996; Quine, 1970). Therefore, theories are logically prior to evidence, since they provide the criteria for relevance in selecting data to support the theory by confirming a prediction, for example. Evidence is, furthermore, expressed in the language provided by the theory, using its definitions and constructs to communicate what has been observed as the result of an experiment. The theories under consideration and others used to set up experiments and tests contain the articulation of conventions that guide the practice of science with approved procedures. All these constitute a set of epistemic values associated with that field of knowledge. In other words, there is a deep intertwining of content and values in the very production of scientific knowledge that enables the set of scientists working in the field to become a community of knowledge (Douglas, 2000; Lacey, 2005).

The details of this interrelation of content and values in scientific knowledge vary in subtle ways from field to field and also from time to time within a field when important shifts in the direction of research occur. A fascinating example of this comes from the field of mental health research. Work by Anthony, Rogers, and Farkas (2003) represents a vigorous effort to respond to the call for rigor from evidence-based medicine with a keen awareness of better-informed theory for assessing the relevance and validity of evidence. They show how a fundamental theoretical shift in mental health research, labeled the "recovery vision," has radical consequences for what counts as evidence in an evidence-based medicine approach to research and clinical practice. According to Anthony and associates, fundamental treatment outcome variables used in the evidence-based medicine approach (e.g., variations in hospital relapse or recidivism, inpatient hospitalization, length of stay, symptoms) become relatively unimportant compared to others that have to do with patients' experiences and goals as indicators of recovery. The development of the new theoretical perspective requires a commitment to develop evidence to explore its implications either to support and improve it or to discard it for better ones. The very content of evidence-based medicine will be different depending on the path researchers decide to follow in their theoretical commitment.

The criteria that guide evidence assessment for relevance and quality are also expected to differ from one field to another. It has been noted that evidence-based medicine has its origin in two particular subfields of clinical medicine—namely, general internal medicine and clinical epidemiology—and that transferring evidence assessment criteria from them to other fields of medicine creates problems (Upshur, VanDen-Kerkhof, & Goel, 2001). In particular, from those fields, evidence-based medicine brings along the emphasis on quantitative measurement and, especially, randomly controlled trials (Worrall, 2002). In fields outside those in which it originated, these aspects of measurement and evidence gathering may not be feasible or as important. Upshur (2001) calls for an inclusive model of evidence in health care to "integrate the epistemologies found in the various disciplines involved in health care" (p. 95). This perspective recognizes that knowledge translation will necessarily be an interdisciplinary endeavor because of the diversity in the communities of knowledge producer-users that make up the delivery of health care. Therefore, the array of epistemic and contextual values that are integral to each must be taken into account for the dynamics of knowledge flow to be assessed.

Since the application or utilization of knowledge is not a simple, passive process of adopting an instrument and following instructions, so to speak, getting involved with new knowledge requires a significant investment of capabilities and resources. In the industrial innovation literature this is widely recognized, and the concept of absorption capacity has been introduced to explain the nature of these efforts to enable the use of external knowledge. Many industrial firms have their own research capabilities, often with the principal objective of being able to absorb external knowledge rather than create their own from scratch (Cohen & Levinthal, 1990).

Scientific publications are not easily understood by untrained persons. The more specialized and novel the content of the research results, the more distant it is expected to be from non-specialists' experience and capabilities. Therefore, there must be an expectation of significant payoff for the commitment of resources to be made. In other words, scientific research will be applied if it is perceived to add value to the user (Landry, Amara, Pablos-Mendes, Shademani, & Gold, 2006). There are several kinds of value: a commercial opportunity, enhanced professional capability, and realization of a social priority, among other things. However, everybody expected to make an investment in the absorption process must perceive the possibility for added value. This may be a challenge in hierarchical systems, such as the health care system, in which the added value is perceived by decision makers, but the burden of absorption is borne by a group of subordinates. A study of the values grounding the professional identity of nurses showed that the actualization of other-oriented values is integral to their provision of nursing care as professionals and that they realize self-oriented values, such as the satisfaction and reward in their work, through the realization of the other-oriented values (Fagermoen, 1997). However, contextual factors stemming from the organizational and administrative levels may be limiting their ability to provide care and increasing their sense of strain, making their work less meaningful. Change in the broader context of work seems to be what should occur, according to McGuire (1990) and Rushmer and associates (2004). McGuire protests the implication that the outcome of evidence-based practice as behavior modification means that the use of experience and craft knowledge in nursing is irrational. Change should be expected at another level in order for nursing practices to change rather than building from the individual up. It is not surprising to read in the conclusions of knowledge translation intervention studies that what the ones that actually work best all have in common is that the interests and values of the users have been taken into account!

The clinical practices of doctors is another area that has received much attention as a critical case for assessing various knowledge translation interventions or knowledge utilization strategies because the lack of consistency across the medical field in diagnosis and treatment of several common conditions is one of the main gaps motivating evidence-based medicine and knowledge translation (Hader, White, Lewis, Foreman, McDonald, & Thompson, 2007). A strategy used to address this issue has been the implementation of clinical practice guidelines stemming from evidence-based medicine. The overall results of this strategy have been lackluster. In a recent study of factors leading to changes in doctors' clinical practices, Hader and associates found that decisions to adopt clinical practices are made in complex networks of consultation and collaboration with colleagues. But the evidence-based medicine guidelines are expected to be followed independently of those networks; thus these guidelines expect the judgment of unknown experts to be trusted. The guidelines acquire meaning for the doctors within the entire network of relations and exchanges that grounds their professional decisions and actions. So they not only provided information but also created questions about their ability to make critical medical decisions and were not sufficient to enable the doctors to produce new medical knowledge in the context of their use.

Knowledge translation processes occur at the boundaries between communities that have different cognitive styles and value frames, even though they may be focused on common areas of social experience (Fallis, 2006). There are many such boundaries since there is no simple duality of producers and users to mediate between. Rather, there are differences among fields of research as well as among various categories of practitioners, service providers, assistive technology firms, policy makers, and administrators, to name some of the obvious groups. These all interact and participate in health knowledge flows and fulfill producer-user roles that create the meaning of health knowledge content at each point in social space and time. Insofar as shared goals of improved health care outcomes are being realized in the process, knowledge translation processes are being successful. However, it is clear that no simple intervention on the basis of fixed knowledge content and the expectation of behavior modification at one point of this system can be expected to ensure success.

KNOWLEDGE VALUE MAPPING: A FRAMEWORK OF KNOWLEDGE TRANSLATION STRATEGY DESIGN

Empirically Based Knowledge Translation: A Knowledge Value Map

The diversity of values of interacting groups of producer-users is often subsumed under the notion of stakeholders (Canadian Institutes of Health Research, 2005; Fixsen, Naoom, Blasé, Frieman, & Wallace, 2005). It is understood that in a collaborative environment or in a negotiated process, the interests of stakeholders have an influence on the choices, decisions, and, ultimately, outcomes. Rarely, though, is the specific set of priorities of stakeholders included in the analytic framework for analyzing knowledge production and use dynamics and their effect on the outcome.

The preceding analysis shows that in order to increase the chances that a knowledge translation implementation will work and that increased knowledge flows will happen up and down the paths linking various communities of producer-users, interventions require detailed understandings of the content–value maps of the network. Since the focus of attention of a knowledge translation initiative could be narrow or broad in its intended reach, strategies might vary in the complexity of content–value combinations they must address. In narrowly focused cases, the size of the communities is small, so there is a high degree of familiarity through a long history of interactions, leading to shared communication patterns and a good understanding of each other's values and goals. Knowledge translation strategies may involve a simple reformulation of knowledge content into media and formats that suit applications and activities that all concerned know quite well ahead of time.

The experience with evidence-based medicine, evidence-based practice, and knowledge translation in the last 20 years reflected in studies and evaluations shows that most cases of interest are not so simple. Even in the case of doctors, who are said to be responsible for one of the main gaps in knowledge use due to inconsistencies detected in their clinical practices, initial knowledge translation efforts have been unsuccessful, and the main reason given is that the patterns of knowledge flow in which they are embedded are much more complicated than was originally supposed and those efforts have not provided adequate combinations of content and value for them to change their practices.

The emphasis on the evidence base for devising guidelines and other normative components in knowledge translation approaches is, ironically, not matched by a similar emphasis on a fully empirical approach to the social phenomena of knowledge flows. The empirical investigation is generally confined to the measurement of outcome variables related to the desired changes in behavior (Sudsawad, 2007). Part of the problem stems from the fact that knowledge translation has been defined normatively first and, as such, is not the natural knowledge frontier of any particular field of research. Efforts to systematize relevant knowledge about knowledge translation have shown that there are numerous social science theories that are relevant to a greater or lesser degree (Estabrooks et al., 2006; Graham et al., 2006). Research in education, diffusion of innovations, organizational behavior, psychology, social communication, management, and political science, among other fields, all have potential contributions. Some authors have attempted a reduction to first principles or a small set of dimensions, virtually creating a new social science field of knowledge translation research. This kind of work may produce useful results but, at least for the time being, will inevitably be subsidiary to the main research in the existing fields. The knowledge translation research questions are not naturally emerging problems from established research streams in the social sciences. Rather, they are social science questions derived from a policy agenda in medicine mostly investigated by researchers trained in the life sciences trying to adapt social science work to their new needs. Not surprisingly, there is much confusion around its development (Straus & Mazmanian, 2006).

An alternative strategy is to begin with a more complete description of the knowledge flows that are the object of knowledge translation. Since the application of a reduced number of categories of knowledge action to explain and predict knowledge utilization has not been very successful, it may be more fruitful to attempt an explicit enumeration of relevant entities involved in the knowledge flow for each knowledge translation problem or field of interest. To use an analogy from mathematical modeling, rather than a closed functional form representation of the relations under investigation, an explicit enumeration of instances of the relation may be needed. Ebener, Khan, Shademani, Compernolle, Beltran, Lansang, and Lippman (2006) used a similar device derived from the knowledge management literature in a developing country to assess the availability of health knowledge in the local context. In this case, the map only accounted for knowledge content without establishing content–value relations.

This description of the knowledge flow would be a knowledge value mapping of the field that the knowledge translation agenda is focused on. As a matter of fact, for the areas in which most of the knowledge translation initiatives have been implemented and evaluated, such as clinical practices of doctors in Canada (Hader et al., 2007) and the studies of evidence-based practice in nursing in the United Kingdom (McGuire, 1990), the elements of such a map already exist scattered in the publications and reports containing that work. A knowledge value mapping approach would aggregate the information on content–value structures from all those studies rather than attempt to condense all that work into a few conceptual categories.

The map describes the relations of all the knowledge producer-users linked to the knowledge flow in a specific field of interest. The relations of interest are only those that have to do with participation in the knowledge flow. These relations of production and use may be indicated by citation in publication, participation in training, request for information, and licensing agreements, among numerous other possibilities. Since the knowledge translation agenda already has an area of knowledge application in view, it will always suggest an initial set of producer-users. Through the use of documentation, surveys, interviews, membership lists, and other materials, it is possible to identify a population of producer-users of interest in a particular field of interest to knowledge translation.

The next step involves studying the specific features of content–value relations of the population that has been identified. Various types of content–value relations will be associated to roles and groups involved in practices. Therefore, it is expected that the number of distinct content–value structures actually detected in the population will be much smaller than the number of individuals. This information will constitute the knowledge value map of the field in question.

Application of the Knowledge Value Map to Determine the Gaps

The three general types of gaps identified in the knowledge translation literature must be closed or bridged with interventions that bring evidence-based medicine or evidence-based practice as the solution. The more detailed investigations of the gap have been directed at doctors' clinical practices and nursing in the context of health service organizations. Some work has also been done on general conditions under which policy makers use scientific knowledge in their deliberations and decisions. However, the potential for content–value structures to affect knowledge flow is much greater. Furthermore, the actual problems may not be in the place where the symptom seems most obvious (for example, the impact of organizational leadership on individual practices of occupational therapy; see, e.g., Welch & Dawson, 2006).

The first immediate analytical application of the knowledge value map is to determine empirically all the points in the map where content–value structures seem to be misaligned or maladapted for the desired knowledge translation outcomes. These are all potential gaps. On the positive side, the map also serves to document the evolution of facilitating content–value structures, which may serve for analytical purposes to make generalizations about them. Most of the cases of knowledge translation interest today are in fields other than those that originated its development. Since the different fields of research and corresponding professional practice will have different content–value structures, the nature of the gaps is potentially different too. In these cases, the construction of a knowledge value map is probably more important and useful, because having had less attention paid to its knowledge flow, the field does not have a set of categories of its own for articulating the main knowledge translation challenges and is in danger of distorting the problems by importing them from the other areas.

For example, Pillemer and associates (2003) studied interventions in the field of social gerontology. In spite of general agreement in the field that theory and basic research findings should be well integrated in the interventions, they maintain that actual connections are often weak or absent. Interventions to support caregivers of elderly family members had badly misunderstood their role, and a close investigation of the mismatch between the nature of the need and the design of previous interventions led to the use of social psychology theories for new designs. The content–value structure of the caregiver role had not been investigated properly, so available research on care of the elderly was not brought to bear on the interventions.

The example of the change in prevalent theory in the field of mental health is also applicable here. The work of Farkas, Gagne, Anthony, and Chamberlain (2005) points out the need for articulating the value frame of patients in order for evidence-based practice to be implemented. Interestingly, this work presents the challenge of developing services that take into account the values of patients with severe mental illness. Before a recovery vision of mental health problems was developed, patients were thought not to be able to have coherent values or priorities. Farkas and associates argue that consideration of those values has an effect on the agenda and approaches of research in mental health, the managerial tasks of administrators of mental health services, and the ability of advocates and consumers to assess how well available services fit their needs.

In sum, the nature of the gap detected from analytical application of knowledge value mapping will guide the selection of appropriate intervention strategies that take advantage of the facilitating features of the knowledge value structure of the field revealed in the map.

Reflexive Statement of the Knowledge Translation Agenda: The Portfolio Level

Since each type of content–value structure will require different knowledge translation strategies, it may seem natural to conclude that researchers in each field are their natural implementers. As a matter of fact, since most of the literature on knowledge translation assumes that the results of research keep their meaning and implications intact as they flow to the utilization context, extending their responsibility to ensure the usability of their results seems to be a logical conclusion. However, the perspective developed in this chapter argues against it. Researchers are not in control of the transformations that their research results undergo as they flow to other communities of producer-users. Furthermore, their research specialty is almost certainly quite different from what is required to understand the details of contextual phenomena that take place as knowledge flows through the other communities. Charging them with the responsibility of analyzing knowledge translation phenomena and implementing strategies to achieve its goals creates another case of content–value misalignment that doesn't favor knowledge flow.

Actually, the need for knowledge translation is generally perceived by decision makers who have responsibilities over several teams of researchers in multidisciplinary fields who actually or potentially interact with or affect a large number of complex constituencies (involving, among others, practitioners, health organizations, policy makers in other agencies, industry in assistive technology or pharmaceutical fields, patients and their families, and advocacy groups). In such a situation, a knowledge translation strategy based on the efforts of individual researchers would probably not have much impact, nor would it contribute significantly to desired outcomes, and it would result in frustration and wasted resources for those called to implement knowledge translation programs. The reasons are clear by now. In a complex system such as this, which is typical of many research funding or health service agencies in the United States and other industrialized nations, the assumptions of immutability of the meaning of knowledge content and of the alignment of values and priorities of interacting producer-user communities break down completely. The demands of knowledge translation are too great for single teams without the interdisciplinary experience with social sciences, and it is even suggested that it is too big a problem for a single agency to tackle on its own (Kerner et al., 2005a).

At this level, it seems invaluable to develop knowledge value maps in all the areas covered by the portfolio in order to diagnose the gaps and understand their nature. This should be an ongoing endeavor carried out by interdisciplinary teams with experience in studying the social dynamics of knowledge. From the results available at any stage, work can be commissioned to address the gaps and aim to ensure that the best research knowledge flows to the relevant communities of producer-users.[1]

Sustainability of Knowledge Translation Strategies for Realization of Desired Outcomes

The most common statement of measurable effects of knowledge translation interventions is behavior change or changed practices of health care providers, be they doctors, nurses, or other practitioners (Davis et al., 2003; Grimshaw et al., 2001; Lavis, 2006; National Health Service, 1999). Some studies have indicated that the observed behavior change of individuals may not be sustained in time if further conditions that are not part of the original intervention are not in place (Plastow, 2006; Welch & Dawson, 2006). These observations call into question whether the ultimate outcomes of knowledge translation can rest on the measured behavior change of one individual practitioner at a time. Welch and Dawson insist that the context of work set by the organization within which nurses, occupational therapists, and other practitioners provide care is highly determinant of their sustained practices.

Knowledge value mapping should be used to determine which producer-user roles are in a position to ensure the long-term sustainability of desired practices. It may require a rethinking of the roles that practitioners perform in their organizations. The new knowledge may demand such a content–value structure that not only will assumed patterns of work no longer be adequate in their clinical aspects as the research findings may indicate, but also other relational and hierarchical patterns may be challenged.

As some of the authors we have cited have already indicated, the level of change at stake is, more often than not, organizational, not individual. In the business world this challenge has been confronted for a long time now, and a large body of literature on organizational change and its management exists (Weick & Quinn, 1999). Change of practices at the individual level usually follows, but it is not assumed that the aggregate level is a simple outcome of individual behavior changes one by one. Organizational structures are known to have significant effects on the patterns of knowledge flow (Carlile, 2004; Gopalakrishnan & Santoro, 2004).

Since the changes in practice that knowledge translation interventions aim for are based on the acquisition and appropriation of knowledge, the very notion of behavior change as a result seems inappropriate. It suggests a necessitated or logical response to instructions rather than the reasoned decisions of an empowered knower. It is not surprising that evaluations of evidence-based medicine interventions have often been caught off guard when the target practitioners challenged the content of the knowledge and expressed disagreement with its claims (Hader et al., 2007). The knowledge value mapping framework proposed here recognizes the active engagement of the targets of knowledge translation interventions, who play producer-user roles rather than mere user ones. In knowledge processes, this is akin to expressing "informed consent" regarding risk, for example. In the context of risk communication, policies aiming at behavior modification to reduce risk exposure have also been proposed. The point has been forcefully argued that seeking informed consent is the appropriate policy to recognize people as moral agents and contribute to a more sustainable outcome in response to risk (Bostrom, 2003).

CONCLUDING REMARKS: DO WE NEED A NEW INSTITUTIONALIZATION OF THE HEALTH CARE PROFESSIONS?

This chapter presented an analysis of knowledge translation and its implications from the point of view of the social dynamics of knowledge flows and proposed a framework to empirically establish the specific knowledge translation issues in a field of knowledge. The argument and the framework are based on the recognition that there is a deep intertwining between the attribution of meaning to knowledge content and an array of values of all participants in the knowledge flow. As a result, there are no clear-cut producers or users of knowledge. Rather, there are many communities of producer-users who use and transform knowledge at every stage. Therefore, knowledge translation problems cannot be studied with abstract categories that apply equally to all fields. The content–value structure for each member or community of participants in the field must be determined, and the nature of a potential gap or other challenges to the desired outcomes of knowledge translation established empirically. For that, a knowledge value mapping approach is suggested.

The widespread sense that there is a gap between knowledge produced in research and the practices that could be informed by this knowledge in almost every field of health care raises a deeper and more general question about the overall institutional arrangement on which health care is generally based. After several decades of efforts dedicated to these issues with dissemination and utilization programs, evidence-based medicine and evidence-based practice, knowledge translation, and other such initiatives, we should not conclude that all these approaches have failed. Rather, the situation seems to be that many different things could work under different circumstances, but each time, success is met with radical questioning by practitioners regarding what the changes mean for their roles as health care providers and whether what they do has the same meaning (Hader et al., 2007; Hancock & Easen, 2004; Welch & Dawson, 2006).

Taking a cue from studies of the patterns of everyday life and emergence of structure in social systems (Bourdieu, 1977; de Certeau, 1988; Giddens, 1986), we know that most common social practices are embedded in routines. These routines become the informal structures on which everyday social life rests. Many professional practices are acquired by intense training that allows for the routine application of complex skills. Furthermore, the model of explicit, conscious, rational decision making at every step is so much more prone to error and demanding of energy that these routines are essential to both high performance and efficiency. Social roles are assumed and embodied in the context of such routine social activities (Bourdieu, 1977). These facts of social existence go a long way in explaining why change is very difficult and that constant change is probably so disruptive and stressful that it cannot be sustained in human society.

From the evidence gathered in the knowledge translation–related studies, it seems plausible to hypothesize that the dynamics of knowledge creation and flow in the contemporary knowledge society are putting the established institutional arrangements under stress, and the routine performance of health care roles is under pressure to change too much and too rapidly for this to occur within the current structures. The ordinary forms of communication of researchers, doctors, nurses, therapists, patients, pharmaceutical industries, health care agencies, policy makers, administrators, and insurance providers, among others, are no longer adequate for the quality of care to match the availability of knowledge without the creation of new facilitating roles and the implementation of changes to the current ones. It is not possible to offer a clear path ahead for this process here. The detailed analysis of content and value of knowledge using knowledge value mapping may be a way to develop evidence to test the hypothesis.

NOTE

1. Translational research programs such as the one at the U.S. National Institutes of Health appear to be efforts in that direction (see Office of Portfolio Analysis and Strategic Initiatives, n.d.). The systematic elaboration of knowledge value maps does not seem to be a part of this program. It probably relies on informal versions of such maps.

REFERENCES

Amara, N., Ouimet, M., & Landry, R. (2004). New evidence on instrumental, conceptual, and symbolic utilization of university research in government agencies. *Science Communication, 26*(1), 75–106.

Anthony, W., Rogers, S., & Farkas, M. (2003). Research on evidence-based practices: Future directions in an era of delivery. *Community Mental Health Journal, 39*(2), 101–113.

Ball, K., Wadley, V., & Roenker, D. (2003). Obstacles to implementing research outcomes in community settings. *The Gerontologist, 43*(Special Issue), 29–36.

Bostrom, A. (2003). Future risk communication. *Futures, 35*(6), 553–573.

Bourdieu, P. (1977). *Outline of a theory of practice.* Cambridge: Cambridge University Press.

Bozeman, B., & Rogers, J. (2002). A churn model of knowledge value: Internet researchers as a knowledge value collective. *Research Policy, 31,* 769–794.

Canadian Institutes of Health Research. (2004). *Knowledge translation strategy 2004–2009: Innovation in action.* Ottawa, ON, Canada.

Canadian Institutes of Health Research. (2006). *Evidence in action, acting on evidence: A casebook of health services and policy research knowledge translation stories.* Ottawa, ON. Canada.

Caplan, N. (1979). The two-communities theory and knowledge utilization. *American Behavioral Scientist, 22,* 459–470.

Carlile, P. (2004). Transferring, translating, and transforming: An integrative framework for managing knowledge across boundaries. *Organization Science, 15*(5), 555–568.

Choi, B. (2003). Bridging the gap between scientists and decision makers. *Journal of Epidemiology and Community Health, 57,* 918.

Choi, B. (2005). Understanding the basic principles of knowledge translation. *Journal of Epidemiological Community Health, 59,* 93.

Cohen, W., & Levinthal, D. (1990). Abosrptive capacity: A new perspective on learning and innovation. *Administrative Science Quarterly, 25*(1), 128–152.

Conner, R. (1980). The evaluation of research utilization. In M. Klein & K. Teilmann (Eds.), *Handbook of criminal justice evaluation* (pp. 629–653). Beverly Hills, CA: Sage.

David, P., & Foray, D. (2002). Economic fundamentals of the knowledge society. *Policy Futures in Education: An E-Journal, 1*(1), 20–49. Retrieved September 22, 2007, from http://www-econ.stanford.edu/faculty/workp/swp02003.pdf

Davis, D. (2006). Continuing education, guideline implementation, and the emerging transdisciplinary field of knowledge translation. *Journal of Continuing Education in the Health Professions, 26*(1), 5–12.

Davis, D., Evans, M., Jadad, A., Perrier, L., Rath, D. Ryan, D., et al. (2003). The case for knowledge translation: Shortening the journey from evidence to effect. *British Medical Journal, 327*(7405), 33–35.

Dawid, R. (2006). Underdetermination and theory succession from the perspective of string theory. *Philosophy of Science, 73*(3), 298–322.

De Certeau, M. (2002). *The practice of everyday life.* Berkeley: University of California Press. Originally published in 1974

Douglas, H. (2000), Inductive risk and values in science. *Philosophy of Science, 67*(4), 559–579.

Ebener, S., Khan, A., Shademani, R., Compernolle, L., Beltran, M., Lansang, M. A., & Lippman, M. (2006). Knowledge mapping as a technique to support knowledge translation. *Bulletin of the WHO, 84,* 636–642.

Estabrooks, C., Thompson, D., Lovely, J., & Hofmeyer, A. (2006). A guide to translation theory. *Journal of Continuing Education in the Health Professions, 26*(1), 25–36.

Fallis, D. (2006). Epistemic value theory and social epistemology. *Episteme, 2*(3), 177–188.

Farkas, M., Gagne, C., Anthony, W., & Chamberlain, J. (2005). Implementing recovery oriented evidence based programs: Identifying the critical dimensions. *Community Mental Health Journal, 41*(2), 141–158.

Farkas, M., Jette, A., Tennstedt, S., Haley, S., & Quinn, V. (2003). Knowledge dissemination and utilization in gerontology: An organizing framework. *The Gerontologist, 43,* 47–56.

Fiske, J. (1990). *Introduction to communication studies.* London: Routledge.

Fixsen, D., Naoom, S., Blasé, K., Frieman, R., & Wallace, F. (2005). *Implementation research: A synthesis of the literature.* Tampa: University of South Florida, Louis de la Parte Florida.

Mental Health Institute, The National Implementation Research Network (FMHI Publication #231).

Forrest, J. (1991). Models of the process of technological innovation. *Technology Analysis & Strategic Management, 3*(4), 439–453.

Gertzler, E. (2001). *Contemporary translation theories* (2nd ed.). Multilingual Matters Limited.

Giacomini, M., Hurley, J., Gold, I., Smith, P., & Abelson, J. (2004). The policy analysis of "values talk": Lessons from Canadian health reform. *Health Policy, 67*(1), 15–24.

Giddens, A. (1986). *The constitution of society: Outline of a theory of structuration.* Cambridge: Polity Press.

Graham, I., Logan, J., Harrison, M., Straus, S., Tetroe, J., Caswell, W., & Robinson, N. (2006). Lost in knowledge translation: Time for a map? *Journal of Continuing Education in the Health Professions, 26*(1), 13–24.

Grimshaw, J., Santesso, N., Cumpston, M., Mayhew, A., & McGowan, J. (2006). Knowledge for knowledge translation: The role of the Cochrane Collaboration. *Journal of Continuing Education in the Health Professions, 26*(1), 55–62.

Grimshaw, J., Shirran, L., Thomas, R., Mowatt, G., Fraser, C., Bero, L., et al. (2001). Changing provider behavior: An overview of systematic reviews of interventions, *Medical Care, 39*(8 Suppl. 2), II2–II45.

Grimshaw, J., Thomas, R., MacLennan, G., Fraser, C., Ramsay, C., Vale, L., et al. (2004). Effectiveness and efficiency of guideline dissemination and implementation strategies. *Health Technology Assessment, 8*(6), 1–72.

Gopalakrishnan, S., & Santoro, M. (2004). Distinguishing between knowledge transfer and technology transfer activities: The role of key organizational factors. *IEEE Transactions on Engineering Management, 51*(1), 57–68.

Hader, J., White, R., Lewis, S., Foreman, J., McDonald, P., & Thompson, L. (2007). Doctors' views of clinical practice guidelines: A qualitative exploration using innovation theory. *Journal of Evaluation in Clinical Practice, 19*(4), 601–606.

Hancock, H., & Easen, P. (2004). Evidence-based practice—an incomplete model of the relationship between theory and professional work. *Journal of Evaluation in Clinical Practice, 10*(2), 187–196.

Hofer, J., Chasiotis, A., & Campos, D. (2006). Congruence between social values and implicit motives: Effects on life satisfaction across three cultures. *European Journal of Personality, 20,* 305–324.

International Development Research Center. (2005). *Knowledge translation: Basic theories, approaches and applications,* Retrieved from http://www.idrc.ca/en/ev-90105-201-1-DO_TOPIC.html

Jacobson, N., Butternill, D., & Goering, P. (2003). Development of a framework for knowledge translation: Understanding user context. *Journal of Health Services Research and Policy, 8*(2), 94–9.

Kerner, J. (2006). Knowledge translation versus knowledge integration: A "funder's" perspective. *Journal of Continuing Education in the Health Professions, 26*(1), 72–80.

Kerner, J., Guirguis-Blake, J., Hennessy, K., Brounstein, P., Vinson, C., Schwartz, R., et al. (2005a). Translating research into improved outcomes in comprehensive cancer control. *Cancer Causes and Control, 16*(Suppl. 1), 27–40.

Kerner, J., Rimer, B., & Emmons, K. (2005b). Dissemination research and research dissemination: How can we close the gap? *Health Psychology, 24*(5), 443–446.

Kline, S., & Rosenberg, N. (1986). An overview of innovation. In R. Landau & N. Rosenberg (Eds.), *The positive sum strategy: Harnessing technology for economic growth* (pp. 275–306). Washington: National Academy Press.

Lacey, H. (2005). On the interplay of the cognitive and the social in scientific practices. *Philosophy of Science, 72*(5), 977–988.

Landry, R., Lamari, M., & Amara, N. (2001). Climbing the ladder of research utilization: Evidence from social science research. *Science Communication, 22*(4), 396–422.

Landry, R., Lamari, M., & Amara, N. (2003). The extent and determinants of the utilization of university research by government agencies. *Public Administration Review, 63*(2), 192–205.

Landry, R., Amara, N., Pablos-Mendes, A., Shademani, R., & Gold, I. (2006). The knowledge-value chain: A conceptual framework for knowledge translation in health. *Bulletin of the WHO, 84,* 597–602.

Lavis, J. (2006). Research, public policymaking, and knowledge-translation processes: Canadian efforts to build bridges. *Journal of Continuing Education in the Health Professions, 26*(1), 37–45.

Lavis, J., Lomas, J., Hamid, M., & Sewankambo, N. (2006). Assessing country-level efforts to link research to action. *Bulletin of the WHO, 84,* 620–628.

Lavis, J., Posada, F., Haines, A., & Osei, E. (2004). Use of research to inform public policymaking. *Lancet, 364*(9445), 1615–1621.

Lavis, J., Robertson, D., Woodside, J., McLeod, C., & Abelson, J. (2003). How can research organizations more effectively transfer research knowledge to decision makers? *Milbank Quarterly, 81*(2), 221–248.

Lavis, J., Ross, S., Hurley, J., Hohendadel, J., Stoddart, G., Woodward, C., & Abelson, J. (2002). Examining the role of health services research in public policymaking. *Milbank Quarterly, 80*(1), 125–154.

Mayo, D. (1996). *Error and the growth of experimental knowledge.* Chicago: University of Chicago Press.

McGuire, J. (1990). Putting nursing research findings into practice: Research utilization as an aspect of the management of change. *Journal of Advanced Nursing, 15*(5), 614–620.

Miles, A., Polychronis, A., & Grey, J. (2006). The evidence-based health care debate—2006. Where are we now? *Journal of Evaluation in Clinical Practice, 12*(3), 239–247.

National Center for the Dissemination of Disability Research. (2005). What is knowledge translation? *Focus: Technical Brief, No. 10.* Austin, TX: Southwest Educational Development Laboratory.

National Health Service 1999. Professional Behavior Modification.

National Institute for Disability and Rehabilitation Research. (2005). *Knowledge translation planning panel: Summary of the June 9–10, 2005 panel meeting.* Retrieved from www.ncddr.org

Nelson, R., & Winter, S. (1982). *An evolutionary theory of economic change.* Cambridge, MA: Harvard University Press.

Nutley, S., & Davies, H. (2000). Making reality evidence-based practice: Some lessons from the diffusion of innovations. *Public Money and Management, 20*(6), 35–42.

Office of Portfolio Analysis and Strategic Initiatives. (n.d.). *Re-engineering the clinical research enterprise: Translational research.* Retrieved September 30, 2007, from http://nihroadmap.nih.gov/clinicalresearch/overview-translational.asp

Pillemer, K., Suitor, J., & Wethington, E. (2003). Integrating theory, basic research, and intervention: Two case studies from caregiving research. *The Gerontologist, 43,* 19–28.

Plastow, N. (2006). Implementing evidence-based practice: A model for change. *International Journal of Therapy and Rehabilitation, 13*(10), 464–469.

Quine, W. (1970). On the reasons for indeterminacy in translation. *Journal of Philosophy, 67,* 178–183.

Rogers, E. (1995). *Diffusion of innovations.* New York: Free Press.

Rogers, J., & Bozeman, B. (2001). Knowledge value alliances: An alternative method to R&D project evaluation. *Science, Technology and Human Values, 26*(1), 23–55.

Rushmer, R., Kelly, D., Lough, M., Wilkinson, J., & Davies, H. (2004). Introducing the learning practice—I. The characteristics of learning organizations in primary care. *Journal of Evaluation in Clinical Practice, 10*(3), 375–386.

Savory, C. (2006). Translating knowledge to build technological competence. *Management Decision, 44*(8), 1052–1075.

Steinmuller, W. (2002). Knowledge-based economies and information and communication technologies. *International Social Science Journal, 171*(1), 141–153.

Straus, S., & Mazmanian, P. (2006). Knowledge translation: Resolving the confusion. *Journal of Continuing Education in the Health Professions, 26*(1), 3–4.

Sudsawad, P. (2007). *Knowledge translation: Introduction to models, strategies, and measures.* Austin, TX: Southwest Educational Development Laboratory, National Center for the Dissemination of Disability Research. Retrieved September 21, 2007, from www.ncddr.org/kt/products/ktintro/

Timmermans, S., & Mauck, A. (2005). The promises and pitfalls of evidence-based medicine. *Health Affairs, 24*(1), 18–28.

Upshur, R. (2002). If not evidence, then what? Or does medicine really need a base? *Journal of Evaluation in Clinical Practice, 8*(2), 113–119.

Upshur, R., VanDenKerkhof, E., &. Goel, V. (2001). Meaning and measurement: An inclusive model of evidence in health care. *Journal of Evaluation in Clinical Practice, 7*(2), 91–96.

van Kammen, J., de Savigny, D., & Sewankambo, N. (2006). Using knowledge brokering to promote evidence-based policy-making: The need for support structures. *Bulletin of the WHO, 84,* 608–612.

Van Kerkhoff, L., & Szlezak, N. (2006). Linking local knowledge with global action: Examining the global fund to fight AIDS, tuberculosis and malaria through a knowledge system lens, *Bulletin of the World Health Organization, 84*(8), 629–635.

Weick, K., & Quinn, R. (1999). Organizational change and development. *Annual Review of Psychology, 50*(1), 361–386.

Welch, A., & Dawson, D. (2006). Closing the gap: Collaborative learning as a strategy to embed evidence within occupational therapy practice. *Journal of Evaluation in Clinical Practice, 12*(2), 227–238.

Worrall, J. (2002). What evidence in evidence-based medicine? *Philosophy of Science, 69,* S316-S330.

Zwarenstein, M., & Reeves, S. (2006). Knowledge translation and interprofessional collaboration: Where the rubber of evidence-based care hits the road of teamwork. *Journal of Continuing Education in the Health Professions, 26*(1), 46–54.

International Innovations in Health Communication

14

MUHIUDDIN HAIDER, SCOTT C. RATZAN, AND WENDY MELTZER

Global health and development professionals recently identified new challenges facing the field of health communications. Attendees at "The Rome Consensus," a 2006 conference, also called the World Congress on Communication for Development, identified community ownership of communication by those who's health was most affected by poverty and those who were most underserved as a vital area in need of exploration as health and development communication moves forward. In addition to community participation, knowledge sharing, especially at the local and international level, and evidence-based program planning have been called for in order to ensure the continued success of health communication.

Global innovations in the field of health communication and, more specifically, media landscaping have the ability to address these emerging challenges. Radio and television have been the predominant media channels for health communication in the developing world. However, as computers and other digital technologies become more widely available, innovation in health communication is slowly starting to shift to Web-based and computer-based applications.

Media landscaping may be viewed as a collection of health and development communication phases. Product-based communication, in which

The authors would like to thank Mila Gonzela and Casey Aldrich, who did the background research work identifying and analyzing the case study.

the development or health product (in the form of a program, knowledge, or an actual good) is presented or sold to its audience, is the most recognizable phase of media landscaping. Service-based communication is the phase during which service organizations introduce their services and products not only to the consumer but to each other as well in an act of innovation diffusion. Finally, the organizational-based communication phase can be seen as a public–private partnership of sorts wherein policy makers, administrators, service providers, and development and health professionals at all levels share program design elements, implementation processes, and assessment indicators. Emerging technologies are expanding the reach and utility of health and development communication.

Health communication specialists have long embraced electronic channels as a means of furthering media landscaping. Public service announcements, ads, and serial dramas are the standard forms of media landscaping that have been disseminated via cinema, radio, and television over the past 30 years. However, emerging electronic media technologies are changing the face of media landscaping. Existing media landscaping initiatives take advantage of new technologies to scale up existing initiatives. At the same time, emerging electronic media technologies allow health communication specialists to offer personalized communication messages on a mass media scale. New forms of electronic media create opportunities for health communication specialists to reach new and larger populations while allowing for greater user–message interaction. HIV/AIDS prevention, tuberculosis control, access to clean drinking water, and promotion of improved reproductive health, as well as emerging health issues like the potential avian flu pandemic will benefit from the implementation of new technologies.

However, it should be noted that in developing countries, traditional methods of reaching the population still work and may remain the best option for years to come. If there is access to technology, its use is complicated by rampant illiteracy rates. But technology is still able to play a critical role by expanding the reach of such forms of media.

Despite the changes in media landscaping occurring because of emerging technologies, the best practices study, which has been identified since 1962, still hold true today. This chapter reviews the literature and identifies best practices associated with media landscaping. In addition, the chapter will explore the effects of emerging technologies from a global perspective through case studies describing recent innovations in media landscaping. Change comes with many challenges, which will be further discussed.

Emerging technologies will also play an important role in the nascent field of global health diplomacy in the coming years. Global health diplomacy confronts the developing relationship between international health concerns and politics. Increased movement of people and goods across borders ensures that disease knows no boundaries. Cooperation between sovereign states, international organizations, nongovernmental organizations, and multinational businesses is necessary to confront existing and emerging health pandemics. Widespread threats, such as HIV/AIDS and avian influenza, often require innovative media messaging—media messaging that is adaptable and accessible over long distances and that can be formatted for multiple audiences and technologies. The best practices for electronic media identified in this chapter will prove valuable in meeting the challenges and fulfilling the needs of global health diplomacy.

Technologies such as the Internet, digital broadcasting, and wireless communication have the ability to cut across boundaries and borders in a way that the limited electronic media of the past could not. Older electronic media such as radio and TV were limited in their reach. In addition, program content was often difficult to adapt and did not allow for user interaction. User interaction is a new frontier, as we have seen with the proliferation of blogs, chat rooms, personal broadcasts and wikis, and community interaction on the Internet. This encourages collaboration on a wide spectrum of topics. Health communication will take notes from the business community, where such collaboration is key to expanding the reach of concepts and new ideas, and join the growing field of "wikinomics." Emerging electronic media have the ability to enhance global health diplomacy, as vital health communications can be directed to citizens of multiple countries in real time.

Across health disciplines and geographic locales, certain health communication practices have led to successful behavioral changes among target populations. New best practices are being identified that are specifically associated with new technological media. The combination of best practices identified in the past and the collection of the best practices that are currently being identified will help facilitate media landscaping campaigns in the future.

LESSONS FROM PAST EXPERIENCES

Some media landscaping best practices, such as the development of a multimedia approach, the use of local resources to orchestrate, promotion and delivery of health communication campaigns, and culturally relevant messaging, will be useful no matter what technology is chosen to implement the campaign. These are described below and are summarized in Table 14.1. These practices have laid the foundation for the way the Internet and other digital communication strategies will be developed to address major international health problems.

Population Services International's Condom Promotion Campaign in Rural Kenya

In 1972, Population Services International began a condom promotion campaign in rural Kenya using radio programs and ads (Black & Harvey, 1976). Population Services International wanted to take service-seeking behavior (in this case, the provision of contraception) outside the clinical setting and into the marketplace. The two goals of the intervention were to improve contraceptive knowledge and awareness and to demonstrate how local resources can be utilized to orchestrate, promote, and deliver a health communication campaign. An inexpensive brand of condom called Kinga was developed based on information from survey and interview data. Population Services International used a local marketing company to craft print advertisements and commercials promoting their condom brand and family planning in general to be run at local cinemas. An interactive radio program was aired once a week to answer questions concerning sex, family planning, and condom use. Over the course of the 12-month marketing campaign, 56% of targeted merchants had purchased Kinga condoms and 68% of consumers were aware of the brand.

The Population Services International intervention in Kenya stands as an early example of media landscaping, and its lessons have been utilized by successive generations of health communication campaigns. First, the messaging and materials being promoted were culturally appropriate. Extensive pretesting was conducted to gather the opinions and preferences of shopkeepers and consumers. Second, Population Services International planned ahead and prepared the market for their media landscaping message. Third, Population Services International worked with local agencies to pass along knowledge and ensure sustainability. Finally, the Kinga promotional campaign delivered specific knowledge regarding the price and quality of Kinga condoms, as well as a description, as opposed to messages promoting general family planning. Condom use increased among survey participants, but so did contraceptive knowledge and approval. These best practices have since

Table 14.1

OVERVIEW OF CASE STUDIES AND THE BEST PRACTICES THEY REPRESENT

CASE STUDY	BEST PRACTICES REPRESENTED	LOCATION
Kinga condom promotion campaign	■ Messaging and materials being promoted were culturally appropriate. ■ Extensive pretesting was conducted. ■ The market was prepared for the media landscaping message. ■ Local agencies were involved to pass along knowledge and ensure sustainability. ■ The campaign delivered specific knowledge regarding the price and description of a product, as well as a description of the product, rather than a general health message.	Rural Kenya
Bienvenida Salud	■ *Bienvenida Salud* broadcasts are self-contained and draw subject matter from listeners' letters. ■ The program material was both culturally relevant and created in conjunction with its listeners. ■ Traditional beliefs from the community are incorporated, and both community health workers and traditional shamans act as program advisors. ■ Characters and viewpoints on the program represent older male members of society, leading to a 30% male listenership. ■ Health communication initiatives touted on *Bienvenida Salud* are tied to health services. ■ Community health promoters go back to serve as behavioral models for peers.	Central Peru
Vaccine Day campaign	■ The media campaign was focused on a concentrated population with a high degree of radio and TV access. ■ Health facilities were prepared for an increase in demand ■ Clinics served as partners in the campaign. ■ Workshops and sales conferences we held with clinic workers to ensure buy-in and create partners in the campaign. ■ Specific knowledge (concerning age, location, and cost) was provided, illustrating the importance of behavior-specific messaging.	Philippines

been utilized in similar media landscaping campaigns and will continue to be used in the coming years.

Bienvenida Salud of Central Peru

The radio program *Bienvenida Salud* in Central Peru is another example of successful media landscaping fueled by audience participation and service delivery. The 800,000 residents of Loreto, a region of Central Peru, suffer from high rates of infant and maternal mortality, domestic violence, unsafe abortion, sexually transmitted infections, and poverty (Farrington, 2003). The area lacks paved roads, proper sanitation, and telephone access, but 81% of Loreto residents listen to radio programs and news broadcasts (Inter-American Development Bank, 2004). Eliana Elías founded Minga Peru in 1998 to improve the lives of women in the Peruvian Amazon native communities. Minga Peru's signature product is the radio program *Bienvenida Salud* ("Welcome Health"). *Bienvenida Salud* is broadcast three times a week and, unlike serial dramas, is self-contained and draws its subject matter from listeners' letters. These letters are turned into mini-dramas with educational themes that are performed by a cast of regular characters. Programs touch on the topics of reducing violence in the community, the importance of self-esteem, education for girls, the prevention of cholera, and much more. Over the past 8 years, the program has broadcast over 1,000 episodes, received 5,200 letters, and reached 50,000 listeners (Minga Peru, n.d.).

Bienvenida Salud demonstrates many best practices in the world of health communication. The program material not only is culturally relevant but is actually created in cooperation with its listeners. *Bienvenida Salud* incorporates traditional beliefs from the community and has both community health workers and traditional shamans acting as program advisors. Program listenership is 30% male, thanks in part to characters and viewpoints on the program that represent older male members of society. Health communication initiatives touted on *Bienvenida Salud* are also tied to health services. Some listeners have been chosen to become community health promoters. As an example of diffusion of innovation, these women go back to their communities to serve as behavioral models for their peers (Inter-American Development Bank, 2004). As a locally conceived and produced health communication initiative, *Bienvenida Salud* has a great deal to teach about best practices in the field of media landscaping. The program goes beyond making culturally relevant material and brings listeners into the creative process.

Vaccine Day Campaign in the Philippines

Hundreds of thousands of children die each year as a result of vaccine-preventable diseases. Vaccine delivery is often compromised by poor logistical knowledge on the part of consumers or poor vaccine supply resulting in missed vaccinations. In the Philippines in the late 1980s, vaccination rates among urban children were worse than those among rural children. The government developed a mass media campaign aimed at the mothers of vaccine-eligible children (Zimicki et al., 1994). Radio and television ownership rates among urban households were 73% and 63%, respectively, and 50% claimed to own both. The government created radio and TV ads, which urged mothers to vaccinate their children from the measles. These ads delivered information concerning the age of vaccine-eligible children (38–52 weeks), days on which vaccines could be obtained (every Wednesday), and the cost of vaccinations (free).

After a 7-month campaign, survey results revealed a substantial increase in vaccination rates and knowledge about vaccines. Survey results also revealed a high degree of knowledge concerning the vaccine awareness campaign. Over 70% of survey participants reported seeing an advertisement, could complete campaign slogans, and could recall specific information from the advertisements. Much of the success of the program was due to proper planning on the part of the Filipino government in conjunction with action-oriented messaging. The media campaign was focused on a concentrated population with a high degree of radio and TV access. This population also had easy access to health facilities, which were prepared for an increase in demand. Health communication campaigns must be tied to the direct provision of care, and the Filipino government ensured that their clinics served as partners in the campaign. The workshops and sales conferences held with clinic workers ensured their buy-in and made them active partners in the campaign.

The provision of specific, as opposed to general, knowledge played a large role in the campaign's success. Increased knowledge of the importance of vaccination does not necessarily correspond to service-seeking behavior. It was for this reason that campaign planners decided to provide specific knowledge (concerning age, location, and cost) in an effort to effect service-seeking behavior. Analysis of survey data conducted several years later found that it was service-specific media messaging, above and beyond interpersonal communication or other influences, that drove the service-seeking behavior (McDivitt, Zimicki, & Hornik,

1997). The Filipino Vaccine Day campaign illustrates the importance of advanced planning and behavior-specific messaging in a successful media landscaping campaign.

EMERGING TECHNOLOGIES

Taking the knowledge described above, future communication campaigns will try to address the persisting access barriers to information and communication technologies in many underserved populations, while moving toward more tailored and technology-specific programs. If computer-based technology is the most implemented new technology, the digital divide suffered by vulnerable and underserved populations in developing countries may translate into significant health care disparities. Although developing countries are increasing their use of technology, so are developed countries, and as a result, the divide continues to exist and perhaps widen (Sattelife, 2005). On the flip side, mass media campaigns allow for widespread but potentially incomplete education. A more tailored approach, as is possible with emerging technologies, allows for a more comprehensive learning experience that gives users the opportunity to fill in gaps in their knowledge or dispel myths. Following are some examples of international innovations in health communication utilizing emerging technology.

Scaled-Up Initiatives: Digital Broadcasting Initiative

The Digital Broadcasting Initiative (DBI) is a public–private alliance between USAID, UNDP, the World Bank, WorldSpace, Equal Access, and several Nepalese NGOs. The DBI sought to scale up the utility and popularity of radio media landscaping among the poor and marginalized through the use of emerging technologies (Digital Broadcasting Initiative, n.d.). Realizing that many of the poorest communities are too far from radio transmitters to receive targeted health communication messages, the initiative seeks to deliver these messages via digital satellite broadcasts to inexpensive hand-powered digital radios across Asia. Because the application is digital, it has the ability to stream data, video, audio, and more.

The DBI began an intervention in Nepal to overcome the barriers to communication presented by internal conflict, poverty, and terrain. Nepali-language programming was produced with local input and set to broadcast via satellite to a small number of these digital radios as an experiment in expanding access. The Nepali-language program, named *Aphnai Mato, Aphnai Bato* ("Our Land, Our Path"), would be provided in addition to English-language news and programming. Content for *Aphnai Mato* dealt with early childhood development, HIV/AIDS, human rights, conflict resolution, and safe migration education (for the increasing number of Nepali men who seek work outside Nepal). To date, 400 digital radio sets have been delivered to 400 rural communities, and content is rebroadcast over Radio Nepal and traditional FM stations. The Katmandu office is growing quickly and recruiting local talent to act as program developers and disc jockeys (Westberg, 2006).

Despite a number of logistical mistakes and setbacks, the DBI drew upon best practices in health communication when planning a media landscaping campaign with emerging technologies. Local buy-in was one important aspect of the DBI's program planning. The project worked in conjunction with the Nepali government to gain its input and blessing. Content development and outreach teams worked with local participants to create, produce, and market original programming. Content management sought to incorporate listener input in content development to ensure cultural relevancy while addressing the needs and concerns of the community (Digital Broadcasting Initiative, n.d.). The DBI also succeeded in sharing knowledge and skills with its in-country partners. Local production organizations have sprung up in the wake of the DBI and produce educational and entertaining content for broadcast through digital and FM broadcasters across Nepal. Many of the programs now produced through the DBI better reflect local concerns (such as hygiene, conflict resolution, and women's health issues), as the infrastructure has matured considerably (Westberg, 2006). In addition to these successes, the DBI identified concerns and problems associated with emerging communication technologies.

The DBI health communication intervention adds much to the body of knowledge concerning the upgrading of existing media landscaping with emerging technologies. First, the technical equipment itself poses certain problems. The digital radios, which are produced in India, were held up in customs, which delayed implementation of the program. The digital broadcasting equipment experienced technical glitches associated with inclement weather (Westberg, 2006). In addition, local program administrators of the DBI required training (albeit relatively simple training) in the technical aspects of the program in addition to the various health messages (Digital Broadcasting Initiative, n.d.).

Interventions with emerging communication technologies will require greater advanced planning dedicated to technological aspects of the program in addition to any service or messaging aspects.

Second, communication breakdowns within the DBI drove the program off focus. Because of outside pressures, the project was upgraded too quickly and content began to reflect what *could* be produced as opposed to what was *intended*. Many of DBI's health intervention targets (such as HIV/AIDS and childhood development) were determined by funding priorities, and the feedback channels broke down quickly, leading to very little audience participation in the beginning. Intra-program communication issues may pose particular problems for interventions utilizing emerging technologies because of the need for communication among technology, health, and marketing specialists.

Finally, the financial costs and benefits of emerging technologies cannot be ignored. The digital radios were over $100 each, and technological glitches added additional costs. However, there were cost savings associated with the use of digital broadcasting as well. The physical infrastructure associated with overland communications was eliminated, and much of the DBI equipment was solar or powered by a manually operated crank (Westberg, 2006). The DBI media landscaping experiment can be considered a success, no matter the outcome, because of the valuable lessons it teaches in regards to utilization of new technologies for health communication.

Responsive Messaging

The New Zealand Ministry of Health (2007) made use of emerging technologies to create an adaptive and comprehensive communications platform regarding avian influenza. As a new and potentially deadly communicable disease, avian influenza received extensive media coverage in 2005 and 2006. However, little media attention was given to instructions for preparedness or precautions, and the public was left with little service-oriented knowledge. The government of New Zealand began, in late 2005, to construct a multipronged response to avian influenza suited to actual threat levels and targeted at specific audiences. In addition to commercials, radio announcements, and surveillance activities, the Ministry of Health created a comprehensive Web site to host educational and service-oriented materials. Everything the Ministry of Health created and disseminated in response to avian influenza led back to its Web site, which served as a single portal for the government's information on the potential pandemic. The site provides information on threat levels and definitions and historical background for citizens, travelers, health professionals, and business owners. Links to relevant health care providers, first responders, government services, and hygiene tips are all included on the Web site as well.

The Internet allowed the New Zealand Ministry of Health to create an interactive and adaptive platform for disseminating avian influenza information. Section headings allow specific audiences to find the information and services most relevant to them. Users can also follow links to information on avian influenza for other countries and links to global organizations for tips on preventing the spread and infection of avian influenza. As a platform, the Internet allows for adaptation as the situation changes. The new and alarm-inducing nature of avian influenza almost guarantees that information regarding prevention and treatment best practices will change on a regular basis. Web sites, even more than print, radio, and TV, allow for adaptability and change in the face of new information and situational changes.

In addition to delivering adaptable content, the Ministry of Health's Web site delivers service-oriented information. Much of the information is geared toward specific actions that can be taken in specific situations. The tailored messaging allows for action-oriented instructions. Guidelines and advice for businesses, for example, include recommendations for ventilation control and air recirculation during an outbreak. The business section includes a planning guide for offices and health posters to prevent the transmission of airborne pathogens. Sections aimed at health care workers provide information on how to establish a community-based assessment center for rapid assessment and triage for at-risk populations. This section also includes training guides and exercises for clinic staff. The New Zealand Ministry of Health's Web site provides information aimed at a variety of groups, each of which will have its own distinct concerns and responsibilities in the event of an avian influenza outbreak. In addition, the Web site goes beyond information dissemination and provides tools and services to its users.

Women Connect! The Use of New Communication Technologies for Reproductive and Sexual Health Promotion

The 1994 International Conference on Population and Development in Cairo determined that women's empowerment is essential for sustainable development. The conference acknowledged that issues such as HIV/ AIDS, unintended pregnancy, and gender-based violence require the involvement of women's NGOs and other civil society organizations that have strong links with communities. In 2002, the International AIDS Conference in Barcelona concluded that the lower social position of women and their vulnerability in society contribute directly to the AIDS epidemic. Therefore, women's organizations that address these issues by educating the community and developing grassroots efforts to ensure the protection of women are deemed a good investment.

After the conference in Cairo, the pressing question within the international community was how to increase the dialogue among women about family planning and empower them to make decisions about contraception and other sexual health concerns. A multi-country evaluation conducted by the Pacific Institute for Women's Health and the Global Fund for Women found that women's NGOs have much direct and indirect positive impact in family planning and contraceptive use through well-targeted messages in their communication and outreach work. However, one of the limitations of many of the women's NGOs was that they were in need of technical assistance to improve efficacy. A 5-year initiative to support women's NGOs in developing countries called Women Connect! was created with the aim of improving health communication activities in order to enable the NGOs to be more effective in their impact in the community. Zimbabwe, Zambia, and Uganda participated in this program, but the lessons learned could apply to women's NGOs throughout Africa, Asia, and Latin America. The conceptual framework and design of Women Connect! is based on health from the perspective of a women's NGO, the use of information communication technology, and the need for women's organizations to use traditional media more appropriately.

The UN Economic Commission for Africa, which made NGOs' development of information communication technology capacity a top priority in 1999, emphasized the need for a more appropriate use of traditional media. In fact, most women in the developing world have less access to information technology than do men of the same economic level. Access and use of these technologies are directly linked to social and economic development; thus, it is important to guarantee that women in developing countries understand these technologies and have access to them. The technological limitations of women's NGOs in developing countries also present a barrier, as many of the resources available are not reaching those women in need.

The aim of the initiative was for women's NGOs not only to build information communication technology capacity but also to learn how to use modern media channels strategically in order to improve their impact in the community. Some activities developed to improve their skills in this area were training workshops and technical collaborations. Initially, 29 grants were given out to NGOs that rarely conducted research in order to assess perceptions and behaviors and to evaluate whether people understood the disseminated messages. During the implementation of these initial grants, 12 NGOS addressed these issues through community publications and by developing traditional media campaigns, conducting research, and repackaging information from the Internet for dissemination to low-literacy audiences and translating it into local languages. The other 17 NGOs focused on developing information communication technology capacities in order to increase the reach of health information and the access to technologies by women in these communities. Women's Internet cafés were created in Zimbabwe and Uganda to function as Internet learning centers. The Uganda Private Midwives Association developed a series of health tips from reliable Internet sources on antenatal care, safe motherhood, and infant nutrition and broadcast the tips via radio programs. Web site development was an important step for some of the women's NGOs. Pillsbury and Mayer (2005) found that there was great demand for up-to-date health information and interest in downloading and repackaging women's health information from the Internet. However, introducing new technology into an organization causes changes that place pressure on systems, relationships, communication, and management styles (Pillsbury & Mayer, 2005). Therefore women's NGOs engaged in advocacy and outreach should consider implementing well-researched campaigns using multiple forms of media.

Sattelife Handhelds for Health: Uganda Health Information Network

A collaborative project was launched by the Uganda Chartered HealthNet, AED-Sattelife, Makerere University Medical School, and Connectivity Africa of the International Development Research Center of Canada to expand access to health and medical information and support data collection and analysis through the use of PDAs connected via the local GSM cellular telephone network.

The project attempted to address the fact that although a rural area in Uganda might have a medical clinic, it is less likely that the clinic has access to information that may be necessary for diagnosis or treatment. There are few medical libraries in Uganda, and health workers lack the time to visit them (Sattelife, 2005). A PDA solves that problem by providing a virtual library that can be accessed anywhere and anytime. In addition, these handheld computers provide a mechanism for storing and transmitting information in a country where data collection is difficult to achieve.

Two years from the program's start, more than 120 remote facilities serving more than one million people who lack Internet access and even, possibly, electricity are able to send and receive regular transmissions of information. Uganda has one of the highest burdens of disease in the world and also some of the best cellular telephone coverage in Africa, which makes this project particularly relevant (Sattelife, 2005).

The cellular network was used for both information dissemination and data collection. There were regular broadcasts that provided health information from Sattelife's information services; continuing medical education and health updates on malaria, HIV/AIDS, and tuberculosis; and treatment updates. Field workers also used their PDAs to collect data for routine reporting. The project demonstrated cost effectiveness, contributed to increased compliance in disease surveillance, improved data quality at the point of collection, and allowed for a faster response to emerging situations. The project also allowed health workers access to information and materials without the need for travel to distant headquarters (Sattelife, 2005).

Though there were technical glitches, Uganda Health Information Network had success in creating an effective data network over a mobile telephone infrastructure. It was done in a way that was relatively affordable and sustainable. Uganda Health Information Network was able to combine the power of data collection with continuing medical education, providing information to health workers isolated in rural areas, and may ultimately be able to provide e-mail access via the PDA devices.

Future Trends: Audience Targeting

The Internet allows for sensitive health-related issues to be dealt with privately while opening the door for greater user interaction with health messages. A team consisting of Stanford media, marketing, and health specialists, has put together "Interactive Teaching AIDS" (2007), an HIV/AIDS educational tool aimed at the vulnerable population of those between the ages of 18 and 24 in India. The program is an animated doctor–patient scene addressing what HIV/AIDS actually is, how it works, how it is transmitted, and how to protect oneself from the disease. The educational message is aimed at Indian youths who may be too afraid or ashamed to seek information concerning HIV and its routes of transmission. The program can be delivered to computers and mobile devices to enhance privacy and is a stand-alone educational tool, meaning no human interaction is required. The program content focuses on the biological and clinical aspects of HIV/AIDS and largely avoids sensitive or embarrassing sexual issues. Users control the pace of the presentation and may follow links online to either delve deeper into the issue or find answers to lingering questions.

HIV/AIDS messaging is most often handled in India by mass media outlets, which allows for a widespread but incomplete education. This incomplete education can lead to misconceptions and rumors surrounding the HIV virus and how it is transmitted and create a stigma for those who are infected. "Interactive Teaching AIDS" allows for a more comprehensive learning experience that gives users the opportunity to fill in gaps in their knowledge or dispel myths.

"Interactive Teaching AIDS" makes good use of existing knowledge of best practices in health communication while harnessing the increasing power of the Internet as a communications tool. The program's format is appealing to users and is based upon extensive interviews and an institutional review board–approved study conducted in India. These findings indicated that users were most comfortable with information presented in a cartoon format (Technology, Health and Development, 2006). All content was created and tested to be specific to the target audience. There are "male" and "female" versions of the program with their own specific culturally understandable appearances and expressions, existing in several different languages. The visuals and teaching methods reflect institutional review board survey research findings and are meant to increase user comfort with the material being presented. Each section of the program was created with the help of feedback from students and other potential users.

One of the criticisms that can be made of "Interactive Teaching AIDS" is that it does not build local health communication capacity. There was no transfer of knowledge to in-country institutions, and besides a funding connection for a general Asian version with the South Korean government, no local partners were established (Technology,

Health and Development, 2006). This can be forgiven, however, because of the importance of the subject matter and what it teaches us about the use of emerging technologies for media landscaping.

Teaching modules produced for distribution over the Internet allow for greater diffusion, both geographically and technologically. While "Interactive Teaching AIDS" was originally created for Indian users, a general Asian version has been produced in conjunction with the South Korean government. At the same time, producers are currently working on culturally appropriate versions for Latin American and African audiences as well (Interactive Teaching AIDS, n.d.). Just as "Interactive Teaching AIDS" is not confined to the Indian subcontinent, nor is it confined to computers. The program could be delivered to consumers via a wide variety of electronic networked platforms. Cell phones, PDAs, and portable electronic music platforms such as iPods could download and run the program. "Interactive Teaching AIDS" program managers are currently working with Indian cell providers to make the educational tool available over cellular networks (Technology, Health and Development, 2006). Personal handheld electronics allow for the greatest degree of privacy for users and could change the way in which sensitive educational material is delivered to consumers. The program is worth watching as an example of a new project in emerging technology.

LIMITATIONS OF NEW TECHNOLOGY IN THE DEVELOPING WORLD

The term "e-health" is defined as the application of emerging information and communication technologies, such as the Internet, to improve population health (Eng, 2001). The use of new technologies has a major impact in the media landscape by addressing some of the limitations of traditional communication paradigms. E-health communication offers a unique environment where concepts of customization, interactivity, and mixed media can be successfully applied (Neuhauser & Kreps, 2003). E-health technologies could resolve long-standing global health problems through improved tailoring of information and the expansion of mixed media channels (Eng, 2004; Neuhauser & Kreps, 2003). And e-health technologies can extend the reach of programming already developed, as in the case of online broadcasting of radio interventions (Davis, 2005). In the last decade, computer-based technology has been the most implemented new technology (Suggs, 2006). Today, even telephone technology is dependent on computers, and other new technology applications that are computer based include CD-Roms, PDAs, Web sites, touch-screen computer kiosks, and customized software programs (Noar, 2006; Suggs, 2006).

But where does this innovation leave developing countries, where even if there is access to technology, its use is complicated by rampant illiteracy rates? At the United Nations World Summit on Information Society in 2005, leaders put forth a new level of commitment within the United Nations development agenda that specifically focused on the innovative use of computers, handheld devices, landline and wireless telephones, radio and television, and other technologies in order to address development goals and other challenges such as the improvement of health outcomes. There is evidence to support the idea that reducing access barriers to new technologies is not impossible, as shown by the success of mobile telephony in connecting those previously unconnected as well as the positive impact it has had in the development of telecommunications markets (United Nations Economic and Social Council, 2006). For instance, more than 60% of the increase in telephone access in 2005 happened in developing countries, where wireless phones now outnumber landline connections (Eng, 2004).

It is also worth noting that even if a technology is successfully introduced, it may not result in improved results. A recent example is a pilot study using SMS text messages to increase patients' compliance with TB medication regimens in South Africa. Though both the patients and health care workers liked the service and were able to use cellular technology, a significant number of patients interviewed were not using the service as instructed. As the study's authors put it, "This technology is not a silver bullet to solve the problem of patient adherence: it is all down to the way in which it is implemented" (Hüsler & Peters, 2005).

Despite the excitement surrounding the development of new technologies, it is important to recognize the invaluable role of old technology such as radio and television in promoting health in developing countries. Radio and television are still indispensable in regions like sub-Saharan Africa and the Maghreb, since these are still the main channels of communication that enable poor and marginalized populations to access information and dialogue (World Electronic Media Forum II, 2005). In 2005, Bourem Inaly, Lerneb, and Almoustarat in Mali were 3 of 14 communities that inaugurated new FM radio stations, for which USAID provided the equipment and technical training. For countries such as

Afghanistan, which has illiteracy rates reaching 70%, radio is essential for communication strategies to raise awareness about breast-feeding practices and other issues concerning maternal and child health. That is not to say that new technology cannot enhance older forms. In Mali, about 96% of the population receives information about the dangers of HIV/AIDS through the network of community radio stations. Mali has adopted innovative information communication technology applications such as geographic information systems software as part of the HIV/AIDS surveillance efforts in order to target HIV/AIDS high-risk areas, thus guaranteeing that radio messages on HIV/AIDS prevention reach these areas (USAID, 2004).

Wireless technologies can connect desktop computers to the Internet and provide communities that lack telephone lines with Internet connectivity. Mobile Internet devices target many of the barriers in developing countries, including the lack of convenient access points, lack of access in rural areas, the cost of the technology. Connectivity thus far has varied widely throughout the world. For instance, Ethiopia lacks any telephone infrastructure and has very few mobile subscribers. In contrast, although Madagascar has a poor communications infrastructure, it has experienced an increase in the number of wireless users (Maxfield, 2004).

In rural Bolivia, the introduction of these new technologies in the public health sector has lifted many access barriers to family planning and to reproductive health information and services (USAID, 2004). In addition, Martínez, Villaroel, Seoane, and del Pozo (2005) assert that computer-based systems integrated with a voice system have the potential to improve epidemiological surveillance, emergency management, consultations, and distance training of health professionals in isolated rural communities. Consequently, because of the common limitations between the communication networks in Latin America and those in other developing countries, conditions for success include the use of technology with low operational costs, a simple infrastructure, and low maintenance (Martínez et al., 2005).

CONCLUSION

Proven health communication best practices will continue to drive successful media landscaping initiatives with emerging technologies. Mass media landscaping, developed in 1962, has helped identify which initiatives have proven to work. New technologies will continue to take advantage of these proven techniques. New technologies, however, will run afoul of new pitfalls in the field of health communication. Greater investment in research and the development of emerging communications technology is necessary. It will be necessary to identify what still works, what will work, and what will no longer work when it comes to media landscaping with new technologies. At the same time, research and development must focus on linking these communication messages with health services. Whether or not these new media will lend themselves to more, less, or the same amount of service-seeking behavior is yet to be learned. Finally, utilizing these new technologies for media landscaping will only exacerbate the digital divide unless local capacity is seen as an essential element of health communication efforts. Fortunately, many of these new technologies are proving easier to upgrade than older variations (cellular technology is spreading at a much greater pace than its land-based precursor) and are overcoming the digital divide. Other technologies, however, demand a more conscious effort to expand to poorer, more isolated populations. This expansion not only will require added infrastructure but will also demand increased training to ensure that it is utilized and maintained at the local level.

Media landscaping interventions, developed in 1962, have identified a series of best practices for those utilizing electronic media as a means of health communication. Successful health communication campaigns:

- Produce culturally relevant material
- Involve local stakeholders and pass along valuable knowledge
- Provide specific knowledge rather than general knowledge to affect behavior
- Tie their programs to service delivery
- Engage in advanced planning

The interventions discussed in this chapter drew upon these elements, to varying degrees, in order to build successful media landscaping campaigns. Emerging electronic technologies have the potential to overcome the limitations of older means of communication. However, the lessons learned and best practices identified will continue to be as relevant tomorrow as they are today.

Successful media landscaping programs using emerging electronic media borrow from many of the best practices discussed in this chapter while identifying new areas of concern. In addition to the concerns of all media landscaping programs, emerging electronic media necessitate:

- Technological planning in addition to health and media planning
- Increased communication among multiple organizations (health, technology, and media partners)
- A recognition of both increased costs and cost-savings associated with new technologies
- Awareness of opportunities for greater diffusion of innovations
- Planning for integration in multiple platforms

Fittingly, the examples of media landscaping with emerging electronic media examined above identified both advantages and disadvantages associated with new technology. While nothing concrete may be identified from this small sample of media landscaping programs, the examples give an indication of both the new issues and the possible advantages that arise with emerging technologies.

REFERENCES

Black, T., & Harvey, P. (1976). A report on a contraceptive social marketing experiment in rural Kenya. *Studies in Family Planning, 7*(4), 101–108.

Davis, J. (1995). *Radio for development: discussion paper, exchange lunchtime discussion.* Retrieved February 2007, from http://www.healthcomms.org/comms/integ/ld-radio-oct05.html

Eng, T. R. (2001). *The eHealth landscape: A terrain map of emerging information and communication technologies in health and health care.* Princeton, NJ: Robert Wood Johnson Foundation. Retrieved April 29, 2007, from www.rwjf.org/publications/publicationsPdfs/eHealth.pdf.

Eng, T. R. (2004). Population health technologies: emerging innovations for the health of the public. *American Journal of Preventive Medicine, 26*(3), 237–242.

Digital Broadcasting Initiative. (n.d.). *Equal access.* Retrieved April 29, 2007, from http://www.equalaccess.org/programs/nepal/index.htm

Farrington, A. (2003). *"Family matters" in the Amazon.* Retrieved April 29, 2007, from http://www.fordfound.org/publications/ff_report/view_ff_report_detail.cfm?report_index = 451

Hüsler, J., & Peters, T. (2005). *Evaluation of the on cue compliance service pilot-testing the use of SMS reminders in the treatment of tuberculosis in Cape Town, South Africa.* Retrieved April 29, 2007, from http://www.bridges.org/cell_phones_and_handheld_devices

Inter-American Development Bank. (2004). *Listeners in the heart of the Amazon.* Retrieved April 29, 2007, from http://www.iadb.org/news/articledetail.cfm?artid = 2128&language = en&arttype = ws

Interactive Teaching AIDS. (n.d.). *Interactive Teaching AIDS*. Retrieved April 29, 2007, from http://www.stanford.edu/~sorcar/ita/index.html

Martínez, A., Villaroel, V., Seoane, J., & del Pozo, F. (2005). Analysis of information and communication needs in rural primary health care in developing countries. *IEEE Transactions of Information Technology in Biomedicine, 9*(1), 66–72.

Maxfield, A. (2004). Information and communication technologies for the developing world. *Health Communication Insights*. Baltimore: Health Communication Partnership based at Johns Hopkins Bloomberg School of Public Health / Center for Communication Programs.

McDivitt, J., Zimicki, S., & Hornik, R. (1997). Explaining the impact of a communication campaign to change vaccination knowledge and coverage in the Philippines. *Health Communication, 9*(2), 95–118.

Minga Peru. (n.d.). *Radio soap opera: Bienvenida Salud.* Retrieved April 29, 2007, from http://www.mingaperu.org/proyectos.htm

Neuhauser, L., & Kreps, G. (2003). Rethinking communication in the e-health era. *Journal Health Psychology, 8*(1), 7–23.

New Zealand Ministry of Health. (2007). *Pandemic influenza.* Retrieved April 29, 2007, from http://www.moh.govt.nz/pandemicinfluenza

Noar, S. M. (2006). A 10-year retrospective of research in health mass media campaigns: Where do we go from here? *Journal of Health Communication, 11*(1), 21–42.

Pillsbury, B., & Mayer, D. (2005). Women Connect! Strengthening communications to meet sexual and reproductive health challenges. *Journal of Health Communication, 10*(4), 361–371.

Sattelife. (2005). *Handhelds for health: Satellife's experiences in Africa and Asia.* Retrieved from http://www.healthnet.org/pdaprojects.php

Suggs, S. (2006). A 10-year retrospective of research in new technologies for health communication. *Journal of Health Communication, 11*(1), 61–74.

Technology, Health and Development. (2006). *HIV/AIDS awareness and prevention through animation-based curriculum: An interview with Piya Sorcar.* Retrieved April 29, 2007, from http://thdblog.wordpress.com/2006/12/26/hivaids-awareness-and-prevention-through-animation-based-curriculum/

UNAIDS. (2005). *Getting the message across: The mass media and the response to AIDS.* (UNAIDS Best Practice Collection No. UNAIDS/05.29E). Geneva, Switzerland: Author.

United Nations Development Program. (2006). *Human development report 2006.* New York: Author.

United Nations Economic and Social Council. (2006). *Substantiate session of 2006: Fourth annual report of the Information and Communication and Technologies Taskforce.* Geneva, Switzerland. Retrieved April 29, 2008, from http://www.unicttaskforce.org/perl/documents.pl?do = download;id = 968

USAID. (2004). *Information and communication technology for development: USAID's worldwide program* (USAID Publication No. PD-ABZ-702). Washington, DC: Author.

Westberg, G. (2006). Digital communication for development in Nepal: An evaluation of the Digital Broadcast Initiative. *Global Times.* Retrieved April 29, 2007, from http://webzone.k3.mah.se/projects/gt2/viewarticle.aspx?articleID=57&issueID = 5

World Electronic Media Forum II. (2005). *World electronic media forum.* Retrieved April 29, 2008, from http://www.abu.org.my/public/documents/english%2Epdf

Zimicki, S., Hornik, R. C., Verzosa, C. C., Hernandez, J. R., de Guzman, E., Dayrit, M., et al. (1994). Improving vaccination coverage in urban areas through a health communication campaign: The 1990 Philippine experience. *Bulletin of the World Health Organization, 17*(3), 409–422.

Connecting Cognate Fields: Health Communication and Biomedical Informatics

15

BRIAN K. HENSEL, SUZANNE A. BOREN, AND GLEN T. CAMERON

Collaboration between health communication and biomedical informatics is central to an exciting, cross-cutting future for new media research in health and health care. Health communication and biomedical informatics are both young fields that are "cognate" or fundamentally related in their shared interest in communication of information using technological channels. Here, we introduce each field to the other.

This chapter maps overlapping and related research interests and variables, identifying and illustrating with examples where these fields overlap as well as how each makes unique contributions. The chapter identifies benefits for each in the use of both together in the conduct of research. In these ways we support the call for a more systematic approach in interdisciplinary health services research (Aboelela et al., 2007). These objectives were accomplished through reviews of both bodies of literature for representative self-definitions and operational descriptions, as well as early intimations of what is possible when the fields coordinate effort. Collaboration is occurring; indeed, the National Cancer Institute has a Health Communication and Informatics Research Branch, which reflects the strength of knitting the two domains together to address challenging research and outreach questions. But greater opportunities exist, and growth in productive collaboration between respective scholars starts with a general understanding of the research foci of the other field. The chapter is written for audiences in both fields; thus both are defined and described in some detail. Biomedical informatics is defined and described first, then health communication, followed by a discussion of overlapping research foci with examples of collaborative opportunities.

BIOMEDICAL INFORMATICS

The umbrella label of biomedical informatics evolved from the earlier label of medical informatics in recognition of newer applications in biological sciences (Friedman et al., 2004; Greenes & Shortliffe, 1990). Biomedical informatics includes bioinformatics and medical informatics. For clarity, and because we view health communication's current overlap with each as different, medical informatics and bioinformatics are defined and described separately.

Medical Informatics

Greenes and Shortliffe (1990) define medical informatics as "the field concerned with the cognitive, information processing, and communication tasks of medical practice, education, and research, including the information science and technology to support these tasks" (p. 1115). They identify tasks (cognitive, information processing, communication), broad areas of application (medical practice, education, and research), the general tool (technology), and a primary component discipline (information science) of the field. Shortliffe, Perreault, Wiederhold, & Fagan, (2001) define it as "a field of study concerned with the broad range of issues in the management and use of biomedical information, including medical computing and the study of the nature of medical information" (p. 785). Here, the focus is broader than that of the previous tasks, and we see movement toward bioinformatics in its recognition of both biological and medical information. Another definition is deliberate in its inclusion of health care beyond medical care: "Medical informatics comprises the theoretical and practical aspects of information processing and communication, based on knowledge and experience derived from processes in medicine and health care" (van Bemmel, 1984, p. 175). J. van Bemmel and Musen (1998) include public health in their definition of medical informatics as "informatics applied to medicine, health care, and public health."

Harrison (1984) observed that the word "informatics" is used in the label biomedical informatics at least in part to "encompass [the] conglomerate of knowledge . . . [in] science, engineering, and technology" (pp. 939–940). Informatics, from the French term *informatique* (Greenes & Shortliffe, 1990),

> represents the conjunction of information science and information technology. It is the formal study of information, including its structure, properties, uses, and functions in society; the people who use it; and in particular the technologies developed to record, organize, store, retrieve, and disseminate it. (Reitz, 2004)

This definition identifies what about information is of interest to informatics (i.e., its structure, properties, uses, and functions), and how technologies of interest operate on information (they record, organize, store, retrieve, and disseminate it). Furthermore, it establishes that, in addition to information and technology, informatics is interested in human factors related to their use. According to another definition, informatics is "the science that studies the use and processing of data, information, and knowledge" (van Bemmel & Musen, 1998). Data are "simple facts," information is "an interpretation of data that relates or puts into some context individual data," and knowledge is "information that is true or correct, incorporated into a system of belief, and believed with good reason" (Patrick, 2005, p. 100). (The word "information" will be used generically in much of this chapter.)

Functions of Medical Informatics Technologies

Core functions that medical informatics applications fulfill for their users include information retrieval, decision support, patient monitoring, and image production (Shortliffe et al., 2001). Examples in a clinical context include retrieval of a patient's electronic medical record. Decision-support tools assist health professionals in clinical and managerial decisions and are based on the knowledge of experts in given domains (Musen, Shahar, & Shortliffe, 2001). Patient monitoring applications collect, display, store, and interpret physiological and other health data of patients in institutional settings such as hospitals (Gardner & Shbot, 2001) and even in the home (Demiris, 2005). In imaging informatics, radiological scans of patients use digital images and are used for diagnostic and interventional purposes. Examples of imaging informatics in an educational context include the Visible Human project, which renders digital photographs of human cadaver cross-sections into three-dimensional images (Greenes & Brinkley, 2001).

Component Sciences

Turley (1997) identifies three core component sciences of nursing informatics that are fundamental to other domains of medical informatics: information science, computer science, and cognitive science. She describes information science's central role in developing ontologies and taxonomies to organize information and knowledge. An ontology is "an explicit specification of a conceptualization" (Gruber, 1993, p. 199). Cognitive sciences assist in examining how information should be organized and displayed to best support the ways in which human users process and use it. Friedman and associates (2004) identify the following "basic informational and computing sciences" as important to biomedical informatics: computer science, information and telecommunications science, cognitive science, statistics, decision science, and management/organizational science. These largely mirror Turley's components, while making explicit the related disciplines of telecommunications, statistics, and decision sciences, and adding management/organizational science. This addition recognizes that the management, organization, and leadership of medical informatics' initiatives are crucial to their success (Brown, 2005). Li, Mitchell, Tian, and Rikli (1995) identify the "structure of medical informatics knowledge" as including medical or clinical domains, computer and systems theory, engineering equipment and methodology, and health services management.

Medical informatics must rely on multidisciplinary efforts to bring the necessary expertise to its questions and problems. Greenes and Shortliffe (1990) illustrate this with the doctoral thesis work of a physician student of theirs, the goal of which was to determine how empirical findings from the literature are used by expert anesthesiologists and how that knowledge could serve as the basis for a computerized anesthesiology advice system. This work, and the fields of expertise of members of the student's doctoral committee, involved the use of computer science, clinical medicine, biostatistics, and artificial intelligence.

Musen (2002) assists our understanding of the field in terms of its practical applications as well as what he sees as its uniqueness as a science. The field has contributed greatly in building what he labels artifacts, such as physician software systems. He recognizes the importance of research in the development, deployment, and evaluation of such artifacts and that "satisfying institutional requirements for clinical data management . . . provided the substrate for much of the seminal research in medical informatics" (p. 13). But Musen argues that medical informatics' uniqueness as a separate science lies in its capacity to develop ontologies and problem-solving methods necessary for representing knowledge and reasoning in medicine. He identifies the Medical Subject Headings hierarchy for indexing biomedical literature as an exemplar of ontology construction, and computational algorithms used in genetic sequencing (in bioinformatics) as an exemplar of problem-solving methods. He bases his argument in part on Blois's (1984) contention that the field of medicine is unique as an area of human endeavor in its vast hierarchy of information levels. Clinical knowledge depends on "understanding other knowledge that can be defined only at lower levels of abstraction (e.g., that of organismal biology), which in turn can be understood only in terms of knowledge that needs to be defined at still lower levels of abstraction (e.g, that of biochemistry), and so on" (Musen, 2002, pp. 14–15). Musen's arguments are important for understanding that medical informatics is about more than the artifacts it develops, and that much of its basic work is done "behind the curtain" of these visible technologies.

Application Domains

At its inception, some questioned labeling the field *medical* informatics because, although actually defined more broadly to include "all parts of the health care arena" (Stead, 1987 p. 14), it implied a discipline restricted to physician use and application. With a broader, more inclusive definition in mind, Figure 15.1 reproduces Shortliffe and Blois's (2001) conceptualization of the field, including its application domains.

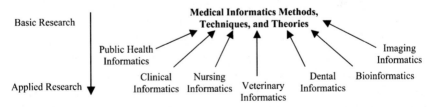

Figure 15.1 Application domains of medical informatics.

Note. From Figure 1.16 in *Medical Informatics: Computer Applications in Health Care and Biomedicine*, 2001, p. 29. With kind permission of Springer Science and Business Media.

Here, medical informatics is the umbrella science whose methods, techniques, and theories are applied to a number of domains, including veterinary and dental sciences. Each domain includes research, educational, and practical applications. Nursing and imaging informatics are ultimately focused on patient care and thus are included under clinical informatics in this chapter. Shortliffe and Blois (2001) include consumer health informatics under public health informatics. We view consumer health informatics (which is consumer driven) as fundamentally different from public health informatics (which is provider driven). In this chapter, clinical, public health, and consumer health informatics are defined and described, followed by bioinformatics.

Clinical Informatics. Clinical informatics is defined as "the application of medical informatics methods in the patient care domain" (Shortliffe et al., 2001, p. 756). Flow and use of electronic information have been predominately within individual health care systems and between providers and payers. Patients' access to their own electronic medical records has been limited (Kukafka, 2005).

Public Health Informatics. Public health informatics is "the application of information science and technology to public health practice and research" (Friede, Blum, & McDonald, 1995, p. 240). It is concerned with epidemiological surveillance of populations, with information gathered through disease registries (especially for cancers) and methods such as periodic surveys and special studies (Brennan & Friede, 2001). Public health informatics is also used in tracking environmental hazards to health, such as air pollution and chemical toxins (Brennan & Friede, 2001); supports public health departments in disease prevention (e.g., immunizations); and can be used in health promotion campaigns (e.g., Internet-based anti-smoking campaigns).

Consumer Health Informatics. Eysenbach (2000) defines consumer health informatics as "the branch of medical informatics that analyses consumers' needs for information; studies and implements methods of making information accessible to consumers; and models and integrates consumers' preferences into medical information systems" (p. 1713). The end user here is not the health care or public health provider; it is the health consumer and the consumer-patient as coproducer of his or her health care (Brennan & Friede, 2001). Information sources outside of clinical and public health informatics are included (e.g., mass media). In an Internet-based survey of members of the American Medical Informatics

Association, 65% of those who responded said that they would "somewhat" to "strongly" "recommend that consumer health informatics be considered a separate discipline within medical informatics" (Houston, Change, Brown, & Kukafka, 2001). To emphasize its consumer (versus provider) orientation, consumer health informatics may benefit from a broader label for its parent field, such as health informatics, a title preferred by some for its inclusiveness (Breslow, 1977).

Bioinformatics

Altman (2001) defines bioinformatics as "the study of how information is represented and transmitted in biological systems, starting at the molecular level" (p. 638). Bioinformatics "uses techniques from informatics, statistics, molecular biology, and high performance computing to obtain information about genomic or protein sequence data" (Mitchell, 2004). Research using new sources of information such as the GenBank database is "revolutionizing our understanding of human biology" (Altman, 2001, p. 639), with clinical informatics and bioinformatics situated "on a collision course as genomics data become used in patient care" (Mitchell, 2004).

HEALTH COMMUNICATION

Health communication is a subdiscipline of human communication. Berger and Chaffee (1987) describe the goal of human communication science as seeking "to understand the production, processing, and effects of symbol and signal systems by developing testable theories, containing lawful generalizations, that explain phenomenon associated with production, processing, and effects" (p. 17). They identify the basic phenomena of interest as the production, processing, and effects of information or messages. "Symbol or signal systems" can take multiple forms, including spoken and written words, nonverbal signals, images, and even physical objects. McQuail (1987) identifies specific acts that can occur in human communication processing, including sending, receiving, storing, and seeking information.

Human communication "occurs when a person responds to a message and assigns meaning to it" (Kreps & Thornton, 1992, p. 14). Communication can differ in its direction (one or two way) and in the timing of responses to it (immediate or synchronous, or delayed or asynchronous). Response may be direct and immediate, as with a patient's response in a face-to-face two-way conversation with his or her physician about diagnosis or prognosis, or indirect and delayed, as with the targeted population's attitudinal and behavioral responses to a one-way media campaign to reduce prevalence of smoking. Meaning is intended by senders of messages (at all levels, including mass media) in their encoding of information and is created by the receivers of messages in their decoding of information. "Meanings are in people. . . . They are in us, not in messages" (Berlo, 1960, p. 175).

Witte and associates (1996) define health communication as "the exchange, transmission, perception, and/or internalization of health-related information, within varying social and physical environments, regarding factors that influence health and/or health-related behaviors" (p. 230). This highlights health communication's central interest in health and health-related behaviors. Health communication is defined by the topic of communication—health or health care—and not by its participants, channel, level of analysis, or setting (except for organizational health communication, which by definition takes place in an organizational setting). It can take place between anyone, anywhere, via any channel.

Risk communication is also incorporated in health communication in that it involves phenomena that ultimately affect health (e.g., communicable diseases, natural disasters, environmental hazards, terrorism) (McComas, 2006).

Levels of Analysis

Human communication can be specified at five levels of analysis: intrapersonal, interpersonal, group, organizational, and mass communication (Berger & Chaffee, 1987; Kreps & Thornton, 1992). Intrapersonal communication "refers primarily to thinking" and is, more broadly speaking, "concerned mainly with the seeking out, reception, interpretation, and further processing of messages or signals from an environment of objects, events, and other people" (McQuail, 1987, p. 334). Interpersonal communication involves the dyad of two participants; small group communication involves three or more participants, up to a size that is reasonable for personal communication (Berger, 1996). Interpersonal communication—indeed any level of human communication—can include verbal and nonverbal information and messages (Burgoon & Hoobler, 2002). Organizational communication is defined as communication occurring within formal organizations and institutional networks

(McQuail, 1987). Finally, mass communication occurs at a societal level through print (e.g., newspapers, magazines, mass mailings) and electronic (e.g., radio, television, Internet) mass media, with the main types of content including news, entertainment, and advertising. With the Internet, a distinction is necessary between level of communication and level or type of channel or medium. The Internet may accurately be labeled a mass communication channel through which different levels of communication can occur (e.g., interpersonal e-mails, group or organizational Listservs, and Web sites aimed at and available to the mass public).

Functions of Human Communication

Although "much communication is either *purposeless* or an end in itself" (McQuail, 1987, p. 328), much communication—and certainly goal-driven health communication—has a function or purpose for its sender and/or receiver. McQuail offers a typology of psychological functions that spans levels of analysis and sender and receiver.

Examples of this typology include, at the intrapersonal level, the function of communication in reducing uncertainty for receivers (McQuail, 1987). Kreps and Thornton (1992) identify two dimensions of information or messages: the content level and the relationship level. Content information is the "basic, tangible information being presented in the message" (Kreps & Thornton, 1992, p. 23), and functions to reduce uncertainty about the object of communication. Cognitive-oriented content information informs receivers about the "facts" involved. An affective function identified by McQuail (1987) is expressing attachment or caring, which fits within Kreps and Thornton's relationship level of communication. Social functions at a group level include developing group consciousness and expressing group identity (McQuail, 1987). Examples of functions of communication at an organizational level include value formation and promoting solidarity, attachment, and integration (McQuail, 1987). Functions at a societal level include relaying information and connecting members (McQuail, 1987).

Related Disciplines

Communication is a social phenomenon, and as such, the field has been built upon other social sciences. The field emerged as a separate discipline with a strong initial focus on mass communication, including the effects of political propaganda and electoral campaigns (Delia, 1987; Kar, Alcalay, & Alex, 2001). Persuasion research remains a strong tradition within communication. The field began and remains strongly linked with social psychology and sociology, and, in political communication, with political science. The field has evolved to include foci at all levels of communication, including the intrapersonal or information-processing level, which has necessitated a strong link to the field of cognitive psychology. Health communication research includes a strong focus on behavioral effects, including their cognitive (e.g., knowledge) and affective (i.e., emotional and attitudinal) antecedents and the influence of social (e.g., norms) and even personal (e.g., personality) factors. This focus builds on theories of social psychology to explain the behavioral effects of health and health-related messages. Consistent with its social science roots, the field examines communication phenomena within their sociocultural context.

OVERLAPPING RESEARCH FOCI AND VARIABLES

Shannon's (1949) model of communication (Figure 15.2) and Weaver's application of it to human communication provide a useful framework within which to identify where and how respective research foci and variables overlap.

Shannon (1949) describes his model as one of "engineering communication" and stresses that the "semiotic aspects of communication are irrelevant to the engineering problem" (p. 3). Weaver (1949) cautions that Shannon's use of information "must not be confused with its ordinary usage . . . [i.e.,] with meaning" (p. 99). Engineering communication involves the encoding, transmission, and decoding of information in the form of binary digits (bits). It is concerned with what Weaver (1949) labels the "technical" problem of technology-mediated

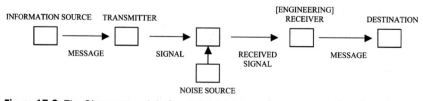

Figure 15.2 The Shannon model of communication.

Note. From *The Mathematical Theory of Communication* by Board of Trustees of the University of Illinois. Copyright 1949, 1998. Reprinted with permission of the University of Illinois Press.

communication: "How accurately can the symbols of communication be transmitted" (p. 4)? This is an engineering communication question addressed by computer science and engineering within biomedical informatics.

Weaver (1949) asks us to "imagine . . . another box labeled 'Semantic Receiver' interposed between the engineering receiver (which changes signals to messages) and the destination" (p. 115). In this way he helps us locate human communication (sending and receiving messages and their meanings) as separate from engineering communication (transmitting and receiving signals). If one views the transmitter and receiver boxes as representing a technology, these boxes and the central portion of the diagram between them describe engineering and computer science work in biomedical informatics. In health communication, such technologies represent channels for human communication.

Weaver focuses on message and on source and destination components. Human communication research, including that within biomedical informatics, focuses on semantic meaning in messages as intended by human sources or senders and as perceived by human destinations, which we will label receivers—not to be confused with the engineering receiver in Shannon's model. This exchange involves what Weaver (1949) labels the semantic problem of communication: "How precisely do the transmitted symbols convey the desired meaning" (p. 4)? This question is pursued by information science in biomedical informatics and cognitive sciences in both biomedical informatics and health communication. It is a question that can also benefit from health communication research on message creation.

Weaver (1949) is also interested in the effects of communication (the effectiveness problem): "How effectively does the received meaning affect conduct in the desired way?" (pp. 4–5). Of Weaver's three questions, this may benefit most from interdisciplinary research with health communication, given its application of multidimensional theories to explain behavioral effects of health-related messages.

Figure 15.3 summarizes overlapping (two middle segments) and separate (two outer segments) research interests, or foci, based on the selected definitions and descriptions and using Weaver's conceptualization of Shannon's model for dimensions of the framework. The figure illustrates a sociotechnical research continuum with the two fields at opposite poles. Its aim is to illustrate relative emphases between the fields in their overlap in human communication variables, not to argue for bright lines of division.

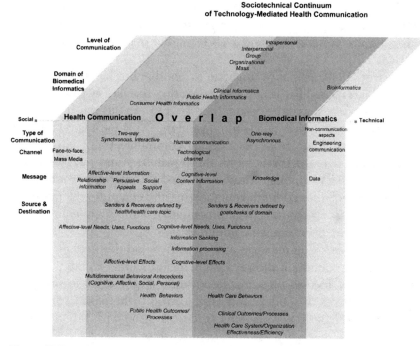

Figure 15.3 Overlapping research foci and variables.

Working down Figure 15.3, the fields overlap directly in research interests that span levels of communication and domains of biomedical informatics, with the exception of bioinformatics, where their overlap is clearly indirect. Bioinformatics is focused on basic biomedical research; its findings are then applied, via routes including technological channels, in clinical, public health, and consumer health settings. Consumer health informatics is positioned somewhat closer to the health communication pole because, as discussed below, neither restricts its research foci in terms of senders and receivers.

In terms of type of communication, there are, of course, noncommunication aspects of biomedical informatics, such as software and device engineering. Indeed, Musen (2002) argues that the distinguishing theoretical contributions of the field lie in the areas of ontologies that organize information and algorithms that act upon it, areas that could be thought of as "pre-communication" endeavors. Moreover, biomedical informatics includes engineering communication, which does not involve human communication.

However, the definitions and descriptions of biomedical informatics also include human communication. Health communication's overlap is in this aspect of biomedical informatics. More specifically, because biomedical informatics by definition includes technology, health communication's direct overlap is in human communication through technological channels such as the Internet, intranets, telemedicine and telehealth, and even telephonic applications. Health communication involves a greater relative focus on two-way synchronous interaction, whereas biomedical informatics includes a greater focus on one-way asynchronous transmission of information. In-person face-to-face communication and non-Internet-based mass media (i.e., television, radio, and print media) are channels unique to health communication. Nonetheless, health communication research that includes these channels contains related research questions that are important to biomedical informatics.

Identifying the overlap in message and source and destination is more difficult. Even so, the definitions and descriptions of biomedical informatics narrow communication variables in these dimensions to those that are of direct interest to it.

Health communication and biomedical research overlap in their interest in cognitive-level "content information" (Kreps & Thornton, 1992), or messages aimed at informing and functioning to reduce uncertainty in health-related decisions. This includes biomedical informatics' strong focus on knowledge. This orientation toward cognitive-level content is clearly the case in bioinformatics (e.g., advances in biological knowledge) and much of clinical informatics (e.g., diagnostic test results). It is also the case with most of the information in public health informatics (e.g., surveillance information) and much of it in consumer health informatics (e.g., information on quality of individual hospitals in HealthGrades.com).

The assertion that these fields overlap in cognitive-level content is also supported in that both include cognitive sciences as component or related disciplines. Biomedical informatics is more interested in how such content can be organized and represented via computer technology, while health communication is more interested in how to develop effective cognitive-level messages. The transmission of data is deemed of interest only to biomedical informatics because, unlike information and knowledge, data does not include context necessary for meaningful human communication. In addition, applications of biomedical informatics to data do not always include the goal of communication. For example, informatics is applied to genomic and proteomic data for molecular analysis and discovery.

In addition to cognitive-level information meant to inform, health communication is interested in affective-level information. This includes relationship information, as defined by Kreps and Thornton (1992), inherent in relational communication (e.g., between physician and patient). In addition, there is an affective dimension in persuasive communication (e.g., a public health campaign), where information is aimed at eliciting emotions and influencing attitudes toward a behavior (e.g., smoking). Social support may also be communicated in, for example, online health support groups.

With the exception of consumer health informatics, the range of senders and receivers in health communication research is broader. Senders and receivers in clinical, public health, and bioinformatics are determined largely by the goals and tasks of these domains and generally include health care providers, patients, public health departments, targeted populations, and biomedical scientists. Senders and receivers in health communication and consumer health informatics are defined by the topic—health or health care—and not restricted to a particular relationship or setting.

Both fields are interested in cognitive-level needs, uses, and functions (e.g., for decision making and to reduce uncertainty) with health communication additionally interested in affective-level needs, uses, and functions (e.g., for emotional support and to express attachment or caring). Information needs, uses, and functions in turn motivate information seeking, a research variable of overlapping interest.

Biomedical informatics and health communication share an interest in examining information processing using cognitive psychology and other cognitive science. Health communication makes an additional contribution in its interest in how a receiver's affect (including mood) influences information processing. A relevant example is the effect of a newly diagnosed cancer patient's fear on learning about the disease.

Consistent with other dimensions in the model, both fields share a research interest in effects at the cognitive level, such as learning. Health communication is additionally interested in affective-level effects such as emotions induced by the message or information. The selected definitions and descriptions distinguish health communication in describing and explaining effects within a multidimensional framework.

Indeed, applying multidimensional theories from social psychology and other social sciences to explain behavioral responses to information may represent health communication's most valuable relative contribution in its overlap with biomedical informatics. In the selected definitions and descriptions, biomedical informatics does not focus beyond cognitive antecedents of behavior. This implicitly assumes a rationalistic knowledge-attitude-behavior sequence, where "knowing better" leads to "better" behaviors, including decisions. This sequence may fit the provider task orientation in clinical informatics, although even here the less-than-universal adoption of clinical guidelines by physicians argues to the contrary. In response, some scholars from fields including psychology, medicine, nursing, and health communication formed an area of study called behavioral informatics to examine associated behavior within a broader theoretical framework (Houston, Bock, Bickmore, & Friedman, 2005).

Given biomedical informatics' strong focus on clinical applications, and health communication's roots in examining personal health behaviors with public health implications, health care behaviors and clinical outcomes/processes are viewed as relatively closer to biomedical informatics, and health behaviors and public health outcomes/processes are viewed as closer to health communication.

Health services research in biomedical informatics is interested in the effects of information technology on clinical effectiveness and economic efficiency, at system-wide and individual organization levels. Organizational communication scholars in health communication are interested in communication's role in these effects.

Focus on effectiveness and efficiencies of informatics applications—Musen's "artifacts"—makes evaluation research important in biomedical informatics. Health communication's interest is in applying sociobehavioral theory in explaining human use and response to these applications.

Identifying Opportunities for Collaboration

An understanding of biomedical informatics' application domains, health communication's levels of analysis, and Weaver's conceptualization of Shannon's model provides a framework within which to identify collaborative opportunities for health communication within biomedical informatics. Table 15.1 shows these dimensions in a matrix, with some examples.

To elaborate on several examples, one that clearly benefits from both the social sciences of health communication and the computing sciences of biomedical informatics is tailored messages. Health communication research has shown that messages that are tailored to an individual user's needs, preferences, and characteristics are more effectively used by the individual than non-tailored information (Kreuter & Skinner, 2000). Through the application of computing sciences, the needs, preferences,

COLLABORATION MATRIX WITH EXAMPLES

Table 15.1

	LEVEL OF COMMUNICATION	SOURCES ↔ RECEIVERS	CHANNELS	MESSAGE/ INFORMATION	RESEARCH PHENOMENA/ QUESTIONS
Bioinformatics	Mass	Journalists. Expert Sources ↔ General public	Mass media	Findings and implications of biomedical research	Effect on public opinion
	Organizational. Group, Interpersonal	Biomedical scientists ↔ Biomedical scientists	E-mail/other electronic forums. Face-to-Face (FTF)	Innovations, progress	Diffusion of innovation
Clinical Informatics	Organizational. Group	Organizational leadership ↔ Employees. Physicians. Other Stakeholders	E-mail/other electronic forums. FTF	Implementation information. Patient care and business function information	Implementation of clinical informatics systems
	Interpersonal	Providers ↔ Patients/Other Providers	E-mail/other electronic forums. FTF	Information about patient care and treatment, disease management, behavioral change	Differential effects of tailored messages

	Level	Participants	Channel	Content	Issues
Public Health Informatics	Mass	Public health agencies ↕ Public	Internet. Other mass media	Disease statistics. Environmental risks. Emergency response. Preventative interventions. Behavioral change campaigns	Emergency response to natural disasters or bioterrorism
	Organizational. Group	Public health agencies ↕ Public health agencies/ Health care providers	E-mail/other electronic forums. FTF	Inter-organizational efforts	Inter-organizational efforts between public health agencies and health care providers
Consumer Health Informatics	Mass	Information providers ↕ Consumers	Internet. Other mass media	Health and health care information	Effect on traditional doctor–patient relationship. Health literacy
	Group	Support group members	Online forums	Personal experiences, encouragement	Health-related virtual communities

Note: ↔ denotes two-way dialogue

and characteristics of individual patients or consumers can be organized, and algorithms developed, so that creation and dissemination of tailored messages to are automated. In clinical informatics, the personal information by which messages are tailored may someday come from the medical record. In Web-based consumer health applications, the user would provide the personal information necessary to individualize content.

Tailored communication provides an example of where the theoretical work of biomedical informaticians and health communication scholars can meet. Health communication theory can inform the content automated by underlying ontologies and algorithms.

Through consumer health informatics applications, including Web sites, health consumers have ready access to health and health care information beyond that of their personal physicians. Someday this will include electronic access for patients from home to their medical records. These changes raise health communication research questions about the effect of such applications on physician–patient interactions and on the traditional physician–patient relationship. Health consumers also have increasing access to provider-specific quality information. Sources, uses, and effects of such information represent another general area of overlapping research. At a societal level, effective use of these new information sources depends on the collective level of health literacy, which represents an area of overlapping cognitive-level research.

Health communication research interests also overlap with those of consumer health informatics in the study of Internet-based "virtual communities" formed in response to shared health problems and experiences. Eysenbach Powell, Englesakis, Rizo, and Stern (2004) call for additional research on peer-to-peer health-related virtual communities, including research on the affective outcomes of social support. Consumer health informatics views the broader area of Internet-mediated communication as a primary opportunity for interdisciplinary research, including health communication: "Understanding how such other disciplines conceive, operationalize and investigate how consumers use health and other sources of information on the Internet should facilitate the development of a coherent field, as long as common conceptual and methodological frameworks emerge" (Bakker, Ryce, Logan, Tse, & Hutcherson, 2005, pp. 24–25).

Before we close, some additional benefits in this collaboration should be noted. One is methodological. Informatics technologies allow an integration of study intervention and data collection. For example, typed responses to Web-based interventions can be captured in real time.

Handheld technologies allow real-time responses to communication interventions transmitted to them or to other everyday real-world phenomena. The methodology of real-time data capture represents an exciting new area of research (Stone, Shiffman, Atienza, & Nebeling, 2007). These new approaches have obvious potential to improve ecological validity in research.

Much of biomedical informatics research takes place in organizations that provide health care and public health services. As we have already argued, this research benefits from the multidimensional and contextual approach of health communication in analyzing human communication aspects. A reciprocal benefit to health communication is facilitated access to research data and opportunities in these patient care and public health organizations.

SUMMARY AND IMPLICATIONS

The fields share a focus on cognitive-level information aimed at informing, including its uses and functions, and on cognitive-level effects such as learning. Health communication contributes an additional focus on the affective dimension of information and the multidimensional antecedents of behavior. Identifying where and how foci of these fields fit together should assist in fruitful collaboration in overlapping and related research.

REFERENCES

Aboelela, S. W., Larson, E., Bakken, S., Carrasquillo, O., Formicoloa, A., Glied, S. A., et al. (2007). Defining interdisciplinary research: Conclusions from a critical review of the literature. *Health Services Research, 42*(1, Part 1), 329–346.

Altman, R. B. (2001). Bioinformatics. In E. H. Shortliffe & L. E. Perrault (Eds.), *Medical informatics: Computer applications in health care and biomedicine* (2nd ed., pp. 638–660). New York: Springer-Verlag.

Bakker, T., Ryce, A., Logan, R., Tse, T., & Hutcherson, L. (2005). *A consumer health informatics (CHI) toolbox: Challenges and implications.* Paper presented at the American Medical Informatics Association symposium.

Berger, C. R. (1996). Interpersonal communication. In M. B. Salwen & D. W. Stacks (Eds.), *An integrated approach to communication theory and research* (pp. 277–296). Mahwah, NJ: Lawrence Erlbaum.

Berger, C. R., & Chaffee, S. H. (1987). The study of communication as a science. In C. R. Berger & S. H. Chaffee (Eds.), *Handbook of communication science* (pp. 15–19). Newbury Park, CA: Sage.

Berlo, D. K. (1960). *The process of communication.* New York: Holt, Rinehart and Winston.

Blois, M. (1984). *Information and medicine.* Berkeley: University of California Press.

Brennan, P. F., & Friede, A. (2001). Public health and consumer uses of health information: Education, research, policy, prevention, and quality assurance. In E. H. Shortliffe & L. E. Perrault (Eds.), *Medical informatics: Computer applications in health care and biomedicine* (2nd ed., pp. 397–420). New York: Springer-Verlag.

Breslow, L. (1977). *Health care versus medical care: Implications for data handling.* Paper presented at international symposium, London.

Brown, G. D. (2005). The role of information technology in transforming health systems. In G. D. Brown, T. T. Stone, & T. B. Patrick (Eds.), *Strategic management of information systems in healthcare* (pp. 1–24). Chicago: Health Administration Press.

Burgoon, J. K., & Hoobler, G. D. (2002). Nonverbal signals. In M. L. Knapp & J. A. Daly (Eds.), *Handbook of interpersonal communication* (3rd ed., pp. 24–299). Thousand Oaks, CA: Sage Publications,.

Delia, J. G. (1987). Communication research: A history. In C. R. Berger & S. H. Chaffee (Eds.), *Handbook of communication science* (pp. 20–98). Newbury Park, CA: Sage.

Demiris, G. (2005). E-health and consumer informatics. In G. D. Brown, T. T. Stone, & T. B. Patrick (Eds.), *Strategic management of information systems in healthcare* (pp. 149–170). Chicago: Health Administration Press.

Eysenbach, G. (2000). Recent advances: Consumer health informatics. *British Medical Journal, 320,* 1713–1716.

Eysenbach, G., Powell, J., Englesakis, M., Rizo, C., & Stern, A. (2004). Health related virtual communities and electronic support groups: Systematic review of the effects of online peer to peer interactions. *British Medical Journal, 328,* 1166—1172.

Friede, A., Blum, H. L., & McDonald, M. (1995). Public health informatics: How information-age technology can strengthen public health. *Annual Review of Public Health, 16,* 239–252.

Friedman, C. P., Altman, R. B., Kohane, I. S., McCormick, K. A., Miller, P. L., Ozbolt, J. G., et al. (2004). Training the next generation of informaticians: The impact of "BISTI" and bioinformatics—a report from the American College of Medical Informatics. *Journal of the American Medical Informatics Association, 11*(3), 167–172.

Gardner, R. M., & Shbot, M. M. (2001). Patient-monitoring systems. In E. H. Shortliffe, L. E. Perrault, G. Wiederhold, & L. M. Fagan (Eds.), *Medical informatics: Computer applications in health care and biomedicine* (2nd ed., pp. 443–484). New York: Springer-Verlag.

Greenes, R. A., & Brinkley, J. F. (2001). Imaging systems. In E. H. Shortliffe, L. E. Perrault, G. Wiederhold, & L. M. Fagan (Eds.), *Medical informatics: Computer applications in health care and biomedicine* (2nd ed., pp. 485–538). New York: Springer-Verlag.

Greenes, R. A., & Shortliffe, E. H. (1990). Medical informatics: An emerging academic discipline and institutional priority. *Journal of the American Medical Association, 263*(8), 1114–1120.

Gruber, T. (1993). A translational approach to portable ontologies. *Knowledge Acquisition, 5*(2), 199–220.

Harrison, A. (1984). Common elements and interconnections. *Science, 224,* 939–940.

Houston, T. K., Change, B. L., Brown, S., & Kukafka, R. (2001). *Consumer health informatics: A consensus description and commentary from American Medical Informatics*

Association members. Paper presented at the American Medical Informatics Association symposium.

Houston, T. K., Bock, B., Bickmore, T. W., & Friedman, R. H. (2005). *What is behavioral informatics?* Presentation at the Society of Behavioral Medicine annual meeting, Boston.

Kar, S. B., Alcalay, R., & Alex, S. (2001). The evolution of health communication in the United States. In S. B. Kar, R. Alcalay, & S. Alex (Eds.), *Health communication: A multicultural perspective* (pp. 45–78). Thousand Oaks, CA: Sage.

Kreps, G. L., & Thornton, B. C. (1992). *Health communication: Theory & practice* (2nd ed.). Prospect Heights, IL: Waveland Press.

Kreuter, M., & Skinner, C. (2000). Tailoring—what's in a name? *Health Education Research, 15*(1), 1.

Kukafka, R. (2005). Public health informatics: The nature of the field and relevance to health promotion practice. *Health Promotion Practice, 6*(1), 23–28.

Li, Z., Mitchell, J., Tian, A., & Rikli, A. (1995). *On the foundation and structure of medical informatics.* Paper presented at the MEDINFO 95: Eight World Congress on Medical Informatics.

McComas, K. A. (2006). Defining moments in risk communication research: 1996–2005. *Journal of Health Communication, 11,* 75–91.

McQuail, D. (1987). Functions of communication: A nonfunctionalist overview. In C. R. Berger & S. H. Chaffee (Eds.), *Handbook of communication science* (pp. 327–349). Newbury Park, CA: Sage.

Mitchell, J. (2004). *What is bioinformatics?* Presentation at University of Missouri–Columbia.

Musen, M. A., Shahar, Y., & Shortliffe, E. H. (2001). Clinical decision-support systems. In E. H. Shortliffe, L. E. Perrault, G. Wiederhold, & L. M. Fagan (Eds.), *Medical informatics: Computer applications in health care and biomedicine* (2nd ed., pp. 573–609). New York: Springer-Verlag.

Musen, M. (2002). Medical informatics: Searching for underlying components. *Methods of Information in Medicine, 41*(1), 12–19.

Patrick, T. B. (2005). Managing data, information, and knowledge. In G. D. Brown, T. T. Stone, & T. B. Patrick (Eds.), *Strategic management of information systems in healthcare* (pp. 99–118). Chicago: Health Administration Press.

Reitz, J. M. (2004). *Online dictionary for library and information science.* Retrieved March 31, 2006, from http://lu.com/odlis/odlis_f.cfm

Shannon, C. E. (1949). The mathematical theory of communication. In C. E. Shannon & W. Weaver (Eds.), *The mathematical theory of communication* (pp. 3–91). Urbana: University of Illinois Press.

Shortliffe, E. H., & Blois, M. S. (2001). The computer meets medicine and biology: Emergence of a discipline. In E. H. Shortliffe, L. E. Perrault, G. Wiederhold, & L. M. Fagan (Eds.), *Medical informatics: Computer applications in health care and biomedicine* (2nd ed., pp. 3–40). New York: Springer-Verlag.

Shortliffe, E. H., Perreault, L. E., Wiederhold, G., & Fagan, L. M. (Eds.). (2001). *Medical informatics: Computer applications in health care and biomedicine* (2nd ed.). New York: Springer-Verlag.

Stead, W. (1987). What is medical informatics? *MD Computing, 4*(14).

Stone, A. A., Shiffman, S., Atienza, A. A., & Nebeling, L. (Eds.). (2007). *The science of real-time data capture: Self reports in health research*. New York: Oxford University Press.

Turley, J. (1997). Developing informatics as a discipline. *Nursing Informatics, 46*, 69–74.

Weaver, W. (1949). Recent contributions to the mathematical theory of communication. In C. E. Shannon & W. Weaver (Eds.), *The mathematical theory of communication* (pp. 95–117). Urbana: University of Illinois Press.

Witte, K., Meyer, G., Bidol, H., Casey, M., Kopfman, J., Maduschke, K., et al. (1996). Bringing order to chaos: Communication and health. *Communication Studies, 47*, 229–242.

van Bemmel, J. (1984). The structure of medical informatics. *Medical Informatics, 9*, 175–180.

van Bemmel, J., & Musen, M. (1998). *Handbook of medical informatics*. Glossary. Retrieved March 31, 2006, from http://www.mieur.nl/mihandbook/r_3_2/handbook/homepage_self.htm

16

New Media: A Third Force in Health Care

KRISTOFER J. HAGGLUND, CHERYL L. SHIGAKI, AND JORDAN G. MCCALL

Digital and electronic media applications are dramatically changing the way Americans do business and enjoy leisure activities. New media and health information technology have been affecting public health and health care more slowly than other areas but can be expected to eventually revolutionize the nature of health service delivery in the United States. The rapid appearance of digital technologies also brings unprecedented challenges in all aspects of health care. Physicians and other health care providers are faced with increasing demands for nontraditional methods of communication and alternative modes of providing care. At the same time, health care systems are stretching to find new ways of providing care to patients who have limited English proficiency, poor health literacy, and limited electronic communication access and skills (see Chapters 3 and 11). Federal and state governments will be challenged to replace outdated health and technology regulations and systems with new laws and policies that allow for innovation in service delivery while protecting patients' safety, privacy, and financial resources.

The United States is unique in that it is the only developed nation to have maintained a health care system involving both the private and public sectors in substantial proportions. Because of the dynamic interplay and inconsistent integration of these two sectors, health care delivery in the United States has been labeled a non-system. For example, a significant percentage of full-time workers and the majority of part-time workers are not offered health insurance and also are not eligible for a social insurance program (e.g., Medicaid). As another example, many health systems are now using electronic health records, but these systems are developed by different vendors and are often incompatible with each other. The consequence is that patients' electronic health records are often only useful if the patient remains in one health care system.

The negative consequences of the U.S. health care non-system include the fact that a high proportion of the population lacks health insurance or is underinsured, as well as accelerating overall health care costs and health care service quality that varies significantly by payment system and geographical region. The positive outcomes of this structure include a well-respected health professions training system, major innovations in health care treatments, and rapid diagnostic and treatment technologic development.

Although the public and private sectors are the two major forces that have historically driven the U.S. health care system, the new media are rising as a third force. Digital and electronic media are rapidly and dramatically changing how people access and utilize information, including information about health and health care. Emerging trends at the interface of digital and electronic media applications and health care delivery include:

- **Multiple formats for obtaining information.** Information in traditional formats (e.g., newspapers, television) are already being augmented or replaced by Web sites, e-mail, and podcasting.
- **Immediacy of information.** The digital and electronic media provide immediate information. In addition, consumers control the extent and timing of the information obtained.
- **Customized programming.** Consumers are able to use digital and electronic media to control the topic, source, and format of the information in the way they most prefer to receive it.
- **Exponential increases in sources.** The number of digital media sources about health and health care is expanding. These sources vary dramatically in their accuracy (a concern for many health care professionals).

It is difficult to foresee the full extent to which the digital and electronic media will affect health care providers, patients, government programs, and the economy. Whether national policy will guide or react to these changes remains a significant question. Market forces are both powerful and nimble, but policy has historically mirrored or followed societal change.

This chapter will review four major health policy issues and how they are being affected by digital and electronic media: health care access, health care quality, health literacy, and the aging of America. The chapter will discuss how health policy might respond as the business of health care struggles to assimilate new modes of communications and service delivery.

ACCESS TO HEALTH CARE

The most pressing bipartisan concern in health care today is the staggering number of individuals who are unable to afford needed health care services. Approximately 48 million Americans have no health insurance, and millions more are underinsured. Debates on how to reduce these numbers have persisted for decades. The American public has rated access to health care as a high priority in polls over the years (NPR/Kaiser Family Foundation /Harvard Kennedy School of Government, 2002), but no consensus has been reached on how to address this challenge. In addition, many of the 59 million Americans living in rural and frontier areas experience geographic burdens and barriers to receiving timely, high-quality care (U.S. Census Bureau, 2000a).

Additionally, more than half (56%) of all U.S. farm workers perform migrant work that requires them to travel or relocate more than 75 miles each year (U.S. Department of Labor, 2000). A large-scale overhaul of the U.S. health care system to guarantee health care access to all Americans remains unlikely. Incremental changes, such as tax credit approaches, may reduce the number of people who lack insurance somewhat but will still leave millions without access to appropriate, affordable health care (Fuchs & Emanuel, 2005).

If digital and electronic media technologies become a first-line source of health information, they will ease the challenges facing the uninsured and/or others who experience difficulty accessing health care services. Telehealth, for example, has demonstrated success in crossing geographic barriers to health care. Digital and electronic media may involve Web interfaces (e.g., WebMD) that allow consumers to find and interact with information about common, uncomplicated, and easily treated medical conditions (e.g., sore throats, colds).

Interactive Health Information Applications

Widespread adoption of digital interfaces will help facilitate safe and effective self-care management because of the ease of incorporating multiple communication modes and links. Information may translate into different languages, include audio and visual features to facilitate understanding, and direct patients to available in-person resources. It is possible that health care kiosks with interactive media will be available in public places, including schools, public libraries, pharmacies, and shopping centers, providing consumer-patients with access to health information, diagnoses, and treatments. City, county, and state health departments may use such interactive media to promote services such as influenza immunizations and other vaccines, sexual health services, and healthy life promotion. This type of health information and treatment station might come in a variety of formats and function much in the way that ATMs are available for banking services. Digital and electronic media will not provide what is traditionally considered health care or have a significant impact on the barriers to care for the uninsured. It will, however, provide cost-effective basic health and health care resources to those who have little access to such information.

Despite the promises of innovation, however, there is an incompatibility between the goals of market-based digital and electronic media products and the health needs of many consumer-patients, especially vulnerable populations and those living in rural areas. Digital and electronic media products are quickly being adopted and even demanded by consumers accustomed to instant information and entertainment, novelty, and stimulation. New product development is notoriously driven by high-end users, with emphasis on multiple formats, graphics, and ever-increasing speed (e.g., Stamm, 2004). Attention must be refocused on inclusion and "universal design" to meet the needs of those with low literacy, low incomes, and inability to access broadband networks.

Improved access is needed for those living in rural and frontier areas and those living in dense and impoverished urban areas. Much of the digital and electronic media has yet to reach these vulnerable populations because of the cost of needed devices (personal computers, MP3 players, high-end cellular telephones, etc.) and because broadband connections are unavailable. Most rural areas in the United States use dial-up Internet services that have such limited bandwidth that most audio and video/animation applications cannot be accessed.

A call for government-supported broadband expansion is gathering interest. Atkinson (2007) argues that the intervention of the federal government for widespread access to broadband is similar to that of the Rural Electric Administration of the 1930s. This government program brought electricity to nearly all Americans despite arguments against such expansion. Atkinson argues that universal broadband is too important to leave to market forces. Its positive applications to health and health care support his argument. For example, universal access would allow for a significant increase in telehealth services. In addition, insurers, health care providers, and health care systems would have dramatically improved ability to reach consumers and patients, and vice versa.

Public Telehealth

Telehealth care grew dramatically in the 1990s (Brear, 2006). In its best form, telehealth allows health providers to deliver care in synchronous audio/visual formats to patients who are geographically isolated or are unable to travel to the providers' health care institutions. The larger telehealth umbrella also includes low-technology modes, such as individual telephone contacts, teleconferencing among multiple providers/consumers, and asynchronously transmitted health information (e.g., radiological images). Telehealth is particularly useful for allowing providers and patients to access specialists who practice only in larger urban areas and academic health centers. In addition, continuing medical education and other health care related education, research, and business are often conducted via telehealth networks.

Telehealth is most often used by patient–provider dyads. As such, it provides a remarkable opportunity to increase patients' reach to services. In this private format, however, telehealth fails to maximize its technological potential. Public applications, where a provider interacts with multiple individuals, could greatly expand access to critical information among patients and facilitate public health initiatives by improving access to preventive health information. For example, a diabetes health team from an academic health center could work with local libraries or senior centers to provide education about nutrition, exercise, blood glucose testing, and weight management. Public telehealth could be extended to such interventions as group motivational enhancement therapy to improve adherence to treatment regimens and health promotion, or to promote basic services such as community information about immunizations. Telehealth will be extremely valuable in facilitating communication and the provision of vital information in the event of a natural disaster or an infectious pandemic. In such cases, rapid and accurate communication among governmental agencies and health care providers is critical to the protection of the health of the public.

Prior to substantial expansion of telehealth, whether it is being used in provider–patient dyads or public format, several legal-regulatory issues need to be addressed. Specifically, the provision of health care across state lines via telehealth is a violation of professional practice acts for most states (Rogers, 2006; Stanberry, 2006). In recent years, there has been substantial legislative action at the state level aimed at overcoming licensure barriers to care based on jurisdiction (U.S. Department of Health and Human Services, 2003). Other barriers must also be addressed, including the legal liability of health care providers/educators working remotely (Akalu, Rossos, & Chan, 2006; Stanberry, 2006) and duties of maintaining privacy and confidentiality (Stanberry, 2006). The duty to maintain patients' privacy is complicated by remote care, or education provided in a group format where individuals may not be acknowledged but are listening and/or watching the participants.

Providers and policy makers will need to address the standard of care for group telehealth. As Akalu and associates (2006) point out, there are tradeoffs associated with telehealth services. Health care and health education provided remotely to individuals and groups are unlikely to be as powerful as face-to-face encounters. But without telehealth access, health care and education may not be provided at all. Legislative and regulatory changes are being undertaken but are unlikely to keep pace with the technologic opportunities to expand access to health care and education.

Additionally, while Medicare has established telehealth reimbursement schedules, many Medicaid programs have not fully embraced reimbursement for health care services provided via telehealth, despite evidence that it is cost efficient (Gray, Stamm, Toevs, Reischl, & Yarrington, 2006). Most providers would be unwilling to offer continuing services without means for adequate reimbursement. For public telehealth, issues of privacy stemming from HIPAA provisions may have to be addressed if multiple telehealth sites are linked at one time. These and other policy issues are likely to have a negative impact on progress in developing adequate nationwide telehealth infrastructure.

Protecting Privacy

The opportunities for digital and electronic media applications to expand access to health care come with additional liabilities. Many of these have been noted above, but protecting privacy in health is essential. Effective privacy protections have been obtained in other sectors of the economy, however, including banking. The establishment of universal health cards with PINs to allow patient-consumers to participate in a variety of digital and electronic media health care services and maintain their privacy is feasible. Current laws may not be sufficient to allow for this type of sweeping change, however, and may need to be changed.

Insurance-Based Digital and Electronic Media

Employer-sponsored health insurance provides health care coverage for approximately half of the nation's citizens (DeNavas-Walt, Proctor, & Smith, 2007). Employers and their insurance providers are realizing the value of digital and electronic media tools to promote and maintain the health of employees. Nearly all major health insurance companies provide electronic access to benefit summaries, claims histories, provider networks, and other basic information. Many are also using digital and electronic media tools, including e-mail and Web site downloads, to offer additional services such as health promotion programs (e.g., smoking cessation, exercise guidelines, health screening reminders). E-mail approaches appear to be successful, at least to the point that employees open health promotional e-mails (Franklin, Rosenbaum, Carey, & Roizen, 2006). Insurance companies are providing information to health care providers about evidence-based practices, available treatment resources, common claims submission errors, and the like (Business Wire, 2007). Similar actions are occurring at the state level with the introduction of electronic health monitoring by patient–provider partnerships. In at least one state, providers are being compensated through Medicaid for the ongoing electronic communication with patients of chronic diseases (Missouri Department of Social Services, 2007).

More controversially, health insurers may use digital and electronic media and/or health information technology to track the health of those they insure, and to intervene to prevent future problems and/or promote health. As of April 2008, Japan requires its health insurers to maintain annual checkups on their beneficiaries (Okomato, 2007). While they are intended to combat chronic disease states, such actions potentially violate beneficiaries' freedom to choose their own behaviors. For example, beneficiaries who choose to smoke or overeat may perceive their individual rights and privacy are being violated if these behaviors are monitored. Outcomes from this reform will certainly play a role in the global approach to chronic disease management.

HEALTH CARE QUALITY

Improving health care quality has been an elusive goal for the U.S. health care system. The largest barrier to improved quality is the complexity of the health care system, especially the discontinuities in financing, payment, and delivery systems created by a dual private-public system. The Institute of Medicine's seminal report *To Err Is Human* (2000) noted that health care errors cause approximately 98,000 deaths each year. The Institute of Medicine's later report, *Crossing the Quality Chasm* (2001), emphasized the importance of inter-organizational cooperation and health system redesign to improve the quality of care. The six goals articulated in this report include making the health care system safe, effective, patient-centered, timely, efficient, and equitable. To obtain these goals, the Institute of Medicine recommended a redesign of health care processes that would be augmented by digital applications. For example, the Institute of Medicine recommended that the patient be seen as "the source of control" and that patients should have "unfettered access to their own medical information and to clinical knowledge."

Consumer-Patient Access to Electronic Health Records

Already, consumer-patients are using digital and electronic media applications, including health-oriented Web sites, blogs, and podcasts to gather information about their health in general and about potential diagnoses and treatments for symptoms in particular. They are also using digital and electronic media to maintain their own health care history. The health care industry has yet to fully embrace the Institute of Medicine's quality recommendations and the digital and electronic media applications that would facilitate the achievement of these recommendations. It is likely that the consumer-patient demand for digital and electronic media will drive changes among health care systems and providers. Consumer-patients are already demanding increased convenience, information, and transparency around health service transaction. Digital and electronic media will be needed to meet these demands.

Adoption of universal electronic health records would profoundly reduce the number of health care errors by improving diagnostic accuracy, reducing unnecessary repetition of lab and other diagnostic tests, reducing administration of contraindicated medications and interventions, and increasing individualized treatments (Kizer, 2007; Menachemi & Brooks, 2006). Electronic health records will be enhanced in that they will allow consumer–patients access to their health records, as recommended by the Institute of Medicine. In addition, using digital and electronic media applications, consumers should be allowed to add to their health records in an unrestricted section of the records. Patient-consumers can provide background context and additional information that has not been recorded and point out perceived errors in their records.

Pay for Performance and Digital and Electronic Media

Pay for performance (P4P, as it is commonly known) is another promising approach to improving health care quality. P4P replaces the usual quantity-based reimbursement protocols with reimbursement based on quality of care. Health care systems and individual providers are rewarded for adhering to quality processes and/or success in improving the health of their patients. P4P is hypothesized to reduce the substantial practice variations in utilization of services that are not supported by evidence (Weinstein, Bronner, Morgan, & Wennberg, 2004; Wennberg, O'Connor, Collins, & Weinstein, 2007).

P4P initiatives are still in their infancy, and critical issues still need to be resolved before they are widely adopted. Among these issues are specific reimbursement models (e.g., penalty versus reward for improving quality) and whether "process" outcome measures (e.g., adopting health information technology) versus health outcome measures (e.g., infection rates) will be accepted (Kuhmerker & Hartman, 2007). Nevertheless, P4P initiatives are using new health information technology such as electronic health records and digital and electronic media applications, like Web-based health information and e-mail. Under these circumstances, patient-consumer interaction may not only help improve quality initiatives but also provide measures of outcome such as satisfaction with services through digital and electronic media applications.

Digital and Electronic Media and Quality Transparency

Unlike most product markets, information on the skill and expertise of the provider, quality of the health service, and indicators of value are essentially hidden from consumer-patients. A modest amount of information about hospital quality is being provided to consumers, but this is only marginally helpful for most consumers. For example, the Leapfrog Group (www.leapfroggroup.org) provides a Web-based ratings system for hospitals across the country. But hospital participation is voluntary, and the ratings are restricted to a few key areas, such as use of computerized physician order entry and performance ratings of high-risk treatments. The Leapfrog Group emphasizes using both purchasing power and public information about quality as leverage to force providers to improve quality. This innovative example of a market-based approach using digital and electronic media applications to improve health care quality holds promise.

Other private-public partnerships are using Web-based applications to enhance consumer-patient awareness of the quality of providers. For example, Hospital Compare (www.hospitalcompare.hhs.gov) provides quality evaluations to consumers about the performance of local hospitals for the treatment of adults. This Web tool was created through the collaboration of the Centers for Medicare and Medicaid Services and the Hospital Quality Alliance: Improving Care Through Information.

Physician ratings are much more controversial, and there is, as yet, no agreed-upon method to rate physicians' quality of service provision or value. Initiatives to rate physicians by insurance companies, private companies, and even a few states have begun to be introduced but are opposed by most physicians and physician organizations. Nevertheless, digital and electronic media applications and patient-consumer demand for information about quality will continue to grow, making physician and other health provider ratings a likely future product for patient-consumers.

Will patient-consumers take rating health provider quality and service into their own hands? The Web-based Angie's List (www.angieslist.com) provides ratings of quality and service for contractors of all types. Consumers join for a relatively nominal fee and are able to review the aggregated ratings from other consumers before choosing a contractor to provide a service. Might Angie's List or another consumer-oriented company (e.g., Consumers' Union) begin to use digital and electronic media applications to collect consumer-patient ratings of physicians and make the data public?

Digital and electronic media applications will reshape health care quality issues in the United States. Already consumer-patients are obtaining information from the Web and other digital and electronic media sources about their health care concerns prior to interacting with their health care providers. It is yet unknown how this will change the relationships between patients and their providers. Clearly, the existence of more informed patients will move health care further away from a paternalistic model of care to a contractual model, where the patient has more control over health care decisions. Many health care providers and health care policy makers lament that patient-consumers are not taking adequate responsibility for their health. Undoubtedly, digital and electronic media applications are starting to change patient-consumers' approaches to health and health care. With appropriate nurturing, digital and electronic media applications will become a critical tool for providers and patients alike. Consumer-oriented patients appear to be enthusiastic users of digital and electronic media to augment their efforts to stay healthy and to effectively interact with health care providers. In contrast, other than initial health information initiatives by health insurers and health systems, providers have not appeared to have the same enthusiasm as consumers for digital and electronic media applications. Their hesitancy may stem, in part, from the failure of policy, regulations, and reimbursement to maintain pace with digital and electronic media application development and adoption. It may also stem, in part, from training in providing care in more traditional formats that do not teach new providers how to effectively use digital and electronic media to enhance their patients' welfare.

The challenges of getting valid and reliable information to patient-consumers are substantial, however. How do consumers know that the information about illnesses and treatments are accurate? Are federal and state governments the arbiters of health and health care information, or will a laissez-faire approach be effective? Is it possible for the marketplace to sort out the useful and accurate information versus inaccurate and potentially dangerous information? The stakes are high in this area; even seemingly modest misinformation can have dangerous and potentially lethal affects on individuals. Of course, those most at risk for accepting and using inaccurate information are also those who are least likely to have good health care access (e.g., populations with low income or low health literacy) (Institute of Medicine, 2004).

HEALTH LITERACY

Low literacy may pose the largest barrier to the effective delivery of care to our nation's citizens. Health literacy—the "degree to which individuals have the capacity to obtain, process, and understand basic health information and services needed to make appropriate health decisions" (U.S. Department of Health and Human Services, 2000)—has been recognized as a serious barrier to high-quality care in the United States today. The lack of ability to understand information about health and to use this information to make choices and change behavior (properly taking medicine, avoiding certain foods or activities, etc.) has drastic effects on the health of the U.S. population. Patients with limited health literacy have higher rates of hospitalizations, know less about their disease management, and are more likely to be in general poor health (Baker, Gazmararian, Sudano, Patterson, Parker, & Williams, 2002; Nath, 2007; Paasche-Orlow & Wolf, 2007). Providers continuously face health literacy issues without being able to identify or correct them (Bass, Wilson, Griffith, & Barnett, 2002). From an economic standpoint, patients with limited health literacy cost the government nearly four times as much as their peers with higher health literacy levels (Weiss & Palmer, 2004). In addition, the total burden on health care resources presented by low health literacy may be between $29 and $69 billion (Friedland, 1998).

Traditional tools are being used to combat health illiteracy. Most of them, however, rely on provider training or printed materials. Digital and electronic media applications provide an expanded set of useful tools. Access to regulated Web sites such as MedlinePlus.gov gives patients streams of information that can help people become more health literate. Unfortunately, many Web sites that present health information are not regulated by experts; nor are the Web sites in language suitable for those with limited health literacy (Greenberg, D'Andrea, & Lorence, 2004). Other health promotion outlets are offering materials in a variety of media, including Web sites, printable documents, MP3 audio lessons, online video, and portable video capability, such as iPods and cell phones (Cassey, 2007). Although these tools serve a great need for the technologically inclined, they present yet another barrier for those who are not.

Indeed, the digital divide, as it has come to be known, is a critical issue for people who are not technologically savvy or have few resources to purchase or use needed digital and electronic media devices. Such a cultural division produces a barrier to digital and electronic media but can also serve to further isolate other vulnerable populations, such as those with limited health literacy, the elderly, and those from rural communities and different cultural backgrounds, from the innovative and informative digital and electronic media applications. For example, elderly individuals with limited literacy skills have a more difficult time learning how to use a keyboard, mouse, and the Internet (Pevzner, Kaufmann, Hilliman, Shea, Weinstock, & Starren, 2005). These setbacks serve to widen the digital divide and will require extra attention as digital and electronic media are developed to address health concerns of the elderly. Broadband availability is a critical issue in rural areas. Many rural areas do not have access to broadband internet capabilities (Horrigan & Murray, 2006). In these communities computer use is markedly different from that in urban areas. The technology is more likely to be used for educational purposes (Horrigan & Murray, 2006). This inclination toward furthering knowledge could play a powerful role in reducing health literacy if greater broadband coverage were to be achieved. Cultural barriers are also present when Web sites and other digital media use only the English language and American customs (Chagrani & Gany, 2005). To reach a wider audience, health information points of access will have to be adjusted to fit the growing immigrant populations.

AGING OF AMERICANS AND DIGITAL AND ELECTRONIC MEDIA

Among digital and electronic media–based health and wellness resource users, older adults comprise a subpopulation with a distinct and unprecedented role in the shaping of policy. Foremost, older adults are the fastest-growing demographic group nationwide and worldwide. Although adults over 65 accounted for 12% of the U.S. population in 2000, this figure is expected to surge to 21% by 2030 (U.S. Census Bureau, 2000b). An increase of this magnitude will have dramatic consequences for public health, health care financing and delivery systems, and caregiving systems ("Public Health and Aging," 2003).

Unique among this cohort is the overwhelming degree to which health care costs are subsidized by government-based programs (Medicare and Medicaid). Older adults have the highest rates of use of inpatient and chronic health care services and incur the highest per capita health care costs (Desmond, Rice, Cubanski, & Neuman, 2007; Thorpe & Howard, 2006). Older adults are disproportionately represented in rural areas, where basic and specialty health care services are notoriously sparse (Haugh, 2005; U.S.Department of Agriculture, 2000). Given these factors, older Americans are poised to become the nation's largest group of technology-dependent health service users.

Only one-third of seniors currently over 70 are actively "wired." Nevertheless, many may be "passive" Internet health care users; that is, younger family members may be visiting Internet sites on their behalf. In contrast, over 50% of seniors in their 60s are active Internet users

(Fox, 2006). As America's technologically savvy baby boomers reach retirement age, the demographics of Internet utilization will become less disparate (Fox, 2006). In emerging health care applications, however, the new media have implications far more widespread than simple online consumer activity. Services and technologies such as monitors or other devices that record information on an individual's chronic condition (e.g., diabetes, heart disease) and relay information across a broadband network also fall under the umbrella of new media. In a study of telehealth-based case management, seniors with diabetes who were provided with in-home videoconferencing equipment and trained to use it demonstrated improved hemoglobin A1C, blood pressure, and cholesterol levels (Shea et al., 2006).

Cost savings and quality improvement are major driving forces in the development of health policy. These factors also will have an impact on the prevalence and use of digital and electronic media in health care. A 2005 report prepared for the New Millennium Research Council projected that accelerated national broadband deployment could lead to very significant cost savings among older adults and individuals with disabilities, the populations most likely to use monitoring devices for chronic conditions (Litan, 2005). The report projects that savings occurring through lower medical costs, lower costs of institutionalized living, and additional output generated by more seniors and people with disabilities in the labor force could potentially exceed the equivalent of half of U.S. annual spending for medical care for all its citizens. (Litan, 2005).

Importantly, Internet marketing has increased its focus on senior consumers. Health-related businesses such as online pharmaceuticals, supplements, health care information, insurers, and homecare services market directly to older consumers. These sites frequently contain links and information on chronic health conditions that can be personalized with entry of personal health data. Senior-oriented special-interest organizations are providing a full array of informational services via Internet communications (e.g. AARP, the Senior Coalition). Digital and electronic media–based products for self-care are proliferating. For example, the Web site of the American Diabetes Association (2008) journal *Diabetes Forecast* includes the 2008 annual resource guide that provides information on 12 software packages that work in conjunction with blood glucose meters to accept and analyze data.

Technology vendors worldwide are becoming increasingly attentive to the needs of senior users and to the economic potential of this market base. As early as 1999, Microsoft reported on the company's initiative to issue guidelines for making Web sites user friendly for seniors (Microsoft, 1999). Microsoft also has commissioned a research report on its product accessibility and use of accessible technology (Microsoft, 2004). Key findings revealed that the majority (57%) of computer users are either likely or very likely to benefit from the use of accessible technology, and that significant growth in numbers of technology users should be anticipated because of the increase in the number of individuals over 65. While awareness of the availability of accessible technology was high among respondents, it was determined that significant development opportunities exist in making accessibility options easier to discover.

The predominant mobile phone operator in Japan, NTT DoCoMo (2006) has introduced multiple digital and electronic media–based products with health applications for older adults, including a cell phone that slows speech to increase comprehensibility without increasing overall communication time. This company has primarily targeted elderly users with hearing loss (AARP, 2005). The company markets a videophone for bedridden elderly individuals and distant caregivers with multiple accessibility and emergency features, as well as the Wellness mobile phone, which is advertised as a hassle-free way of keeping track of their health. The product comes with a motion sensor that detects body movements and calculates calories burned and tracks jogging targets. New and developing features of the phone include a body fat calculator, pulse monitor, bad breath monitor, and caloric intake monitor (Tabuchi, 2007).

Britain-based Vodafone currently markets a minimalist cell phone with larger and fewer buttons and features to older adults, and U.S.-based Safe Guardian markets a one-button cell phone that connects the user to an operator who can contact family, provide directory assistance, or dispatch emergency personnel (AARP, 2005). Siemens is currently preparing to market a multipurpose phone device that can be used as a mobile alarm, a fitness trainer, and an emergency call system for the elderly and disabled. Sensors register sound, temperature, and movement and can be used anywhere in the world. The system can notify caregivers if an elderly person has fallen or is motionless. People with special needs can use the display as an emergency call button to summon rapid assistance (Gizmag.com, 2007). Finally, VeriChip Corporation is test-marketing an implantable microchip for individuals with Alzheimer's disease that would allow medical personnel to access information and medical records quickly in an emergency situation (Business Wire, 2007).

THE NEW MEDIA AS THE THIRD FORCE IN HEALTH CARE

Will the new media become a powerful third force in the U.S. health care system? The early evidence suggests that consumer-patients are already turning to digital and electronic media applications for information about health and health care. Web sites such as WebMD have health news, interactive features (e.g., determining body mass index, symptom-based diagnosis suggestions), and communication features such as blogs and message boards. These Web sites have proven track records and are commercial successes. Consumer-patients are also ordering pharmaceuticals through Web-based companies, finding information about benefits from their health insurance companies, and using Web sites to find information about health care facilities' quality ratings. Consumer-patients are increasingly taking information found through digital and electronic media applications to their appointments and corresponding with their health care providers by electronic mail.

Digital and electronic media have the potential to greatly expand access to health services, especially for those who have been traditionally underserved. Substantial investments in infrastructure are needed if digital and electronic media will be accessible to vulnerable populations, such as the elderly, those living in rural areas, and those without easy access to digital and electronic media services. The investments that appear to be needed include universal broadband Internet access, a wireless or cellular infrastructure that could connect and support remote geographic areas, and increased attention to computer training through public programs. Ambitious universal wireless projects, however, have so far been met with both economical and technical challenges (Associated Press, 2007). These setbacks all but ensure that widespread municipal wireless access is far from being a reality, with rural prospects even further down the road.

How will health care quality be affected by digital and electronic media? Consumers may use Web sites such as Angie's List to rate their health care providers on service and quality. College students are using such applications to grade their professors. Can health care providers be far removed from this type of consumer-based evaluation? What is not known is how providers will respond. Health care systems are beginning to pay attention to their public evaluations and making changes to their practices. If experience from other markets is an indication, health systems and providers who are able to embrace digital and electronic media applications to reach their consumer-patients will find that their consumers respond positively. Health systems and providers who are willing to accept digital and electronic media applications are likely to find improvements in patient satisfaction, market share increases, and perhaps enhanced health among patients.

Digital and electronic media applications will improve the nation's health literacy because they can be used to move away from text-only information to audio and visual information and interactive services. Digital and electronic media applications also provide a means to translate and disseminate health and health care information into multiple languages. Telehealth interpretation services that facilitate communication between providers and patients who speak different languages are growing quickly. These services allow health care facilities to enable interpretation without employing multiple interpreters.

The digital and electronic media have begun to change how health care interacts with aging Americans. Telehealth and remote monitoring allow elderly patients to remain in their homes and communities and have frequent interaction with their health care providers. Substantial improvements in infrastructure are needed to increase penetration of digital and electronic media applications to the aging populations, including a universal broadband network and "universally designed" consumer products (larger numbers, volume assists). Given that elderly Americans account for the use of the majority of health care services in this country, thoughtful application of digital and electronic media in health care systems for this population will reduce costs, improve health, and increase independence.

The digital and electronic media have already dramatically changed the way Americans conduct business and enjoy leisure. It will soon transform the U.S. health care system.

REFERENCES

AARP. (2005). *International: Cell phones go retro to appeal to older users.* Retrieved January 30, 2008, from http://www.aarp.org/international/agingadvances/univdesign/Articles/12_05_intl_cell-phones.html

Akalu, R., Rossos, P. G., & Chan, C. T. (2006). The role of law and policy in telemonitoring. *Journal of Telemedicine and Telecare, 12,* 325–327.

American Diabetes Association. (2008). *2008 resource guide.* Retrieved July 16, 2008, from http://www.diabetes.org/diabetes-forecast/resource-guide.jsp

Associated Press. (2007, August 31). *EarthLink abandons San Francisco wi-fi project.* Retrieved January 2008, from http://www.nytimes.com/2007/08/31/technology/31earthlink.html

Atkinson, R. D. (2007). *The case for a national broadband policy.* Retrieved July 14, 2008, from http://ssrn.com/abstract=1004525

Baker, D. W., Gazmararian, J. A., Sudano, J., Patterson, M., Parker, R. M., & Williams, M. V. (2002). Health literacy and performance on the mini-mental state examination. *Aging & Mental Health, 6*(1), 22–29.

Bass, P. F., III, Wilson, J. F., Griffith, C. H., & Barnett, D. R. (2002). Residents' ability to identify patients with poor literacy skills. *Academic Medicine, 77*(10), 1039–1041.

Brear, M. (2006). Evaluating telemedicine: Lessons and challenges. *Health Information Management Journal, 35*(2), 23–31.

Business Wire. (2007). *25 Alzheimer's patients and caregivers receive VeriMed RFID implantable microchip at Alzheimer's educational conference.* Retrieved January 30, 2008, from http://www.businesswire.com/portal/site/home/index.jsp?ndmViewId = news_view&ndmConfigId = 1000010&newsId = 20070611005651&newsLang = en

Cassey, M. Z. (2007). Building a case for using technology: Health literacy and patient education. *Nursing Economics, 25*(3), 186–188.

Changrani, J., & Gany, F. (2005). Online cancer education and immigrants: Effecting culturally appropriate Websites. *Journal of Cancer Education, 20*(3), 183–186.

DeNavas-Walt, C., Proctor, B. D., & Smith, J. (2007). *Income, poverty, and health insurance coverage in the United States: 2006.* Washington, DC: U.S. Government Printing Office. Retrieved July 16, 2008, from http://www.census.gov/hhes/www/hlthins/hlthin06.html

Desmond, K. A., Rice, T., Cubanski, J., & Neuman, P. (2007). The burden of out-of-pocket health spending among older versus younger adults: Analysis from the consumer expenditure survey, 1998–2003. *The Henry J. Kaiser Family Foundation: Medicare Issue Brief.* Retrieved July 17, 2008, from http://www.kff.org/medicare/upload/7686.pdf

Fox, S. (2006). *Are "wired seniors" sitting ducks?* [Data memo]. Pew Internet & American Life Project.

Franklin, P. D., Rosenbaum, P. F., Carey, M. P., & Roizen, M. F. (2006). Using sequential e-mail messages to promote health behaviors: Evidence of feasibility and reach in a worksite sample. *Journal of Medical Internet Research, 8*(1), e3.

Friedland, R. (1998, October 7–8). New estimates of the high costs of inadequate health literacy. In *Proceedings of Pfizer Conference "Promoting Health Literacy: A Call to Action"* (pp. 6–10).Washington, DC: Pfizer, Inc.

Fuchs, V. R., & Emanuel, E. J. (2005). Health care reform: Why? What? When? *Health Affairs, 24*(6), 1399–1414.

Gizmag.com. (2007). *The ingenious AySystem mobile alarm.* Retrieved January 30, 2008, from http://www.gizmag.com/go/6907/

Gray, G. A., Stamm, B. H., Toevs, S., Reischl, U., & Yarrington, D. (2006). Study of participating and nonparticipating states' telemedicine Medicaid reimbursement status: Its impact on Idaho's policymaking process. *Telemedicine Journal & E-Health, 12*(6), 681–690.

Greenberg, L., D'Andrea, G., & Lorence, D. (2004). Setting the public agenda for online health search: A white paper and action agenda. *Journal of Medical Internet Research, 6*(2), e18.

Haugh, R. (2005). A rural crossroad. *Hospitals & Health Networks, 79*(12), 48–50.

Horrigan, J., & Murray, K. (2006). *Rural broadband internet use* [Data memo]. Pew Internet & American Life Project.

Institute of Medicine. (2000). *To err is human: Building a safer health system.* Washington, DC: National Academies Press.

Institute of Medicine. (2001). *Crossing the quality chasm: A new health system for the 21st century.* Washington, DC: National Academies Press.

Institute of Medicine. (2004). *Health literacy: A prescription to end confusion.* Washington, DC: National Academies Press.

Kizer, K. W. (2007). The adoption of electronic health records: Benefits and challenges. *Annals of Health Law, 16*(2), 323–334.

Kuhmerker, K., & Hartman, T., (2007). *Pay-for-performance in state Medicaid programs: A survey of state Medicaid directors and programs.* New York: Commonwealth Fund. Retrieved July 17, 2008, from http://company.ipro.org/shared/pubs/p4p_state_medicaid_progs_report.pdf

Litan, R. E. (2005). *Great Expectations: Potential economic benefits to the nation from accelerated broadband deployment to older Americans and Americans with disabilities.* New Millennium Research Council. Retrieved July 17, 2008, from http://www.newmillenniumresearch.org/archive/Litan_FINAL_120805.pdf

Menachemi, N., & Brooks, R. G. (2006). Reviewing the benefits and costs of electronic health records and associated patient safety technologies. *Journal of Medical Systems, 30*(3), 159–168.

Microsoft. (1999). *Microsoft issues guidelines for making user-friendly websites for all ages.* Retrieved October 4, 2007, from http://www.microsoft.com/presspass/press/1999/May99/GuidelinePR.mspx

Microsoft. (2004). *A research report commissioned by Microsoft Corporation and conducted by Forrester Research, Inc.* Retrieved January 28, 2008, from http://www.microsoft.com/enable/research/phase2.aspx?v=t

Missouri Department of Social Services. (2007, January 16). Chronic care improvement. *Division of Medical Services Provider Bulletin, 29*(22).

Nath, C. (2007). Literacy and diabetes self-management. *American Journal of Nursing, 107*(6 Suppl.), 43–49.

NPR/Kaiser Family Foundation/Harvard Kennedy School of Government. (2002). *National survey on health care.* Retrieved January 2008, from http://www.kff.org/insurance/20020605a-index.cfm

NTT DoCoMo. (2006, March 6). *NTT DoCoMo Unveils "Raku-Raku PHONE Basic" handset* [Press release]. Retrieved January 2008, from http://www.nttdocomo.com/pr/2007/001323.html

Okamoto, E. (2007). Is health a right or an obligation? *International Journal of Integrated Care, 7*, e03.

Paasche-Orlow, M. K., & Wolf, M. S. (2007). The causal pathways linking health literacy to health outcomes. *American Journal of Health Behavior, 31*(Suppl. 1), S19–26.

Pevzner, J., Kaufmann, D. R., Hilliman, C., Shea, S., Weinstock, R. S., & Starren, J. (2005). Developing computer skills and competencies in seniors. In *AMIA, Annual Symposium Proceedings,* p. 1078.

Public health and aging: Trends in aging—United States and Worldwide. (2003). *MMWR Weekly, 52*(6), 101–106.

Rogers, S. (2006). Multistate nurse licensure in case management. *Case Manager, 17*(2), 43–46.

Shea, S., Weinstock, R. S., Starren J., Teresi, J., Palmas, W., Field, L., et al. (2006). A randomized trial comparing telemedicine case management with usual care in older, ethnically diverse, medically underserved patients with diabetes mellitus. *Journal of the American Medical Informatics Association, 13*, 40–51.

Stamm, B. H. (2004). *Modeling telehealth and telemedicine: A global geopolitical perspective.* 26th annual international conference of the IEEE EMBS. San Francisco.

Stanberry, B. (2006). Legal and ethical aspects of telemedicine. *Journal of Telemedicine and Telecare, 12*, 166–175.

Tabuchi, H. (2007). *New prototype phones gives fitness check.* Retrieved January 30, 3008, from http://www.worldhealth.net/p/new-prototype-phone-gives-fitness-check.html

Thorpe, K. E., & Howard, D. H. (2006). The rise in spending among Medicare beneficiaries: The role of chronic disease prevalence and changes in treatment intensity. *Health Affairs, 25*, w378–w388.

U.S. Census Bureau. (2000a). *Data set: Census 2000 summary file 1 (SF 1) 100-percent data. United States—urban/rural and inside/outside metropolitan.* Retrieved January 31, 2008, from http://www.factfinder.census.gov/servlet/GCTTable?_bm=y&-geo_id=&-ds_name=DEC_2000_SF1_U&-_lang=en&-redoLog=true&-mt_name=DEC_2000_SF1_U_GCTP1_US1&-format=US-1&-CONTEXT=gct

U.S. Census Bureau. (2000b). *International database. Table 094. Midyear population, by age and sex.* Retrieved January 31, 2008, from http://www.census.gov/population/www/projections/natdet-D1A.html

U.S. Department of Agriculture. (2000). *Changes in the older population and implications for rural areas.* Rural Development and Research Report No. RDRR90. Retrieved July 18, 2008, from http://www.ers.usda.gov/publications/RDRR90/

U.S. Department of Health and Human Services. (2003). *Telemedicine licensure report.* Prepared by the Center for Telemedicine Law. Health Resources and Services Administration. Retrieved July 17, 2008, from ftp://ftp.hrsa.gov/telehealth/licensure.pdf

U.S. Department of Health and Human Services. (2000). *Healthy people 2010: Understanding and improving health.* Washington, DC: Author.

U.S. Department of Labor. (2000, March). *Findings from the National Agricultural Workers Survey (NAWS) 1997–1998.* Research Report No. 8. Retrieved July 17, 2008, from http://www.dol.gov/asp/programs/agworker/report_8.pdf

Weinstein, J. N., Bronner, K. K., Morgan, T. S., & Wennberg. (2004). Trends and geographic variations in major surgery for degenerative diseases of the hip, knee, and spine. *Health Affairs (Project Hope).* Web exclusive. Retrieved July 17, 2008, from http://content.healthaffairs.org/cgi/content/full/hlthaff.var.81/DC3

Wennberg, J. E., O'Connor, A. M., Collins, E. D., & Weinstein, J. N. (2007). Extending the P4P agenda, part 1: How Medicare can improve patient decision making and reduce unnecessary care. *Health Affairs, 26*(6), 1564–1574.

Health Communication in the New Media Landscape: A Summary

17

ESTHER THORSON AND MARGARET E. DUFFY

This volume brings together researchers from a wide variety of backgrounds to consider the question of how the digital revolution is affecting and will continue to affect health and health care in the United States and around the globe. By "digital revolution," we mean all the new ways that computers and a vast array of digitally-based electronic devices provide ways for people to experience content.

The Internet, of course, is the centerpiece of the digital revolution because it brings together the features of television, radio, telephone, and print media. It has also changed the meaning of "mass communication" because although the masses use the Internet, they can use it for interpersonal communication (i.e., from one individual to another), as well as for mass communication. In fact, the "mass communicating" can occur in a way that is customized to individuals, which of course the legacy media do not allow. The Internet also allows people to interact both with the source of the mass message and with each other. The "one-to-many" model of mass communication has been profoundly disrupted.

Because it is so inexpensive to create and send messages using digital media, it has democratized communication in terms of who may be a source of communication. It is no longer just those with deep pockets (e.g., government, corporations, politicians, policy makers) who can send messages now that anyone with a computer, e-mail capacity, or the ability to create a Web site can reach thousands of people.

Of course, the digital revolution has also meant the emergence of many communication devices, including wireless phones, PDAs, digital still and video cameras, laptops, and pagers. The proliferation of these devices and constantly falling prices, miniaturization, and increases in speed and capacity have revolutionized how people communicate with each other, get information, are entertained, and acquire goods and products.

It is clear that the digital revolution is changing—and will continue to change—just about every aspect of human behavior. This volume has focused on how it changes health and health care. The chapters have looked at the impact of telehealth, e-mail, individual health care records, health and clinical informatics, cell phone health information delivery, Web sites, chat groups, social networks and many other products of the digital revolution. With each of these products we see huge possibilities for change in health and health care. Greater message impact, specialization to individuals, increased message efficacy, more social support, and the potential to promote healthy behaviors and growth in health literacy are all outcomes that we can expect from the digital revolution. Our challenge is to use the tools technology is offering to accomplish health outcome goals.

A central assumption is that health communication can become far more effective in the digital world than it is now. It is also assumed that health communication is a crucial process in relating all elements in the health and health care world. In a simplified way, Figure 17.1 represents the units in that world. At the center is health. Chapter 1 defined health as "a state of complete physical, mental, and social well-being, not merely the absence of disease or infirmity." Intervening between health and non-health conditions (both acute and chronic) is prevention. Notice that for both prevention and acute and chronic non-health, there are five variables to consider: access to health care, quality of health care, social support, health literacy, and self-care. These can all be thought of as interventions that either keep people healthy or return them to health.

Surrounding this central core of health and non-health are the vectors that influence the movement between health and non-health. First, there are health policies. These emerge from two sources: private enterprise (hospitals, pharmaceutical companies, and insurance corporations) and public organizations, primarily government and government agencies, but also nonprofit organizations.

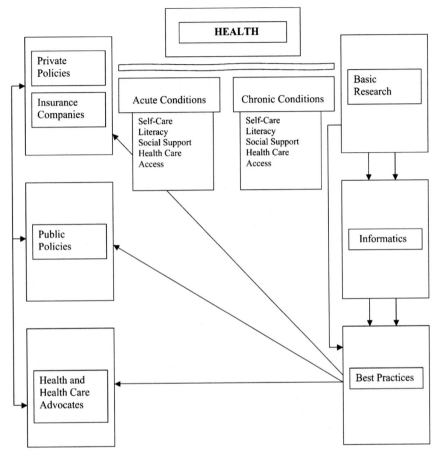

Figure 17.1 Health care providers

Health care advocates have specific perspectives on the prevention/intervention processes and act mostly on private and public policy sectors. However, they often attempt to act on individual citizens, who are located in the central health/nonhealth circle.

On the right side of the figure is basic research (which can come from academic or corporate sources); bioinformatics, which is defined as the management of complex data sets that represent the outcomes of research of various types; and best practices, which is the collection of information on how best to execute all acts of providing health care, formulating policies, informing the public, and managing the flow of information in the system. At the top of the figure are providers—doctors, nurses, therapists, insurers, and all others who are involved in delivering health care directly to citizens.

The pattern of information flow is the key aspect of the health system represented. This information flow is best visualized in terms of a number of elemental stages. When information needs to be moved from one component of the system to another, the first stage is encoding. This involves representing the information so that it is expressed in a message. For example, if the information is about a best practice, it needs to be described in a way that is understandable to its target audience. Here is an example of such a message: "It is best to put babies in their cribs on their backs because this is the best way to avoid crib deaths." That message can be transmitted interpersonally (by a medical professional to a patient) or in brochures, in 30-second television videos, or as online learning modules for nurses. Any message is delivered through some sort of channel, whether it is speech, cell phones, laptops, television, or social networking sites.

When the messages are received (if indeed they *are* received), several more important processes have to occur. The receiver must decode the message and make decisions about what, if any, action he or she should take based on the complexity of the message. For example, when the baby has a cold, should she be placed on her back? Is this true just for newborns or for 12 month-olds too? In some situations, more advanced "re-analyses" are needed. Another key vector involves the strategy for disseminating statistics and data sets from bioinformatics sources. These are key data that help us understand how statistics and other mediating information help health information specialists arrive at beliefs about practices.

A critical point is that communication among all elements of the system represented here is complex and fraught with chances for miscommunication. In fact, we want to make it clear that much communication is "translation," from idea to encoding and from message through the decoding process. This translation is in and of itself a science—the science of health communication.

Chapter 5 offers the media choice model as a useful framework for thinking strategically about how messages should be formed and targeted toward audience needs. It further shows how communicators can send appropriate messages through the best channels at the best time to reach targeted audiences. As represented in the model, where there is a double arrow, the media choice model is operationalized.

The system represented in Figure 5.1 captures the elements of what has always had to happen to maximize health. But the digital revolution has greatly increased how the flow of communication can and should operate. It holds the promise of far more effective relationships among the elements shown here.

The chapters in this volume explicate many of the critical connections shown in the model. So that readers can make best use of the book, we outline how each chapter contributes to improving health communication and, thus, health outcomes.

Chapter 1, "The Challenge of Health Care and Disability," outlines the current state of health in the United States and the world. It discusses the three determinants of health: access to health care, health policies, and intervention. These processes are represented as vectors in Figure 1.1. The chapter is important because it provides a sense of how great the challenge of chronic disease is (accounting for two-thirds of all U.S. deaths). It also shows that much of chronic disease could be prevented because it is caused by tobacco use, too little exercise, and poor diet. The chapter chronicles the challenge that people have accessing health care and how cultural disparities influence access.

Another topic discussed in chapter 1 is the challenge of health care quality. A significant portion of health care is flawed and results in loss of life, long-term health problems, and heightened costs. Health care is represented in Figure 1.1 as a critical intervention in health and acute and chronic disease. Finally, there is the question of skyrocketing health care costs in recent years. Costs are represented in terms of all the interventions—self-care, health literacy, social support, health care, and health care access—although the chapter argues that the most significant impact of cost is for care and access.

Chapter 2, "Emerging Demographics and Health Care Trends," examines how people's demographic features have a profound impact on their health. This chapter distinguishes societal, community, and individual indices of health, marking the impact of most of the vectors surrounding the center of Figure 2.1, individual health and non-health. The chapter shows how race and income are important considerations that must be taken into account when one is attempting to find effective ways to deliver health, nutrition, and exercise messages to people. It further elaborates how communicating with the elderly, females, those living alone, those with disabilities, and those for whom English is a second language requires considerable attention in order for effective communication to occur. Indeed, the diversification of ways to communicate enabled by the Internet and digital devices may lead to a marked increase in communication about the five kinds of intervention that affect health and non-health status.

Chapter 3, "Communication Strategies for Reducing Racial and Cultural Disparities," continues the examination of how differences among individuals affect how health interventions must be designed and executed. While the literature shows that advertising is effective for all groups, combining advertising through traditional media channels with those that employ the Internet and new digital devices is clearly superior. This chapter also reviews how selection of media channel becomes even more critical when individuals of various racial and cultural minority groups are targeted.

Chapter 4, "Health Communication: Trends and Future Directions," examines many of the media choice model aspects of Figure 1 illustrated in the double-arrow relationships. It elucidates what makes physician–patient communication effective and how use of digital media can make a difference. It explores how community-based communications, those that come from private and public organizations, and those that come from health communication advocates influence all five of the interventions affecting health and non-health. Most importantly, the chapter looks at how the digital interface among all these messages and individuals has been directly and drastically influenced by digitization. Examples of the digital interfaces discussed in the chapter include health lifestyle tools, personal health records, more effective delivery of health news, improved health literacy, and the impact of health social networks.

Chapter 5, "Emerging Trends in the New Media Landscape," introduces a simple but powerful model for understanding the process of health communication and how it should be conceptualized in a media environment to which digital media have been added. The media choice model suggests that every use of a medium is motivated by one of four needs: connectivity, information, entertainment, and shopping. The choices people make to satisfy their communication needs are determined by individual differences like demographics (e.g., race, income, education, gender) or psychosocial variables (e.g., subculture, lifestyle). The choices are also determined by "aperture," that is, the natural ebb and flow of various motivations across the day, week, month, or life stage. Before the digital revolution, the main features that the communication channels provided were print, sound, moving images, portability, and scannability. In recent years, the Internet and digital devices greatly expanded the media features available (e.g., immediacy, customizability, interactivity, search, and mobility). The chapter goes on to provide an array of examples of how this digital world of media choices has changed and will continue to change almost every aspect of health communication.

Chapter 6, "Enhancing Consumer Involvement in Health Care," explores how health care information on the Internet has changed how people become involved in their own care and how they find and purchase products such as pharmaceuticals and services usually provided by doctors and hospitals. It further examines how these changes may slow the rise of health care costs. The chapter analyzes whether individuals are ready to become even more involved in their own health care interventions. Opportunities made possible by the digital environment include online personal health records, greater and more convenient access to health care, more help for people looking for high-quality health information on the Internet, and more networking among different providers of health care for individuals.

Chapter 7, "E-Health Self-Care Interventions for Persons With Chronic Illnesses: Review and Future Directions," offers a complete report on research focusing on how people try to provide health care for themselves when they have diabetes, heart disease, or mental illness, all common chronic conditions. The authors conclude that telecommunications approaches are becoming more critical in fulfilling the need for self-care information. The Internet and the telephone both greatly increase the number of alternative information sources. In fact, research shows that experiments on the combination of routine care with telephone- and Internet-delivered information demonstrates how media-enhanced communications are more effective. The authors conclude that the main advantages of the media-enhanced conditions are the opportunities for tailoring and individualizing messages.

Chapter 8, "Increasing Computer-Mediated Social Support," develops the argument that the support of others is crucial for people coping with chronic health problems and for preventing health problems. Communicating with others reduces stress and provides people with increased ways to cope, a process called "buffering." Of course, just as suggested by the media choice model, the Internet brings vast increase in the number of opportunities to communicate with others. The advantages of gaining social support through digital communication include fewer in-group/out-group biases, largely because there are fewer individual difference cues on the Internet. It appears that expressing one's problems in writing is efficacious for individuals. Distant others can be brought closer. There is evidence that people feel better about asking for help when they are in an interactive environment where they can also provide help to others as well. Disadvantages to the Internet environment include the fact that sporadic and short-term use may not be sufficient to fill social needs. Marketers can also be a disruptive force in social support sites. This chapter clearly explains the increased potential for social support that will be available as digital approaches continue to develop.

Chapter 9, "Engaging Consumers in Health Care Advocacy Using the Internet," focuses on what makes advocacy efforts effective in the digital landscape. The chapter demonstrates how the principles of effective health advocacy translate from the pre-Internet environment to the current one. It suggests that the four most important principles are leveraging assets of the advocacy organization, using marketing campaign strategies, bringing together as many allies as possible, and framing health issues in terms of their social rather than individual benefits. The chapter demonstrates how to translate these principles to the Internet.

Chapter 10, "Improving Physician–Patient Communication," examines the complex world of this relationship and how it has been changed by significant digital developments. Of course, the complexities of the physician–patient relationship are significant: how the disease and illness experience is communicated; treatment of the "whole person"; management of medications, treatments, side-effects, and on the like; focus on prevention; and ways to improve the physician–patient relationship. Research has shown that these challenges have been mitigated by new media interventions like e-mail, telemedicine, online health information, wireless handheld devices like PDAs and cell phones, blogs, and laptops.

Chapter 11, "Health Literacy in the Digital World," elaborates on how many Americans have low health literacy and what this means for their health and non-health. The chapter introduces the concept of "health literacy load," that is, how much complexity there is in terms of vocabulary, concepts, and total amount of information needed. The chapter then applies the concept to two experiments, one on geographic information systems that instruct people about where to go and what to do in an emergency, the other on the problems of developing electronic medical records. In both cases, it is clear that the concept of health literacy load is important in the development of better ways to communicate critical health care information to those with low health literacy.

Chapter 12, "Making the Grade: Identification of Evidence-based Communication Messages," begins by showing how new research on mental health has not effectively reached people. A central problem is that it is not clear how to measure the quality of mental health research. The chapter points out that a number of organizations have been involved in this effort and have tried to come up with rating scales and criteria for quality. For example, the federal Agency for Healthcare Research and Quality identifies three criteria: how well the study is carried out, the number of studies carried out and the number of people represented in those studies, and finally the consistency of findings across all the studies. Unfortunately, consumers are generally not informed about these dimensions of quality and therefore can be misled by generalizations based on poor research.

Chapter 13, "New Strategies of Knowledge Translation: A Knowledge Value Mapping Framework," is concerned with identifying and getting best practices knowledge to health care providers. Integrating best practices into the routines of providers is a process called knowledge translation. Only by making routines consistent with best practices can health care be optimized. This is particularly critical for treatment of chronic disease. Clearly communication occupies a central role in knowledge translation. Unfortunately, evidence is clear that there is a significant gap between known best practices and the routines of providers. The chapter extensively reviews problems related to effectively fostering knowledge translation. It concludes by suggesting that an important step involves mapping the values of providers and patients and using that map as a guide to effectively translating best practices into caregiver routines. For example, there might be a mismatch between the needs of caregivers and the elderly, and these differences may call for a reanalysis of the caregiver's role. This can lead to new and more effective interventions. Given the complexity of determining the relationship of needs to care, it is clear that the Internet, databases, and other digitally enabled approaches can be important tools.

Chapter 14, "International Innovations in Health Communications," outlines best practices in using electronic and digital media to serve the needs of global health diplomacy. The chapter discusses blogs, chat rooms, radio broadcasts, wikis, and social networks in terms of their utility in meeting international health challenges. A number of case studies highlight how these new media communication approaches have been applied. In a condom promotion campaign in Kenya, satellite broadcasts to digital radios created local acceptance and made the issue of condom use culturally relevant. In New Zealand, a Web site was developed to make information about bird flu immediately available to anyone with Internet access. Another plan involved handheld computers being connected with a geographic information system network.

Chapter 15, "Connecting Cognate Fields: Health Communication and Biomedical Informatics," develops a model of how these two fields relate and complement each other. Biomedical informatics is defined as the management and use of biomedical information based on information technologies such as computer-based databases. At its heart, the model suggests that the power of bioinformatics lies in enabling translation of complicated data and information about the needs, preferences, and demographics of health consumers and patients. Computer algorithms can then organize the information so it is possible to generate individualized messages. In the model presented in Figure 15.1, biomedical informatics is represented as a translational system between basic research and best practices. Chapter 15 elaborates on how informatics provides an interface between basic research and best practices and thus can inform all the other sectors in the chart: individuals, nonprofit and for-profit health organizations, government, and health advocates. Biomedical informatics is thus a cornerstone of health communication in the digital environment.

Chapter 16, "New Media: A Third Force in Health Care," posits that the media created by the digital revolution can be thought of as a third force, together with private and public sectors of health care. Examples of this new area include telehealth, access to electronic health records, and health literacy approaches enhanced by the Internet and digital devices. Similarly, systems of "pay for performance," which reward quality health care and thus improve the health of patients, show promise. The chapter focuses on how these approaches can be combined to deal with the rapidly increasing number of seniors and the accompanying health challenges of this demographic.

SUMMARY AND CONCLUSIONS

The study of how the Internet and digital-based devices and systems can be used to improve both prevention and care of chronic and acute health conditions is in its infancy. The broad brushstrokes painted in these chapters offer a picture of our current knowledge about the impact of this new media landscape on all the components of health care shown in Figure 17.1. The goal of this effort is to help practitioners, administrators, and policy makers understand more about the promise of new media tools and services for improving health. It is also our hope that these ideas will serve as a launching point for more innovative ideas and the research necessary to test their effectiveness.

Index

AARP, health care advocacy by, 275

Advertising, mass media channels for, 94

African American women, mass media health campaigns and
for cardiovascular disease and, 45
for domestic violence prevention, 46

AMA. *See* American Medical Association

American Indians, influenza vaccination and, mass media health campaigns for, 46

American Medical Association (AMA), 295

Americans for Quality Health Care Campaign, 275

Americans with Disabilities Act, 10

Aperture concept
health communication media choice model and, 105–106
for target audience, 111–112

"Augmenting Human Intellect: A Conceptual Framework" (Engelbart), 122

Autonomy
assaults on, 131–132
connective journalism and, 134
health portals and, 133–134
need for, 130–135
new media landscape and, 132–135
personal health records and, 133
self-help tools for, 132–133

Behavior modification
health care outcomes via, 345–347
knowledge gap and, 344–345

Bienvenida Salud radio program, 377
health communication by, 378

Biomedical informatics, 396–401
cognitive-level content of, 407–408
collaboration opportunities for, 409–412
benefits for, 412–413
health communication and, 445–446
medical informatics and, 396–398
multidimensional theories for, 408–409
noncommunication aspects of, 406
summary/implications of, 413

Braintalk Communities, 272–273

Canadian Institutes of Health Research, 342

Cancer
cervical, mass media health campaigns for, 46
self-care intervention for, 168–169

Cardiovascular disease
mass media health campaigns for, African American women and, 45
prevention for, 164
self-care intervention for
telephone-based results, 164–165
Web-based results, 163–164

Celebrities
as entertainment, 104–105
health communication and, 104–105

Center for Medicare and Medicaid Services, 426
on health care expenditures, 11–12

Center of Medicare and Medicaid Services, 296

447